COMPLETE NU

HOW TO LIVE IN TOTAL HEALTH

The Author

Dr Michael Sharon is a nutrition consultant to health food companies with his own private practice and is the author of the best-selling *Eat to Live* and *Nutrients A–Z*.

His first career was engineering, until ill health made an active life impossible. Finding that orthodox medicine only exacerbated his problems, and on one occasion nearly killed him, he turned to nutrition as a means of cure. After much trial and error, and having devoured every book, article and research paper on the subject, his health improved.

Realizing that a great deal of ill health is caused and maintained by poor eating habits, he decided to make nutrition his career. In 1983 he received his Ph.D. from Donsbach University in Huntington Beach, California, which later became known as IUNE, International University for Nutritional Education. Dr Sharon now divides his time between a busy nutrition practice, lecturing, writing for newspapers and magazines, advising various official bodies and keeping abreast of the latest developments in nutrition research.

Dr Sharon is a superb communicator, a gifted translator of complex nutritional data into terms which the general reader can understand. He does not overwhelm the reader with the intricacies of biochemistry, but he does not duck necessary explanations and definitions either. Every statement he makes is meticulously referenced.

COMPLETE
NUTRITION

HOW TO LIVE IN TOTAL HEALTH

Dr Michael Sharon

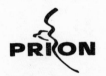

This revised edition published 2002 in Great Britain by
Prion Books Limited,
Imperial Works, Perren Street,
London NW5 3ED
www.prionbooks.com

Reprinted with updates 2002

A catalogue record for this book is available from the British
Library.

ISBN 1-85375-435-8

Cover design by Bob Eames
Text artwork by Tamasin Cole
Printed by Bookmarque

*The publishers, author and editors do not imply or intend
that this book should in any way replace the services of a
physician. Its contents are informative and are not diagnostic
or prescriptive.*

TO MY DAUGHTERS,
WITH AFFECTION AND APPRECIATION

Medicine will turn one day to the prevention of diseases rather than their cure. Man was born to be healthy and the best medicine I know is an active and intelligent interest in nature

Charles Darwin

A truly good physician first finds out the cause of the disease, and having found that, he first tries to cure it by food. Only when food fails, does he prescribe medication.

Sun-Ssu-Mo,
Tang Dynasty (A.D. 600)

Thy food shall be thy medicine.

Hippocrates (460-377 B.C.)

CONTENTS

FOREWORD

The intent of a book about health should be to inform the reader, not to testify to the superior knowledge of its author. Michael Sharon has admirably accomplished that in this book which discusses the part nutrition plays in our daily lives and concisely evaluates the various factors involved in good nutrition. Although it is difficult to write a book on nutrition which nobody will challenge, the author is, in my opinion, 'right on' in his major premises.

I believe the thrust of this book can be best summarized by the author himself: 'The art of healing is, to a great extent, the ability to cooperate with biologic processes in fortifying the natural immune system. Basic and logical as this principle is, medicine still finds it hard to adjust to recent biological and biochemical findings which emphasize the great role which natural, balanced nutrition plays in helping the body heal itself and prevent disease.'

Enlarging on this premise, he gives valuable insights into most of the common conditions which respond readily to nutritional care. Whether he is discussing allergies or premature aging, he gives sound reasons for the nutritional approach.

Readers cannot fail to be impressed with this comprehensive and logically sequenced volume. Writers such as Michael Sharon are a much-needed catalyst for the introduction of nutrition ideas to the public.

Kurt W. Donsbach, Ph.D.

PREFACE

Modern supermarket food is becoming daily poorer in vitamins, minerals and trace elements and richer in water and chemical additives. The latter are intended to increase eye appeal and taste appeal and extend shelf life. During growing, picking, shipping and storage, vegetables and fruits are sprayed with chemicals – pesticides, herbicides and fungicides – and stripped of their vitamins and minerals.

At the same time generic medicines have been developed, some of which are highly toxic. Their toxicity, adverse interactions and side effects can, and do, cause complications which are often more severe than the original disease. To quote A. Turnau, a former regional pharmacist with the Israeli health ministry in Tel Aviv: 'If, in the past, we had dumped large quantities of medicines into the sea, the fish would have laughed. Today, with the high toxicity of new drugs, they will not have time even to smile. Prescription drugs should be strictly dispensed and used only according to a valid prescription. Any deviation from the prescribed dosage can be fatal.'[1] In fact the toxicity of many modern drugs is so critical that no precautions can guarantee complete safety. In the past the U.S. Food and Drug Administration (FDA) has made mistakes and approved bad drugs. Thalidomide, which caused physical defects in the children of mothers for whom it was prescribed, is a classic example of such a mistake. Benedictin, another drug commonly prescribed for nausea in early pregnancy, has also been found to cause birth defects. Its manufacturer, Merrel Dow Pharmaceuticals, in one of the largest lawsuit settlements in history, has agreed to pay $120 million to at least 678 deformed children.[2]

As a direct result of poor nutrition and over-reliance on medication, health in the Western World is declining. Heart disease and high blood pressure have reached epidemic proportions. In the United States alone, over 100,000 coronary bypasses are performed annually at an average per capita cost of $50,000. Billions of dollars are spent on expensive rescuing surgeries. Every day 1,000 Americans die of cancer. Leading medical insurance institutions, like Medicare in the U.S. and the NHS in the U.K. are constantly grappling with critical financial difficulties. These huge costs are taking their toll on the national economies. Improving nutrition, could help save many lives at a much lesser cost. An official American study estimated that improved nutritional status of North Americans might reduce the U.S. national health bill by one-third.[3] Over $40 billion a year could be saved in such areas as dental care, diabetes, heart disease, alcoholism and digestive diseases. Less serious health conditions that do not require hospitalizations are pandemic. Many people are considered 'healthy' by their doctors even if they suffer from low grade sicknesses, like fatigue, nervousness, depression or low sexual potency. The sources of *joie de vivre*, natural pep, vitality and energy are drying up in too many people.

Cancer is the bogeyman of Western medicine. In a recent official address, Dr Sanford Miller, Director of the Bureau of Foods at the U.S. Food and Drug Administration, said: 'Nutrition and cancer are interrelated, in etiology [cause] as well as in its reversing mechanism. Ten to fifteen years ago, we thought that it was enough to identify and remove carcinogenic [cancer-causing] substances from foods. Today, we know that it is not that simple. Today, we understand that the connection between nutrition and cancer is related to modern food processing and technology, in food preservation and in marketing. A balanced diet with moderate protein and fat and plenty of fruits and vegetables, which supply vitamins A and C, is the best guarantee for health.'[4]

Anyone who reads newspapers and watches TV knows that certain drugs and food additives once considered safe are now known to cause adverse effects. In the United States cyclamates and saccharin are now banned. Saccharin, 300 times sweeter than sugar and the most widely used sweetener in the world, has been shown to cause bladder tumors in laboratory animals when taken in large doses.[5]

The general trend today is 'back to nature'. Highly processed foods are increasingly being rejected in favour of simple, natural foods. There is general awareness that health foods and sensible eating habits can prevent and even cure nagging ailments safely, conveniently, and without harmful side effects. The health food market is booming, offering an abundance of whole foods (natural foods which contain richer concentrations of nutrients than ordinary foods) and dietary supplements. More and more people are turning to a vegetarian or macrobiotic way of life. But even among people who prefer a more traditional mix of foods there is growing interest in natural, holistic, or what we shall call 'biologic' nutrition.

Biologic nutrition does not mean sticking to a boring, restricted diet. Quite the contrary. It means eating a great variety of natural foods, raw or with a minimum of cooking, and supplementing the diet with necessary nutrients (vitamins and minerals). In this way optimal levels of all necessary nutrients can be achieved with minimal contamination of the body. Every person is an individual, in the biological and metabolic sense. Diets and supplements should therefore be adjusted to the needs, weaknesses, allergies, hereditary traits and lifestyle of the individual.

Our educational system does not yet include nutrition education. Most people know much more about cars and car maintenance than they do about their own body and its nutritional needs. According to a recent survey, 92 per cent of supermarket shoppers in the United States do not understand the nutritional information on the packaging of foods they buy; 41 per cent of those surveyed were on various diets, and 38 per cent were trying to lose 10 pounds or more. One in every four frequently skipped both breakfast and lunch. And 61 per cent were not aware of the need to eat a balanced diet at all.[6] One of the results of being nutritionally naive is a weakened immune system and low resistance to disease, even in youngsters. The average health level of young people today continues to decline. U.S. Army recruits today are less healthy and fit than those of a generation ago.

This book was written to encourage you to explore various interesting aspects of nutrition and to enable you to take maximum responsibility for your own health. It will help you to get acquainted with the most suitable health foods, herbs, nutrients and diets to nourish your body and mind. It will also help you to lengthen the odds against disease and ill health and enjoy greater vitality and well-being. I truly hope that the interest in nutrition which this book tries to inspire will prove a blessing to all its readers.

My acknowledgments go to my good friends, the research biochemists, Dr Zvi A. Sidelman of A&M University, Texas, and Dr Stephen Levine, leader of the Allergy Research Group (Nutricology) in San Leandro, California, who both contributed valuable remarks to the manuscript; to the nutrition researcher and author, Dr Kurt W. Donsbach who helped me through my nutritional path; to Dennis R. Clark for his continuous assistance; to my publisher Mr Barry Winkleman whose enthusiasm was the driving power behind this edition, and finally, to my editor Mr Andrew Goodfellow, who spared no effort in editing the manuscript. May they all be blessed.

Dr Michael Sharon

CHAPTER 1

A NEW START IN LIFE

You are what you eat, drink and think. This ancient proverb should be repeated time and again until its inner truth is engraved on the mind. Nutrition can largely determine how we look, feel and work; whether we will be nervous, tired and pessimistic, or joyful, comfortable and happily active. Nutrition can also determine whether we will age prematurely or enjoy our lives to the full. To a great degree our nutrition determines whether, after a long day's work, we will drop exhausted into the nearest armchair or walk home with a light step. In short, nutrition can determine our quality of life.

The definition of nutrition in general, and of 'biologic nutrition' in particular, is that it is the study of foods, both plant and animal, and their influence on our bodies and feelings. Nutrition is a fascinating subject because it deals with you personally – with your own health, feelings and fitness. So why is the importance of good nutrition not universally recognized? There are many reasons. First of all, nutrition is a relatively young science. Secondly, for a long time it was the domain of a minority of people who were labelled, by the majority, as eccentrics. A person who avoided 'junk' foods and emphasized health foods, or vegetarianism, was labelled a 'food faddist' or a 'health nut'. Moreover, out of sheer ignorance, nutritious foods were considered unpalatable. It was generally agreed that raw, simple, unprocessed food could not be tasty or even tolerable to a normal person. And until recently the media supported the food processors, for commercial reasons.

There is no point in forcing yourself to eat foods that revolt you, but it makes sense to include as many natural, raw foods in your diet as possible, while gradually developing a taste for them. At one time I really hated avocados. After studying their great nutritional value, particularly for hypoglycemics (people with low blood sugar levels, a common condition which often manifests itself in fatigue, nervousness, depression and allergies), I started nibbling avocados now and then. After a while, I got used to them. Now I love them! The benefit is an additional fine natural source of fats, proteins, vitamins, minerals and carbohydrates. Avocado contains a special type of sugar (mannoheptulose) which depresses secretions of insulin (preventing hypoglycemia) instead of stimulating it, like ordinary sugar.[1]

It is important to emphasize that most common diseases are caused by deficiencies of nutrients in the body. These deficiencies develop gradually, over years of eating an unbalanced diet. So the nutritional knowledge contained in this book will be of considerable value to your health and your life.

NATURAL AND UNNATURAL FOODS

Human beings are a part of nature. Many minerals from the earth's crust, as well as nutrients from vegetable and animal sources, are represented in our bodies. It is therefore logical to assume that only those natural, wholesome foods which occur in nature are suitable for human consumption, both as food and medicine. All synthetic compounds are foreign to our nature.

With the rise of industrialization since the last century, people living in affluent societies have gradually detached themselves from their natural roots. Somehow the idea evolved that scientists could outdo nature in their ability to manufacture foodstuffs. In fact, as soon as scientists started 'handling' (or rather 'mishandling') vegetables and animals as food sources, a nutritional deterioration set in. Chemical industries started 'imitating' nature in the laboratory, producing chemical pesticides and fertilizers. Chemistry also began to provide the modern food industry with a variety of synthetic additives, preservatives, food colourings, artificial flavours and smells, texturizers and taste enhancers, many of which were subsequently found to have adverse effects on human health, or to be factors in the development of cancer in laboratory animals.

A classic example of the use of additives is commercial ice cream, to which some manufacturers add CMC (carboxymethyl cellulose). The sole purpose of this chemical in ice cream is to stabilize and inflate it. Thus, since ice cream is sold by volume, you receive less real ice cream per scoop when it is puffed up. (CMC, by the way, is also used in soap powders to hold dirt in suspension). And that is only the tip of the iceberg! All commercial ice cream flavours can be produced artificially – natural strawberry flavour is created by amyl acetate (a plastic solvent), pineapple flavour by ethyl acetate (another solvent), and vanilla flavour by piperonal (which also kills lice).[2]

A misguided concern for 'hygiene' has further alienated food from its natural state. Scientists have over-extended certain concepts of hygiene with respect to food processing, publicizing the idea that the more refined or processed a food is, the safer, tastier and healthier it is, the message being that raw foods are in some way unsafe. A classic example is white cane or beet sugar, carefully converted into a health hazard by sugar refineries. It all started in the early days of industrialization, when dark, raw sugar was used sparingly. This sugar contained molasses, a sticky residue of cane juice, highly concentrated in vitamins and minerals, with a specific taste, which could cause diarrhoea when eaten to excess. To promote the consumption of white sugar, a rumour was initiated by the newly built sugar refineries and some biased scientists that raw sugar was unclean and therefore unsafe to eat. Eventually, the concept was accepted, paving the way for the wide use of super-refined white sugar in Western countries.

SUGAR: PURE WHITE AND DEADLY

I am often asked what is wrong with refined sugar, a food derived from plants. The answer is that in nature all raw foods contain nutrients (vitamins, minerals, etc.) which are necessary for their assimilation into the body. Each nutrient has a role of its own in the body's chemistry. During the many thousands of years of human evolution, the human digestive system has adapted to these natural, complex compounds and learned to use them efficiently.

For the digestion of sugar, our bodies need several B vitamins, minerals such as chromium and zinc, fibre, and other nutrients. These occur naturally in sugar cane or sugar beets, from which table sugar is derived. However, white sugar, which has all of its component nutrients refined out of it, contains nothing but 'naked' sucrose. When we eat it, we force our digestive system to secrete vitamins, minerals and excesses of insulin out of its own stores in order to digest it. Eating small amounts of white sugar now and then may not do much harm, but eating large amounts day by day depletes the body of beneficial nutrients, and causes insulin production to rise to deleterious levels. In addition, a depletion caused shortage of the B vitamins is almost sure to lead to nervousness, indigestion, constipation and fatigue.

Chromium deficiency has been found to be a major culprit in atherosclerosis (hardening of the arteries) and heart attacks.[3] Zinc deficiency will not only harm one's sex life, but cause an increased craving for sugar. (According to Dr Alexander Schauss, a psychologist and Director of the American Institute of Biosocial Research in Washington, one way to reduce a 'sweet tooth' is to take extra zinc[4]). Moreover, excessive secretions of insulin can trigger the development of atherosclerosis, obesity, diabetes, hypoglycemia and several other diseases. It can also inhibit the release of growth hormone, which not only helps children to grow but also stimulates the multiplication of cells which ensure immunity against infection and other disease processes.[5] Since a considerable amount of growth hormone is released during the first 90 minutes of sleep, it is particularly important not to eat any refined sugar within a few hours of bedtime.

Furthermore, sugar is implicated in the yeast infections which plague literally millions of people, particularly women. Yeast (*Candida albicans*) germs, like tooth decay germs and meningitis germs, thrive on sugar. To grow germs in the laboratory, sugar is almost always added to the culture medium to aid growth. Yeast is present in everyone, but when it thrives more than it should due to excess consumption of sugar, it puts out a toxin which is detrimental to health. According to Dr William Crook, author of *The Yeast Connection*, who has done much research on the subject, the major group of symptoms caused by this toxin affects the nervous system – headache, fatigue and depression. The second group of symptoms affects the reproductive organs, especially in women – abdominal pain, menstrual irregularities, premenstrual tension, persistent vaginitis, bladder problems, loss of sex drive and infertility. The third group of symptoms affects the digestive system – constipation, flatulence, diarrhoea and intestinal problems.

It was therefore most appropriate for Dr John Yudkin of London University to entitle one of his books on sugar *Pure, White and Deadly*. Since it is well known that, as a population, we consume very much more sugar than we actually need,[6] it is not surprising that our national health is declining seriously.

BIOLOGIC NUTRITION

Biologic nutrition – growing and consuming foods of the highest possible nutritional value – is rapidly expanding in popularity. The word 'biologic' denotes compliance with the biological processes of the body. A 'biologic' diet is a natural, wholesome diet, supplemented by vitamins, minerals and health foods. All natural foods are recommended – vegetables, fruits, nuts, seeds, legumes, grains, eggs, milk and dairy products, fish and seafoods, and meat. It is important, however, that all of these be as fresh as possible, and free of residual pesticides, hormones, antibiotics and synthetic fertilizers, what is termed today as 'organic'. As far as possible, foods should be eaten raw or with a minimum of cooking or processing.

Bread should be baked from whole grain flours, preferably without commercial additives to lengthen its shelf life or improve its taste, smell and texture. Rice should be of the unpolished brown variety. As for sweetening, one should use small amounts of sorbitol, malt extract, maple syrup, powdered dates, molasses or honey. A sweet tooth can be satisfied largely with fresh fruits and modest amounts of dried fruits and fruit juices. White sugar and white flour, as well as all foods containing them, should be strictly avoided. The same goes for commercially preserved and processed foods high in hazardous chemicals and poor in natural, health-promoting vitamins. In short, biologic nutrition emphasizes whole, fresh foods which contain all the elements that promote vitality.

The versatility and variety of biologic nutrition ensures a varied and balanced supply of all the many nutrients – macronutrients and micronutrients – needed for optimal functioning of all body processes. By including animal and vegetable foods, it supplies an abundance of high-quality protein, in addition to carbohydrates, fats, vitamins and minerals, trace elements, enzymes, fibre, etc.

The concept of biologic nutrition holds that the body needs all of the nutrients found in natural foods. A deficiency in even one of them can damage biochemical processes and result in imbalances which may develop into clinically recognizable diseases. That is why biologic nutrition, unlike strict vegetarianism, does not impose limitations on any nutritious foods. The exceptions are foods which cause allergies, which should be given up completely.

The modern food industry causes varying losses in nutrients through processing, preserving, canning, freezing, drying and storing. Take, for example, common white flour. According to the Food and Nutrition Board, National Research Council of the Academy of Sciences, 24 nutrients

– including vitamins A, B, E and the mineral elements zinc, magnesium and chromium – are largely removed from grains during milling and refining, by separating the germ and bran from the grains.[7] Four nutrients are sometimes added to flour: vitamins B1, B2 and B3 and iron. This flour is then called enriched! How ironic! If I took a $100 bill from your pocket, returned $10, and then claimed that I had enriched you, you would probably call the police.

Adelle Davis cites the case of Denmark in World War I,[8] when, because of food shortages, the Danish government decided to forbid the milling of grains, among other dietary prohibitions. Nutrition was so improved during these years that the death rate fell by 34 per cent. The incidence of cancer, diabetes, high blood pressure and heart disease 'dropped markedly'. Evidently, public health was greatly benefited by the milling prohibition.

Biologic nutrition also recommends supplementation of the diet with vitamins and minerals, proteins, fibre or digestive enzymes in accordance with individual needs. Dr Roger Williams, the well-known biochemical researcher, teaches that nutritional needs vary greatly from one person to another. This is called 'the principle of biochemical individuality'. Calcium and protein requirements, for example, may vary among different people up to a factor of five.[9]

A few words about meat. In the above list of natural foods recommended for biologic nutrition, meat may appear as the least desirable. Today, many nutritionists consider meat as one of the most contaminated of foods. It is true that lean meat is a valuable source of complete protein and vitamin B12 that is not available from plant sources. However, this advantage has been counteracted by the modern, profit-seeking livestock industry which uses force feeding and a great variety of drugs, hormones, antibiotics and tranquillizers to shorten animal life spans and increase weight. Meat weight means dollars; meat quality means nothing! The slaughtered animals are, in fact, fatty reservoirs of dangerous toxins. The drug diethyl stilbestrol (DES), for example, administered to animals to develop fat and speed up weight gain, is a synthetic female hormone known to have caused vaginal and uterine cancer in girls whose mothers took DES during pregnancy.[10, 11] The recent Mad Cow Disease scare can well be seen as the result of such long standing abuse of beef.

Today's meat cannot, therefore, be considered a safe source of protein. A growing number of scientists are coming to the inevitable conclusion that a meat-centred diet is a very risky business today. Says Gary Null, Director of the Nutrition Institute of America and a well-known nutrition author: 'The accelerating incidence of heart disease in America has been linked with increased beef consumption.'[12] All scientists who dare to protest against the growing risks of excessive meat consumption, particularly when such consumption is not balanced with fibrous plant foods, are in fact justifying biologic nutrition.

THE ROOTS OF DISEASE

There are, in broad terms, four main causes of disease: nutrient deficiency; contamination of the body (toxaemia); a negative state of mind; hereditary disease.

Biologic nutrition can prevent and reverse the first two, nutritional deficiency and body contamination. These conditions can be rectified by increasing the consumption of natural, wholesome foods in a balanced diet properly supplemented with nutrients to meet individual needs, and by avoiding commercially processed foods. In many instances, biologic nutrition can also improve the third cause, a negative state of mind. What is a negative state of mind like depression, anxiety, memory loss or irritability? In many cases it is the symptom of an undernourished nervous system. Specific vitamins, minerals and amino acids are needed by the brain to synthesize neurotransmitters, special chemicals that transmit nerve impulses between nerve cells and influence our moods. Disturbances in body chemistry can warp thinking and distort emotions.[13]

Scientists are now using megavitamin (or orthomolecular) therapy in various institutions. As the name implies, very high doses of vitamins and minerals are used to reverse diseases caused by severe deficiencies. These deficiencies can be either congenital (due to high metabolic requirements) or accumulated over long years of malnutrition. In cases of schizophrenia and depression, impressive results have been achieved by injecting high doses of certain B vitamins. However, megavitamin therapy is by no means confined to mental disorders. Good results have also been achieved with certain physical disorders, such as cardiovascular diseases, which responded most favorably to high doses of vitamin E, and arthritis attacks, which responded well to megadoses of vitamin C and pantothenic acid. However, such megadoses should only be taken under the supervision of a nutrition-oriented physician.

As for hereditary conditions, here again biologic nutrition can lend a hand. Although ability to repair defective genes is obviously limited, it is well known that a well-balanced and properly supplemented diet can improve certain hereditary conditions such as diabetes, allergies and male pattern baldness. As Dr Carlton Fredericks says in his *Nutrition Handbook*, 'Heredity can be modified by nutrition.'

In *The Secret of Healthy Life*, Dr Everson Tilden claims that the basic cause of disease is the development of toxaemia (a state of poisoning) in the body. Toxaemia develops gradually and is the result of prolonged malnutrition. A malnourished body is less efficient at excreting its waste products, and so they build up and gradually contaminate the body. In a contaminated body, pathogenic (disease-causing) bacteria will easily propagate. Common tonsillitis is, in fact, a symptom of toxaemia. Inflamed, enlarged tonsils are the body's attempt to rid itself of toxins, allergens or microbes which have accumulated in excess of the neutralizing capacity of the weakened immune system.

It is well known that contagious diseases spread through pathogenic bacteria. However, we all know that some people do not catch the flu, even during an epidemic. They are as much exposed to the viruses as anybody else, but their immune systems are strong enough to kill the invading, disease-carrying organisms. Pathogenic viruses cannot easily gain a foothold in a clean, strong body.

DO YOU SUFFER FROM NUTRITIONAL DEFICIENCIES?

It is worthwhile developing an awareness of nutrient deficiency symptoms as reflected by your own body language. Are you overweight or too skinny? Is your skin pale, puffy or flabby? Many people age prematurely from deficient diets and develop face wrinkles from the depletion of collagen, the sub-skin tissue protein. Eyes, lips and hair 'speak' deficiency as well. All mucous membranes, from throat to bladder, are deeply influenced by the quality of the diet. Dark, hollowed eyes with blue rings around them are well-known deficiency signs. Cracks around the mouth, a purple or fissured tongue, white nail stains and lustreless hair also reflect deficiencies.

Other signs are tooth decay, foul body odour, poor posture, constipation and indigestion. Nervousness, restlessness, tension, depression, fatigue and apathy, as well as a multitude of infections from tonsillitis to prostatitis may also be deficiency symptoms. (Detailed deficiency symptoms are listed under each nutrient discussed in Chapters 3 and 4).

The art of healing is to a great extent the ability to cooperate with biologic processes in fortifying the natural immune system. Basic and logical as this principle is, orthodox medicine still finds it hard to adjust to the recent biological and biochemical findings which emphasize the great role that natural balanced nutrition plays in helping the body heal itself and ward off disease.

The idea that all diseases are caused by micro-organisms is simply not true. The common degenerative diseases of aging, such as cancer, atherosclerosis, high blood pressure and senile dementia, are caused by highly reactive oxidized particles from our metabolism, called superoxides or free radicals, which accumulate through lack of antioxidant vitamins, not by excess of microbes. Even Louis Pasteur, the first to perceive that microbes carry diseases, never claimed that all diseases were caused by microbes.[14] The late Dr Tom Spies, professor of nutrition at Alabama's Northwestern University Medical School and Director of the Nutritional Clinic, Hillman Hospital, Birmingham, Alabama, has said: 'Today, germs are not our principal enemy. Our chief medical adversary is what I consider a disturbance of the inner balance of constituents of our tissues, which are built from, and maintained by, necessary chemicals (nutrients) in the air we breathe, the water we drink and the food we eat.'[15]

Indeed, we know today of a whole list of critical diseases caused by nutrient deficiencies: scurvy (lack of vitamin C); beriberi (lack of vitamin B1); pellagra (lack of vitamin B3);

pernicious anaemia (lack of vitamin B12). Curing these diseases, which in the past were national epidemics, is very simple. Once the missing nutrients are restored, the disease disappears as if by magic. Although these acute and fatal diseases are now hard to find in our affluent society, most people unknowingly suffer from milder forms of them, because of milder deficiencies. Such deficiencies are not severe enough to cause an outburst of the disease itself, but are enough to cause many secondary symptoms from nervousness and fatigue to constipation and eczema.

After Pasteur, science had a hard time accepting the concept of deficiency diseases. It took twelve long years for Dr Christian Eijkman, the Dutch doctor who was sent to Batavia (Indonesia) in 1886 to study beriberi, to realize that it was a lack of vitamins (discarded with the rice husks), not an excess of microbes, that was causing the disease. Thirty-one years later he received the Nobel prize in medicine for the discovery of vitamin B1.

Many doctors who cannot diagnose deficiencies tell their patients, 'It's all in your mind' or 'It's just your age' or 'Take a vacation' when they complain of minor aches and pains for which no pathological reason can be found. These patients leave the doctor's office feeling frustrated and sometimes even humiliated. They lose hope for improvement through conventional medicine. Is it any wonder that such people are crowding the health food shops?

DRUGS AND YOUR HEALTH

Instead of cooperating with nature in healing and preventing diseases, most doctors prescribe synthetic drugs to alleviate symptoms and pains. A classic example is aspirin, which, in the United States, is sold at the rate of 15 tons a day. [16] Aspirin is used to eliminate all the aches and pains that doctors do not know how to cure, including arthritis and migraines. It is obvious that arthritis is not caused by aspirin deficiency because aspirin was not available before 1893, when it was introduced into medicine by Dr Hermann Dreser in Germany. Aspirin does not cure; it only mitigates or alleviates pain. In so doing, it disguises symptoms and makes it harder to diagnose their underlying causes. In spite of its popularity and its image as a harmless drug, aspirin is still a drug and as such has side effects. It can deplete vitamin C,[17] and its ability to cause stomach haemorrhages and ulcers is well known. In a recent study it was found that oral administration of large doses caused intestinal lesions.[18]

Prolonged use of certain popular tranquillizers, the phenothiazines (Mellaril, Thioridazine or Compazine), for example, can cause as side effects diseases such as tardive dyskinesia, Parkinson's disease and breast cancer in postmenopausal women.[19,20] Many people who depend on benzodiazepine drugs such as Valium or Librium for their tranquillity can substitute much safer nutrients such as vitamin B3, choline and the amino acid GABA, taken in high daily doses.[21]

Steroids, or adrenal cortical hormones, are chemicals produced naturally in the body by the adrenal glands situated over each kidney. They are vitally important to many bodily functions, in metabolizing carbohydrates, fats and proteins, for example. They also help us to handle stress, both emotional and physical, as well as infections and inflammations.

In the late 1940s, laboratories started producing synthetic steroids (cortisones). These were hailed as wonder drugs when it was found that they could suppress allergies and inflammations, especially rheumatoid arthritis. Today, after extensive studies, they are used by doctors to treat a much larger variety of conditions, from allergies, asthma and eczema to haemolytic anaemia, acute leukaemia and serum sickness.

Using steroids for a long list of disorders resulted in nearly as long a list of side effects. While steroids suppress inflammations, they disrupt the natural hormonal balance in the body. They impair healing, aggravate wounds, weaken the body and cause depression. One has only to glance at a pharmaceutical pamphlet for any steroid drug to be confronted with a frightening list of possible side effects and contra-indications. Steroids, like aspirin, do not cure diseases; they merely alleviate symptoms. Joints swell and ache less, but cartilage and bone destruction goes on.

Confronted with this information, a doctor might defend himself or herself by retorting, 'Tell that to someone screaming in agony from arthritis.' These days, doctors believe in the usefulness of steroids as a general tool to combat critical diseases. It is, however, in our best interest to try other natural therapies, including megavitamins, before using steroids in acute conditions. Steroid users must make sure that they are getting the lowest dosage required. And they should discuss the problem of side effects openly with a specialist.

The spreading use of yet another type of steroid by over-zealous athletes – remember the Seoul Olympiad? – is a classic example of health abuse. The drugs commonly used by sports people are androgenic-anabolic steroids, synthetic versions of the male (androgenic) hormone testosterone. 'Anabolic' means that they enhance the build-up of tissue, especially muscle tissue.

Anabolic steroids were first used during World War II, when they were given to German troops to increase muscle strength and aggressiveness. In the 1950s, physicians began using androgenic-anabolic steroids to treat patients with muscle-wasting disorders, for some types of anemia, for burn patients, and for stunted growth in children. It is commonly believed that the Russians were the first to use steroids in sports. And once it was known that the Russians were using steroids to build bigger muscles and increase strength and endurance, athletes all over the world began using them in massive and unsafe doses.

Huge doses of anabolic steroids damage health, as is becoming evident as more athletes become ill or even die. First, it was observed that steroid users become much more aggressive, ready to fight at the slightest provocation. In young athletes steroids cause premature hardening of the cartilage-like plates (epiphyseal plates) at the end of the long bones, resulting in stunted growth. In men anabolic steroids raise circulating levels of the male hormone testosterone, with the result that the pituitary depresses the body's own testosterone production, causing shrinking of the testicles, lower sperm count, sterility and prostate cancer. Women using steroids lose their breasts and develop deepened voices, altered menstrual cycles and body hair. Impaired liver function and jaundice are also prevalent among steroid users, as well as high blood pressure and heart palpitations and irregularities. Conditions related to heart disease, such as hardening of the arteries, are also worsened by anabolic steroid use.

The Medical Commission of the International Olympic Committee, aware of these health hazards, added steroids to its list of banned substances and started drug-testing in 1968. However, it was not until recently that tests became sensitive enough to detect anabolic steroids in urine. In 1987, prednisone (an anti-inflammatory drug) was added to the list of banned substances, because some athletes were using it to block the detection of steroids. It is to be hoped that these revelations will help to halt the use of steroids in sport.

The use of antibiotics, the commonly used 'wonder

drugs' of our century, is starting to decline. The cover story of the March 28, 1994 issue of *Newsweek,* 'Antibiotics: The End of Miracle Drugs?' was a sobering report on the failure of antibiotics, once thought to eradicate all infectious diseases. More and more members of the healing professions are beginning to have doubts about their safety. They are causing more sensitivities in people than ever before and their efficiency is decreasing. Many strains of bacteria have developed immunity to antibiotics and therefore resist antibiotic treatments. It is estimated that roughly 20 per cent of infections contracted in hospitals fail to respond to antibiotics, and that in the United States alone 100,000 people die each year of such infections.[22] Only 10-20 per cent of staphylococcus infections contracted in hospitals are now susceptible to penicillin.[23] There is now a growing tendency to prepare patients for operations by fortifying their immune system, over a period of time, with a carefully balanced and supplemented diet. Originally, antibiotics were highly powerful. They were used only in emergencies and certainly saved the lives of people who would otherwise have died. They also simplified complicated treatments. Gradually, however, antibiotics were misused by overuse. Doctors developed a growing tendency to make it easy on themselves by prescribing antibiotics without a second thought for future infections. The result was that within a few years most bacteria learned to resist antibiotics. It became necessary to prescribe higher doses, so antibiotics were manufactured in much higher potencies, up to 50 times the original ones. New types were also developed to keep one jump ahead of the bacteria. And so a vicious cycle was set up. Included in this cycle were more and more side effects, the most common of which were weakness and depression. In many instances, the side effects were worse than the original infection.

One of the main drawbacks of antibiotics is that they do not distinguish between friend and foe. They kill the friendly intestinal bacteria (which are vitally needed to help food absorption and to synthesize certain vitamins) along with the pathogenic bacteria. When friendly germs are wiped out, body yeasts (*Candida*), which are present in everyone, multiply. It is estimated that 50 per cent of women who have taken tetracycline or one of the broad spectrum drugs develop a vaginal yeast infection (candidiasis).[24] Antibiotics were also found to neutralize the action of the contraceptive pill. Many teenage girls who develop a few pimples and manage to get tetracycline from their skin doctors are also vulnerable. Men can suffer from intestinal yeast infection, particularly if they take antibiotic drugs for long-term prostatitis. That is why it is highly recommended that you eat plenty of live yogurt when you are on antibiotics. Yogurt and other soured milks, such as acidophilus milk or *kefir*, replenish beneficial bacteria in the intestines. (People allergic to dairy products can use lactobacillus-acidophilus tablets instead, or FOS powder.)

Over 2,000 types of antibiotics exist today, and sometimes they are present, in small amounts, in over-the-counter preparations. Instead of using them sparingly, for emergencies, they are being used freely, sometimes in anticipation of an illness, as a 'preventive' measure, before the need exists.

The tide is slowly turning, however. More doctors are now using antibiotics as a last resort, and the idea that immunity can be maintained and enhanced through biologic nutrition principles is gaining ground. We are returning to basics. The indisputable trend, in medicine as well as diet, is 'back to nature'.

CHAPTER 2

BUILDING BLOCKS:
THE MACRONUTRIENTS

Macronutrients, as the name implies, occur in bulk quantities in the body. They are proteins, carbohydrates, and fats and they are generously provided by the foods we eat.

All foods contain varying amounts of different macronutrients. We have all heard about high protein foods or low carbohydrate diets. As already noted, macronutrients, like any other nutrients, never occur alone in nature; each is accompanied by other macronutrients and micronutrients (vitamins and minerals). Every macronutrient has its own specific duties and deficiency symptoms. In many instances, the roles of macronutrients overlap, as we shall see in the following pages. Proteins, for example, can be converted to carbohydrates (sugar) while sugars can be converted to fats; they are mutually dependent, not only in their natural state but in our systems as well.

Each one of us needs the same basic macronutrients, although not in the same proportions. Our needs vary according to our individual metabolic requirements, age, occupation and heredity.

PROTEINS

Protein is the most plentiful substance in the body after water. In fact, the Greek word *protos* means 'first'. Proteins are the building blocks of the body, not only of the muscles and tissues of the skin, as most people know, but also of hormones, enzymes, antibodies and blood. You cannot build a wall with just mortar and sand; you need bricks. The same is true with the human body. The body uses proteins like building blocks, to build up muscle and blood, skin and bone, heart and brain.

Why are proteins so important after the growth years? They act as 'spare parts' for the wear and tear of living. Each instant of our lives, cell proteins throughout our body – red blood cells, immune cells, hormones, enzymes – are being broken down. Proteins build up and regenerate vital hormones such as insulin, adrenalin and thyroxine, which control weight, sexual activity and metabolism. They also serve as a source of heat and energy when there is a shortage of carbohydrates, providing 4 calories per gram.

The constituents of protein are the amino acids. To create the many forms of protein in the body, amino acids have to be linked together to form chain structures. These give each kind of protein – whether it is a protein in bone, hair or nails – its specific characteristics. The supervisors of these complex protein-forming processes are the nucleic acids DNA and RNA, often described as the 'blueprints' of heredity. DNA (deoxyribonucleic acid) in the cell nucleus contains the master code and RNA (ribonucleic acid) is a messenger form of DNA which conveys the instructions contained in DNA to the cytoplasm of the cell, where protein synthesis takes place. Damaged or disturbed DNA or RNA is now believed to impair protein synthesis, causing faulty cell function, premature aging[1] and cancer.[2]

The symptoms of protein deficiency are many and varied. Poor growth and development of body cells is a common consequence of protein shortage. These are reflected mainly in falling hair, brittle nails and rough skin, as well as poor muscle tone and anaemia. Greater or prolonged deficiencies can lead to glandular malfunction, poor sexual drive, susceptibility to infections, fatigue, depression and slow healing of wounds. Other protein deficiency symptoms, in children, include stunted growth and swelling of the joints. In adults, protein deficiency can cause face wrinkles and signs of premature aging. Says Dr Kurt Donsbach, founder of Donsbach University School of Nutrition in California: 'Protein is a rejuvenator'. [3]

A growing number of researchers think that people who suffer from repeated infections, such as tonsillitis, may have a poor immune system due to a poor protein metabolism.[4] Since protein enables the body to synthesize new immune cells, an adequate protein supply is obviously needed to build up a strong resistance to infectious diseases. The traditional Jewish mother used to feed clear chicken soup (a fine source of easily digested protein) to her child whenever he or she caught a cold or had a sore throat. Is it any wonder that many people still call chicken soup 'Jewish penicillin'?

When a diet is low in protein, or high in refined carbohydrates, little bile is produced.[5] When there is little bile, food fats are poorly dissolved in the digestive tract. Parts of the undissolved fats combine with the calcium and iron in the food we eat, and form insoluble soaps (fatty acid salts). These soaps do two things, both harmful to health: they harden the stools, causing constipation, and they prevent the gut from absorbing calcium and iron. If a low protein diet is eaten for long enough, deficiencies of iron and calcium may develop, causing anaemia, porous bones and tooth decay.

The proteins present in food break down during digestion into simpler components, amino acids, and it is thanks to amino acids that cells are maintained and repaired and replaced throughout the body. Dr Paul C. Aebersold, former head of the United States Atomic Energy Commission, said: 'Your body may seem much the same to you as it was a year ago . . . but in a single year, 98 per cent of the old atoms will be replaced by new atoms, which we take into our bodies from the air we breathe, the food we eat and the water we drink.' [6]

The life span of most cells is up to about 120 days. Then their amino acids are recycled to make new cells, and the unwanted products of cell breakdown are converted to waste products by the liver and excreted through the kidney.[7]

AMINO ACIDS

Proteins are the most complex of all food compounds. They are made up of any one of thousands of combinations of just 24 amino acids, which consist of carbon, hydrogen, oxygen, nitrogen, sulphur and iron. The key factor is nitrogen, the crucial ingredient in the formation of amino and nucleic acids (nitrogen–containing compounds). Eight amino acids are 'essential amino acids', ones which the body cannot manufacture (synthesize) itself, but must acquire from food. Without them, no synthesis of protein can take place. The essential amino acids are: leucine, isoleucine, valine, methionine, threonine, lysine, phenylalanine and tryptophan.

From biochemical studies we know that all of the eight essential amino acids must be simultaneously present in food – in the same meal and in the right proportions[8] – for protein synthesis to take place. If even one is absent or disproportionately low, protein synthesis is halted or reduced.

Various amino acids have recently been found to have special beneficial effects in many specific conditions. They are now used like vitamins in the treatment of certain disorders. Studies have revealed that the essential amino acid LYSINE, for example, can very efficiently suppress the *Herpes simplex* virus (mouth blisters, cold sores).[9] Lysine, which is lacking in vegetables and grains, plays an essential role in calcium absorption. Its supplements are therefore important to prevent calcium deficiencies among vegetarians.

TRYPTOPHAN, another amino acid which is plentiful in milk, is converted into a brain chemical called serotonin. Serotonin is a neurotransmitter (a chemical that conveys brain messages) which calms nervousness, puts insomniacs to sleep and alleviates depression. Its effect was found to be of longer duration than the popular antidepressant drug imipramine.[10]

Tryptophan supplements were banned in the late 80s, when a few contaminated lots, produced with a new bacteria caused an outburst of a rare disease called eosinophilia myalgia syndrome (EMS). Hundreds of people contracted the disease and 24 died.[11] Although tryptophan itself was not to blame, only the new manufacturing process, tryptophan supplements were not available until recently, when a new form of tryptophan, 5-hydroproxy Tryptophan (5-HTP) was found in the beans of an African bush (Griffonia simplicifolia). Various studies showed that 5-HTP can cross the blood brain barrier, making its tryptophan available to the body, increasing serotonin levels. Tryptophan–rich foods include milk, turkey, bananas, soya beans, pumpkin seeds, tofu, almonds, peanuts and brewer's yeast.

PHENYLALANINE and TYROSINE, abundant in meat and cheese, are converted into a brain chemical which transmits nerve impulses, norepinephrine (noradrenalin). Norepinephrine (the brain's version of adrenalin) promotes mental alertness, improves memory, alleviates depression and suppresses appetite very effectively, thus assisting weight loss.

Phenylalanine deserves a special mention. Various studies have highlighted its ability to relieve chronic pain and depression in a safe, non-toxic, non-addictive manner, and without the devastating side effects of pain-killing and antidepressant drugs. Phenylalanine (PA) comes in two basic forms, which are mirror images of each other: L-phenylalanine (LPA) which has a nutritional value and D-phenylalanine (DPA) which has the painkilling and depression-alleviating properties. A third form, DL-phenylalanine (DLPA), which is a 50/50 mixture of these two forms, is both nutritional and therapeutic.

Studies conducted by Dr Seymour Ehrenpreis, a pharmacologist at the Chicago Medical School, Dr Reuben Balagot, a neurosurgeon at the Chicago Veteran Hospital, and others, have shown that DLPA alleviates pain by protecting endorphins (natural pain-blocking hormones secreted by nerve cells) from destruction by enzymes. It is this enzymatic action that prevents endorphins from exerting their natural narcotic effect, which is many times more powerful than morphine or aspirin. DLPA provided long-lasting relief for people suffering from the chronic gnawing pains of osteoarthritis and rheumatoid arthritis, and also from headaches, lower back pain and other disorders.[12]

Dr Arnold Fox, an internist and cardiologist from Beverly Hills, explains in his recent book entitled *DLPA*[13] that this amino acid also protects endorphins in those parts of the brain concerned with emotions, particularly with feelings of euphoria and elation. DLPA can also relieve depression by raising brain levels of beta phenylethylamine (PEA) and norepinephrine, shortages of which are known to be associated with depression. Roughly 2 grams brought relief in most cases that responded. Many users find that they can cut back on their doses of DLPA or even discontinue them entirely when full relief has been achieved.

CAUTION: Excessive doses of DLPA may cause irritability, insomnia and elevated blood pressure. People with hypertension should start with a low dose (100 mg daily), then raise it gradually while checking their blood pressure frequently.

Incidentally, chocolate contains PEA, which explains why many people eat chocolate as a mood elevator in times of mental distress, such as a broken love affair. Overweight people would be well advised to use PEA salt rather than tuck into a box of high-calorie chocolates!

Another amino acid, GLUTAMIC ACID (or its more usable form, glutamine), is known as 'brain fuel'.[14] It improves mental functions, memory for example, relieves fatigue and helps to control alcoholism, schizophrenia and migraines. It can also curb excessive cravings for sweets.

ARGININE and ORNITHINE (abundant in home-made chicken soup!) stimulate the secretion of growth hormone by the pituitary gland in the brain.[15] Growth hormone is not only essential for children's growth, but equally important for adults since it promotes the repair of worn tissues, helps to heal wounds and strengthens the immune system.[16] Growth hormone stimulates the growth of lymphocytes, the immune cells in our blood stream that identify, engulf and destroy invading viruses, bacteria and carcinogenic chemicals. In larger quantities, through higher supplementation of arginine or ornithine, growth hormone is reported to stimulate weight loss, by causing one to burn fat while developing muscle.[17] Finally, arginine is abundant in seminal fluid. No wonder that supplements can increase sperm count and motility. Low levels of spermine (a simple polyamine) in blood were found by Dr Carl Pfeiffer to be correlated to poor memory and senility.[18] A combination of arginine, ornithine and methionine can thus help to improve memory.[19] Arginine is closely related to ornithine. In fact, all ingested arginine is converted in the body to ornithine. Ornithine costs about twice as much as arginine, but is required in half the dose.

CAUTION: Arginine and ornithine should be used by adults only, but not by pregnant or lactating women. It should not be used by youngsters who have not reached their full height. Arginine is contra-indicated in cases of herpes, where ornithine can be used instead.

CYSTEINE, a sulphur-containing amino acid plentiful in eggs, is a vital ingredient of reduced glutathione, an antioxidant enzyme, which helps to neutralize dangerous peroxides and free radicals (toxic waste products of metabolism and radiation that oxidize and damage body cells). Through this antioxidant enzyme, cysteine contributes to an increased life span and prevents age-related diseases such as atherosclerosis, heart attack and cancer.[20] In recent years, it has also been reported to discourage degenerative diseases like osteoarthritis and rheumatoid arthritis. Hair is 8 per cent cysteine by weight. Cysteine supplements can therefore accelerate hair growth, while cysteine deficiency can enhance male pattern baldness.[22] Finally, cysteine can block the harmful effects of excess insulin (as in hypoglycaemia) and of atherosclerosis,[23] another reason for sugar-lovers to eat eggs rather than sweets.

A recent form of cysteine is available as NAC (N-acetyle cysteine). NAC is a powerful antioxidant which increases immunity to diseases, infections and colds.[24] It is being studied for its ability to inhibit the AIDS virus and is normally prescribed for bronchitis and liver detoxification.

CAUTION: Diabetics should not experiment with cysteine.

METHIONINE is another sulphur-containing amino

acid. Like cysteine, it is a chelator, which means that it combines with toxic elements such as lead, mercury and cadmium and eliminates them from the body. As these toxins are known to cause a plethora of symptoms, including hypertension, depression, hyperactivity in children, impaired memory and kidney damage, methionine can assist in the treatment of these conditions. Methionine is abundant in dairy products and meat, but is lacking in vegetables and legumes. Vegetarians are therefore susceptible to deficiencies and may benefit from methionine supplementation.

The amino acid HISTIDINE is the precursor of histamine in the body. It stimulates stomach acid secretion and also has a calming effect on the nervous system. Histidine supplements have been found to alleviate allergies, unblock nasal passages, and reduce redness and swelling.[25]

CARNITINE is an amino acid which is made up from lysine and methionine. Biochemically, it helps transport fat into the mitochondria, the tiny power plants in every cell, which 'burn' fat into energy. Carnitine capsules can therefore be helpful as energy boosters in muscles before strenuous activities, like gym workout.

Several studies indicate that carnitine can lower cholesterol and triglyceride levels.[26] In this way, carnitine can help reduce the risk of heart attack. Carnitine can even help protect the heart during a heart attack, by reducing the toxic effects of fatty acid derivatives, which are produced in oxygen-deprived hearts.[27]

Since carnitine helps 'burn' fats, it is assumed that carnitine supplementation can help dieting.[28] In fact, carnitine can help protect dieters from ketosis, a life-threatening condition which is usually a consequence of crash diets, semi-starvation diets or low carbohydrate diets. Daily doses of 1,500 mg of carnitine are also thought to improve sexual performance.[29]

GABA (Gamma-Aminobutyric Acid) is an amino acid which is currently gaining popularity for its anti-anxiety effect. GABA is derived in the body from glutamic acid and was found to be an inhibitory neuro-transmitter.[30] That is, it slows down the activity of the neurons in the brain's lymbic system. The lymbic system is our emotional alarm bell. It is deeply buried in the brain, and, once provoked, sends stress signals to higher brain centres.[31] By dampening the emotional effects of the lymbic system, GABA can help reduce stressful feelings like anxiety, fear and panic.

TYROSINE is the amino acid needed by the thyroid gland to produce one of the major hormones, thyroxine. This hormone regulates many functions, such as growth rate, metabolic rate and hence the efficiency with which fat is burnt to energy, skin health, mental health, and many more. Tyrosine is also a precursor of epinephrine and dopamine, brain chemicals which transmit nervous impulses and which are essential to prevent depression.

People who are interested in using specific amino acids for their beneficial effects will be glad to know that they are now available in most good health food shops. They are usually marked with an L prefix – L-Arginine, L-Lysine, L-Phenylalanine and so on. The role of amino acids is one of the most promising areas in nutrition research today.

MAKING SURE THAT PROTEIN IS 'COMPLETE'

The importance of preventing protein deficiency cannot be overemphasized, especially when many protein foods do not contain all of the essential amino acids. Such foods are 'incomplete protein' foods. Only a part of their protein content can be utilized by the body. Only when a food contains all eight essential amino acids is it a 'complete protein'. Such foods are obviously ideal sources of protein.

Complete protein foods usually come from the animal kingdom: eggs, milk, dairy products, fish and meat. A few plants contain complete protein too, but the majority cannot compete with animal foods for high-quality protein. Examples of high protein plant foods are: soybeans, nuts, seeds, whole grains, legumes, soya bean sprouts, wheat germ, pollen, spirulina (lake algae) and brewer's yeast. These are considered the best non-animal sources of complete protein.

Since incomplete protein is poorly synthesized by the body, it is difficult to subsist on strictly vegetarian foods for long without risking deficiency symptoms. Therefore, it is always better to include some animal protein — cheese, milk, egg — in any vegetarian meal in order to 'complete' the incomplete plant protein. As for meat eaters, biologic nutrition advises eating 'organic' meat, from animals reared in natural, spray-free pastures, free of hormones, antibiotics and other synthetic chemicals. Some complete plant proteins, such as brewer's yeast and spirulina, can be used to 'complete' proteins in strict vegetarian dishes.

Health food manufacturers are aware of the need for simple sources of complete protein. Accordingly, they produce a variety of high protein powders, made of concentrates of soya, brewer's yeast and milk solids. These powders can be used to supplement the deficient diets of children and adolescents, vegetarians, convalescents, busy people who need to balance a low protein intake, and athletes (particularly body builders) who need extra protein. They can be sprinkled on soups or made into protein drinks which, when made with milk can occasionally replace breakfast for the late riser.

CAUTION:These protein powders should not be confused with protein dieting aids. Strict diets based almost exclusively on these are harmful. They cause severe dietary deficiencies and have led to several deaths.

Biologic nutrition, like vegetarianism, recommends making the most of plant protein by learning how to combine different incomplete protein plants in one meal so as to increase protein value. This is done by picking the food combinations (usually grains and legumes) which supplement each other's missing amino acids. Such combinations often form the traditional staples of regional cuisine. The beans and rice of Latin America, Middle Eastern rice and lentil dishes and Chinese sticky rice with soybean paste are all examples of complete protein combinations. In a similar vein, new types of bread are being baked which offer higher protein value by combining incomplete plant proteins. Two such breads are 'cotton' bread, baked from high protein cottonseed flour, and seven-grain bread.

Typically, health food snacks such as 'trail mix' also provide a convenient combination of plant proteins. These nut-soya bean-dried fruit-seed mixtures usually have a high protein ratio. They can, and should, replace all sugary sweets.

Most nutrition publications recommend about 1 gram of protein a day for every 2 pounds of body weight. A man weighing 200 pounds would therefore need about 100 grams of protein a day. However, new studies show that this dosage is too generalized. Some people stay healthy and vigorous with lower protein consumption. In fact, there are studies which warn that consistently high protein meat-centred diets can lead to a toxic condition caused by amino acid waste products in the body. Excessive consumption of protein, especially meat protein, has been found to contribute to heart disease,[32] cancer of the colon[33] and arthritis.[34] A high protein

intake can increase loss of calcium and also tends to be con-
stipating, promoting the growth of putrefactive bacteria in
the intestines.[35] So high meat diets should always be balanced
with supplementary fibre, from fruits, vegetables, whole
grains or fibre tablets to increase stool transit time and counteract their undesirable effects.

Clearly, optimal protein consumption (as with consumption of any other nutrient) varies with the individual. Some
people may need four times as much as others.[36] Stress conditions (mental or physical) can increase protein requirements
by as much as 30 per cent.[37] So if you care about your health
you should check whether your daily protein intake meets
the average figures and then adjust it to your personal
requirements. If you have difficulty doing this, ask a nutritionist for guidance.

CARBOHYDRATES

Carbohydrates supply the body with energy. Like fuel in an
engine, they 'burn' in the presence of oxygen, providing 4
calories per gram. They are plentiful in the plant kingdom
and are abundantly found in fruits and vegetables, grains and
legumes, honey and sugar.

Sugar, the most abundant source of carbohydrates (carbos
for short), is a multifaceted substance. The name is applied scientifically to a group of substances that are similar but not
identical: simple sugars or monosaccharides, such as glucose
(blood sugar) and fructose (fruit sugar); double sugars or dis-
accharides, such as sucrose (table sugar) and lactose (milk
sugar); and complex sugars or polysaccharides, such as cellulose (fibre) and starches. Among the natural foods most plentiful in simple and double sugars are dried fruits. Dates, for
example, contain 78 per cent sugar and raisins 54 per cent.

Simple and double sugars are the most concentrated sources of energy.

However, the body can only use the simple sugar GLUCOSE to provide energy. This means that all sugars and starches, and to a lesser degree proteins and fats, must be converted to glucose by digestive enzymes before they can be used. Glucose is subsequently metabolized and regulated by the hormone insulin. FRUCTOSE (abundant in fruits) is readily converted to glucose by the liver and absorbed from the intestines into the blood, without the need of insulin,[38] making it a fine quick-energy sugar. That is why it is best for people who wake up drowsy in the morning to have a glass of fresh fruit juice rather than coffee. This is also the reason why fructose can be consumed moderately by diabetics (who lack insulin). As it is 50 per cent sweeter than table sugar and causes less tooth decay,[39] it is also safer. Another related sugar which does not trigger insulin release is SORBITOL, most popular among diabetics. Most of it is converted to carbon dioxide. Only a small part is converted to glucose, which is absorbed through the intestines over a longer period of time than table sugar,[40] making it a much more desirable sweetener than ordinary sugar, even for healthy people. Its slow metabolism does not tax the sugar-balancing glands and causes much less tooth decay. Sorbitol also increases assimilation of certain vitamins such as B12, which explains its presence in many multivitamin tablets. MANNITOL is another non-insulin-releasing sugar.

BLOOD SUGAR LEVELS

It is important to remember that our energy level is highly dependent on the specific type of sugar that we regularly consume. And energy is the factor that most influences our physical and mental activity. Keeping a consistently adequate blood sugar level is imperative for a feeling of well-being.

Any excess sugar that we consume is converted to glycogen and stored in the liver and muscles for future use. Some glucose is always present in the bloodstream to supply quick energy to the brain, muscles and organs. A complicated hormonal balancing mechanism is in charge of keeping blood sugar at a fairly constant level. This mechanism involves gluco-receptor cells in the brain which send impulses to the pituitary gland, the brain's main controlling gland. The pituitary then sends hormones to the adrenal glands, the liver and the pancreas.[41] The pancreas is the final blood sugar regulator. When the blood sugar level rises too high for our own good, the pancreas secretes insulin, a hormone which converts excess glucose to glycogen; when the blood sugar level is too low, the pancreas secretes glucagon and the adrenal glands secrete adrenalin, two hormones which convert glycogen back to glucose.

However, when this complicated mechanism is incessantly overstimulated by enormous surges of sugar from candies or soft drinks, the pancreas may gradually become exhausted to a point where insulin secretion diminishes, producing diabetes; or its secreting cells may become so sensitized that they overrespond by secreting far too much insulin, drastically lowering the blood sugar level and causing hypoglycaemia.[42] Excess insulin is also known to contribute to atherosclerosis.[43]

A proper blood sugar level is somewhere between 90 and 100 mg glucose per 100 cc of blood. At this level, we are energetic and feel good. When the level drops to 70 mg, hunger, fatigue and irritability set in. At lower levels exhaustion, dizziness, heart palpitations and nausea are common.

How can we consistently keep a proper blood sugar level

without overstressing our regulating glands? Surprisingly enough, not by eating more candy or drinking more soda pop. Table sugar is a concentrated form of energy which rapidly raises the blood sugar level immediately after ingestion, but the level soon falls to an even lower level than before. Irritation and fatigue are thus aggravated.

Many studies have been made of the factors influencing blood sugar levels. In one study, a high protein breakfast was found to be effective in keeping a consistently optimum level.[44] Unlike sugar metabolism which occurs quickly, protein metabolism is complicated and results in a much slower release of sugar over a much longer period of time. With protein, the adrenal glands and the pancreas easily control the sugar level, as they do not have to overcome sudden surges of sugar. Some nutritionists, such as the well-known naturopathic physician and author Dr Paavo Airola, advocate eating plenty of natural grains, legumes and seeds. These foods provide a combination of protein and starch, which maintains a consistent blood sugar level. The dangers attendant upon excessive consumption of animal proteins are also avoided.[45]

Another effective way to prevent low blood sugar is to eat frequent small meals. This is not only kinder to your pancreas, but also improves metabolism and helps you to diet by avoiding that starving feeling.

Overconsumption of refined sugar and flour foods is one of today's greatest health hazards. In spite of all the warnings by nutritionists, dentists and doctors, average consumption is still rising annually. People find it hard to attribute such bitter properties to such sweet products. They accept the advertized notion that sugar is necessary to supply energy. If we take seriously the key statement made by nutritionist John Yudkin that 'there is no physiological requirement for sugar,' the annual per capita consumption in the United States of

102 pounds of sugar in soft drinks, ice creams and countless sweets is nothing short of appalling. Professor Yudkin also observes: 'If only a fraction of what is already known about the effects of sugar were to be revealed in relation to any other food additive, this material would promptly be banned.'[46]

In fact, many independent scientists have performed studies which link sugar with an endless line of human afflictions. Gout, diabetes, atherosclerosis and obesity have been shown by Dr William Ishmael of the University of Oklahoma to be related to dietary sucrose.[47] Nutritionists Dale Alexander, Carlton Fredericks and others have noted that primitive ethnic groups in isolated regions of the world who do not use refined sugar do not suffer from tooth decay. The high consumption of white sugar is the scourge of the civilized world.

The dangers of refined sugar repeat themselves in the case of refined complex carbohydrates. Instead of supplying the body with natural wholesome starchy foods such as whole grain breads and cereals, bananas, potatoes, brown rice and legumes, we use an overwhelming array of refined starch products such as white breads and rolls, polished rice, and pasta made with white, refined flour. White flour and polished rice are lifeless foods, devoid of the bran and germ, the life-carrier of the grain. We eat a carbohydrate stripped of its nutrients, which mostly supplies empty calories.

Unrefined complex carbohydrates, on the other hand, are the best suited carbohydrates for healthy nutrition. Whole grain breads and pastas, brown rice, jacket potatoes and yams, beans and sprouts should be made the chief source of calories.

The high bulky fibre of these foods satisfies hunger with fewer calories.[48] Their energy supply is readily available causing a reduced need for fat, lowering cholesterol levels. They are also rich in potassium, vitamins and minerals. In contrast, a low bulk, high calorie, sugary diet, encourages hunger and gorging. Such a diet promotes consumption of far more calories before satiety is achieved. No wonder that obesity is uncommon in most primitive cultures who subsist on natural staple foods. Indeed, experimental studies with animals confirm that high bulk diets prevent obesity, while low bulk diet encourage it.[49] Moreover, people on rich, unrefined complex carbohydrate diets also feel better, because these foods supply energy to the body in the least stressful way.

THE EFFECTS OF ALCOHOL

Alcohol is another common source of empty calories. Along with sugar, it is rated as the strongest contributor to high blood cholesterol levels.[50] It is, however, worse than sugar because of its depleting and toxic effects. The 2.5 calories per gram that it supplies deplete the body of several B vitamins, vitamin C, vitamin K, zinc, magnesium and potassium, and promote obesity. Also the liver's ability to metabolize glucose and eliminate waste poisons is compromised, even by what many would consider moderate drinking.[51] Higher consumption of alcohol has been found to result in brain damage,[52] ruptured blood vessels, and agglutinated blood (clumped blood cells), leading to the formation of varicose veins and thrombosis (blood clots); damage to sexual glands (prostate) and sterility; and psychological disorders such as anxiety, depression, mental retardation and distorted emotions.[53]

Alcoholism is a chronic behavioural disturbance which is mostly caused by a metabolic defect, not, as is generally believed, by weak character or lack of morality. During alcohol metabolism, a harmful chemical called acetaldehyde is formed. This chemical gives a drinker a bad feeling which can be overcome by drinking more alcohol, which of course causes more acetaldehyde to be formed, creating a vicious cycle of addiction. It has been found that alcoholics have much more acetaldehyde in their bloodstream after a drink than normal people do.[54] In fact, acetaldehyde is now believed to give rise to dangerous peroxides and free radicals, reactive particles which attack various cells and cause DNA mutations and cancer, atherosclerosis and heart attacks, joint stiffness and skin wrinkles, brain damage and eye cataracts (free radicals are discussed in detail in Chapter 15).

Alcohol cravings have been found to yield to nutritional supplementation. In one study with rats, which were given lethal doses of acetaldehyde, a supplement containing vitamin B1, vitamin C and the amino acid cysteine proved to be a lifesaver.[55] The amino acid glutamine was found to be very effective both in reducing alcohol consumption and preventing alcohol poisoning.[56] It is assumed that glutamine protects the brain cells which control appetite, which is often impaired in drinkers. Other beneficial nutrients are magnesium, which prevents withdrawal symptoms,[57] and large doses (megadoses) of vitamin B3, which can also help to control a sweet tooth.

Sometimes we tend to forget that the plant kingdom offers a great bounty of natural whole sugars and starches – enough to satisfy a reasonably sweet tooth. They contain all of the nutrients needed for their own assimilation. Two apples, which contain everything necessary to digest their own sugar, are the equivalent of one teaspoon of sugar, which doesn't. Carbohydrates are an essential macronutrient. However, if we care about our well-being, sugars and starches should be selected wisely from natural, whole, unrefined and unadulterated sources.

FATS

Fats (lipids) provide the most concentrated form of energy. When they are burned in the body, they supply 9 calories per gram, more than twice the energy available from carbohydrates. But in the affluent West, where so many people are already overweight, this abundance of calories is not seen as an advantage. Therefore many people tend to avoid fats altogether. Is this justified?

All macronutrients are vitally important. Fats are no exception. Despite their bad reputation as a cause of obesity and a source of cholesterol, fats play a vital role in bodily functions. Fat, for example, is the only substance that stimulates gallbladder activity,[58] without which gallstones are likely to form. In fact, crude vegetable oils such as olive or sunflower are known to help prevent gallstones.

Fats help transport through the digestive system and also help to absorb vitamins A, D, E, and K, and the mineral calcium.[59] Certain types of fat insulate the nerves, ensuring a healthy flow of nerve impulses, without which irritability and nervous disorders occur. All cell membranes contain fat. And most important, fats are needed to form hormones, absolutely essential to a vast range of body functions, including sexual activity. Fats are also important for good looks, maintaining soft skin and glossy hair. Therefore all diets, including weight-loss diets, should contain at least some fat, especially of the unsaturated type.

Fats are broken down by digestion into glycerol and fatty acids. These fatty acids give various fats and oils their specific flavour, texture and aroma. Most fatty acids can be manufactured (synthesized) by the body, with the exception of three, known as 'essential fatty acids' (also as vitamin F). These have to be supplied by the food we eat, and they are linoleic acid, linolenic acid and arachidonic acid.

Essential fatty acids (EFAs) are vital substances and have numerous duties. They help to prevent the formation of blood clots in arteries. They also prevent atherosclerosis by helping to form prostaglandins, hormone-like substances which control and regulate many important physiologic processes. Arachidonic acid, for example, is the precursor of the prostaglandins which regulate such diverse reactions as stomach secretions, hormone release and pancreatic function.[60]

SATURATED AND UNSATURATED FATS

There are two types of fatty acids: saturated and unsaturated. Unsaturated fatty acids come from vegetable oils (coconut oil and palm oil are the only saturated vegetable oils) and fish oils. Saturated fats, as a rule, are solids, and most are animal fats. Lard and butter are saturated fats. Margarine or vegetable shortening is saturated (hardened) by hydrogenation (a process which involves forcing hydrogen gas through vegetable oil).

Vegetable oils are the best sources of the essential fatty acids, particularly if they are unrefined (crude) and cold pressed. Soybean, cottonseed and corn oils, for example, are 35–70 per cent essential fatty acids. Safflower and sunflower oils are the richest, containing up to 90 per cent. The more vegetable oils are processed and refined, the lower their essential fatty acid content. That is why margarine is inferior, even compared with butter, in this respect. Butter contains 4–6 per cent of the essentials, while margarine contains only 2–5 per cent.[61]

The basic structure of fatty acids is a chain of carbon atoms, each having one or more free arms (bonds) to link with other atoms. When a fatty acid has one or more free arms, it is called unsaturated, the most desirable form of fatty acid. It is able to participate in metabolic processes by linking with other atoms to transport nutrients to cells and help build cell membranes. A fatty acid with only one free link, such as olive oil, is called mono-unsaturated, while a fatty acid with more free links, such as sunflower oil, is called poly-unsaturated. When all the free 'arms' are engaged (as happens in the hydrogenation process), the fatty acid is saturated and can no longer perform metabolic duties. The more unsaturated the fat, the easier it is for our bodies to process it into heat or energy rather than stockpile it as adipose (fat) tissue.

Polyunsaturated oils contain two main families of essential fatty acids: omega-3 fatty acids, found in ocean fish oils, flaxseed oil and green leafy vegetables, and omega-6 fatty acids which are found in vegetable oils like sunflower, safflower and corn oils. The omega families are vitally involved in the body's biological activity: they regulate cholesterol level by helping its conversion to bile acids; they strengthen cell membranes and thus increase resistance to disease; and they provide the raw material for the synthesis of prostaglandins, hormone-like substances which regulate most physiological functions, including brain, heart and immunity functions.[62] Most studies however were done with omega-3 fatty acids in marine oils, which showed that a rich omega-3 diet can reduce LDL (bad) cholesterol.[63] The omegas are not only very active; they are also very reactive: they oxidize easily and are best protected by antioxidant vitamins like vitamin E.

The reactivity of fats is very significant not only to dieters but to all those who use oils in the kitchen. Unsaturated oils can be converted to saturated by improper storage. Unsaturated fatty acids readily oxidize when in contact with the air. It is therefore important to close oil bottles tightly immediately after use, and to store them in a cool, dark place. In this way, the oxygen in the air is less likely to oxidize the free links and make the oil rancid. Rancid oil is very dangerous. Among other things, it deactivates vitamin E in the body and may cause thrombosis.[64] During prolonged frying, oils become more saturated as oxygen combines with their fatty acids. Fried foods are therefore more difficult to digest and often cause heartburn in susceptible people. They should be avoided by anyone who has digestion problems.

Rancid oils are not only toxic in their own right, but also when contained in stored grains, legumes, nuts and seeds. Recent studies have correlated the consumption of old rice with stomach and duodenal ulcers.[65] The oxidation of the oil in rice bran was found to produce ketoaldehyde, a toxic substance which depletes the stomach and duodenum of a protective enzyme called glutathione and also speeds up lipid peroxidation. It can therefore damage the digestive tract and cause ulcers.

In addition, each fatty acid has a specific decomposition temperature at which it breaks down, producing irritating substances. Overheated fats have been reported to cause cancer in laboratory animals. When fresh, good kitchen oils are overheated, they decompose to cancer-causing substances.[66] Olive oil, for example, decomposes at 347°F (175°C) and butter at 226°F (108°C), but margarine and corn oil have to be heated to 450°F (232°C) before they break down. So if you wish to eat fried foods, at least adjust the frying temperature to the kind of fat you are using. With fresh oil, lower frying temperatures and shorter frying times, irritation of the stomach lining is reduced. Never reuse oil already used for frying – it will be hyper-saturated and contain the dangerous products of hyperoxidation.

Mineral oils, such as liquid paraffin, should not be used as kitchen oils or taken medicinally on a frequent basis. They decrease calcium absorption and drain the body of vitamins A, D, E, and K.[67]

The importance of essential fatty acids to health cannot be overemphasized. Dr Benjamin Colimore, the well-known nutritionist and author, has called fat 'the most abused nutrient in our diets.'[68] People under the influence of the recent cholesterol scare impulsively put themselves on low fat diets, not realizing the consequences of essential fatty acid deficiency. Adelle Davis lists eczema, psoriasis, fatigue, menstrual difficulties, ankle oedema, infertility, scaly skin, dry hair and obesity as common signs of essential fatty acid deficiency.[69] These can all be corrected with only 2 tablespoons of natural vegetable oil a day, or alternatively 4 tablespoons of raw sunflower seeds or 9 whole unroasted pecans. Dieters should realize that, far from being anathema, polyunsaturated oils are essential for shedding extra pounds. And once these extra pounds have been shed, polyunsaturated oils can help to maintain lower weight because they assist in burning rather than stockpiling saturated fats. A word of warning, however. Overindulging in unrefined oils as a general answer to various health problems is not advisable either. As already explained, oil oxidizes easily and becomes rancid. When used in excess, it increases the formation of peroxides and free radicals. These highly reactive substances attack and damage various body cells, contributing to premature aging, arthritis, heart attacks and cancer.[70] In reaction to excessive oil intake, the body uses up its stores of vitamin E to counteract fat oxidation. Oils should be consumed in modest quantities and supplemented with vitamin E [71] and other anti-oxidant nutrients like vitamin C, vitamin B6, selenium and zinc. The amount of oil ingested should not exceed 20 per cent of total fat intake.[72]

It is wrong to think that saturated fats should be totally avoided. The important thing is to balance them with polyunsaturated oils. The lipase enzymes in our digestive system which metabolize body fats to heat and energy are well able to handle modest amounts of saturated fat. They dissolve them into less saturated forms.[73] We can do our share by balancing our intake of saturated and unsaturated fats. A mixture of equal quantities of three polyunsaturated crude oils (safflower, soy and peanut) is highly recommended for use in salad dressings and cooking. These oils are among the richest sources of each of the essential fatty acids.

A good example of fat balancing is Dr Kurt Donsbach's recipe for 'super butter'. Add 2 fluid ounces each of safflower, soy and peanut oil to 1 pound of melted butter. Blend them and refrigerate. The resulting butter is 'super' in flavour, 'super' in fatty acid balance and less fattening than regular butter.

COME BACK CHOLESTEROL ALL IS FORGIVEN

A few additional words about cholesterol. For various reasons, public opinion has cast cholesterol in the role of scapegoat – it clogs arteries (as in atherosclerosis) and causes coronary heart attacks, doesn't it? As a result, some people go to extremes in avoiding fatty foods. But the body needs cholesterol to make sex and steroid hormones, to produce bile, to synthesize vitamin D, to form cell membranes, and to insulate nerves. In fact, it is so crucial to the body that all nucleated cells are capable of synthesizing it, particularly the cells of the liver, adrenal glands, skin, intestines, testes and aorta.[74] The liver produces most cholesterol, up to 1 gram a day. Only about 0.3 gram a day is provided by the average diet.[75] What is more, if we eat less cholesterol, the liver will increase its own production by as much as eight times![76] It is not cholesterol that should be blamed for furred up arteries and heart attacks, but our diets, which are deficient in the nutrients needed to metabolize cholesterol properly. To deal with cholesterol our diets should be fortified with choline and inositol (two B vitamins that have been shown to reduce cholesterol levels in the liver[77]) or with lecithin, a fine fat emulsifier[78] which contains both these B vitamins. Other nutrients which lower cholesterol levels are: niacin (vitamin B3); vitamin B6, which helps to convert linoleic acid to arachidonic acid (a more active form); bran and fibrous vegetables, which improve excretion of cholesterol through the bile; vitamin E;[79] raw wheat germ; vitamin C, which accelerates cholesterol transformation into bile acids;[80] chromium, magnesium and manganese from brewer's yeast; and nuts and seeds.

Substituting polyunsaturated oils for some of the unsaturated fats has also been shown to lower cholesterol levels. Natural oils which have a cholesterol-lowering effect are peanut, cottonseed, corn and soybean. Butter and coconut oil have the opposite effect.[81] Margarine, often advertized as being made from polyunsaturated oils, is produced by saturating vegetable oils with hydrogen gas and so a new type of solid, saturated fat is formed. Although some margarines do contain small amounts of liquid polyunsaturated oil added to the hydrogenated base, the bulk of fat in margarine is saturated or magarine would be liquid, like any other polyunsaturated oil. A recent statistical study in England found that there was a positive correlation between heart disease and the consumption of hydrogenated fats. In areas where margarine was used in significant amounts, there was a greater number of heart attacks than in areas where it was used sparingly.[82]

Additional factors considered to play a part in elevated cholesterol levels and atherosclerosis are smoking,[83] lack of exercise,[84] obesity, hypertension, and drinking soft as opposed to hard water.[85] A recent study not only correlated sugar and alcohol consumption with atherosclerosis, but also suggested that, of all foods, these are the strongest contributors to high cholesterol levels.[86]

Cholesterol needs to be transported by the bloodstream to those cells and tissues which need it rather than depositing itself on artery walls. The blood contains special proteins, lipoproteins, which transport cholesterol. Now cholesterol in the blood behaves differently according to the type of lipoprotein present. Low density lipoproteins (LDL), which carry about 80 per cent of blood cholesterol, are known to be correlated to cholesterol deposits and heart attacks.[87] High density lipoproteins (HDL), which carry about 20 per cent of blood cholesterol, have the opposite effect and act as scavengers of cholesterol.[88] Moreover, HDLs were also found to provide protection against cerebral strokes even in people with normal levels of cholesterol.[89] HDLs are made up mostly of lecithin (choline and inositol), which emulsifies cholesterol into tiny particles, enabling it to pass through the smallest arteries without forming deposits in them. Obviously, higher HDL (or lecithin) levels lessen the risk of atherosclerosis and coronary heart disease.

We now know that LDL levels are more important than cholesterol levels. If your LDL level is less than 100 mg per decilitre, your chances of developing cardiovascular disease are small. If it is 200 or more, you are at considerable risk and should eat a carefully balanced diet, well supplemented with cholesterol-reducing nutrients such as those mentioned above. Ninety per cent of the population have LDL levels between 100 and 200, and should be more concerned about eating foods that will increase their HDL level rather than cutting out cholesterol foods altogether and creating devastating deficiencies of fatty acids. In fact, the only people who should eliminate cholesterol from their diets are individuals with hyperlipoproteinemia, an inherited condition in which the body synthesizes excessive amounts of cholesterol. Such individuals constitute less than 5 per cent of the population, but even they can greatly benefit from the use of lecithin.[90] We must not totally ban cholesterol. After all, we do not ban strawberries just because a few people get a rash from them. Indeed, a growing number of doctors now recommend 25 grams of fat a day in low fat diets, such is the importance of fatty acids in general body condition.

Eskimos in Greenland used to have low rates of coronary heart disease even though they subsisted almost exclusively on fish, seal and whale, abundant in cholesterol and fat. This is because certain factors in fish oils were found to have protective effects which reduce the risk of heart attacks and atherosclerosis.[91] Ocean fish are rich sources of special polyunsaturated fats called eicosapentaenoic acid (EPA). EPA is synthesized in the fish from omega-3 fatty acids and is the precursor of prostaglandins (PG), hormone-like compounds which regulate many body processes.[92] In adequate amounts, EPA has a stabilising effect on blood clotting cells, the platelets.[93] This reduces the tendency of the blood to form blood-clots and cause heart attacks. Salmon, halibut and other ocean fish are good dietary sources of EPA. In supplement form, EPA is marketed by several brands as 'MaxEPA' capsules.

Eggs are a wonderfully balanced food, but during the cholesterol scare, they were much maligned. However, the 200 mg of cholesterol which the average egg contains is naturally balanced by 1,700 mg of lecithin which serve to emulsify the cholesterol. Some studies did show that eggs contributed to higher cholesterol levels, but these studies were done with 'average', i.e. deficient, diets. If you want to lower your cholesterol levels, instead of avoiding eggs – a fine source of protein, sulphur, and magnesium as well as lecithin – why not adhere to a balanced, low sugar diet, fortified with the cholesterol-lowering nutrients and dietary aids mentioned above? An emphasis should be put on fibrous vegetables, soybeans, grains, eggplant, yogurt, pectin (in apples and citrus rind, and in tablet form), fish and turkey. Garlic and onion have also been found to be effective in lowering levels of cholesterol and triglycerides.[94] Smoking, coffee, alcohol, soda, ice cream and candies should be avoided. If you are a woman, do not use contraceptive pills. As Dr Donsbach predicts: 'We shall shortly see butter, cheese, eggs and other cholesterol-containing foods returned to their rightful place in the dietary habits of man.' [95]

CHAPTER 3

AUXILIARIES:
VITAMINS AND ENZYMES

Vitamins are micronutrients found in small and varying amounts in all natural vegetable and animal foods. Each food has a different concentration of its own specific vitamins. About twenty vitamins are known to be vital to human nutrition. They are functionally interrelated and complement each other to maintain health. Apart from a few vitamins which can be synthesized to a certain degree by the body, most are provided by the food we eat. If food is like fuel in an engine, then vitamins are the spark plugs.

The recognition that vitamins play a role in preventing disease has existed since the Scottish physician James Lind published his *Treatise on Scurvy* in 1754. This naval doctor successfully eliminated scurvy from the British Navy with an Admiralty order prescribing the use of fresh lemon juice, a natural source of vitamin C. Later, in 1890, the Dutch doctor Christian Eijkman produced beriberi in chickens by only feeding them white (polished) rice. A comprehensive theory connecting diseases to deficiencies of nutrients was finally formulated in 1912 by Casimir Funk in *The Etiology of*

Deficiency Diseases. Between 1926 and 1948, all of the vitamins we know today – A, B complex, C, D, E, and K – were identified and isolated from food sources.

WHAT DO VITAMINS DO?

Vitamins do not contain calories and do not supply energy. In other words, they do not contribute to weight gain. They are, however, most important as constituents of enzymes, those organic catalysts which enable biological processes to take place. This is why vitamins are sometimes called co-enzymes.

It is totally impossible to imagine our lives without vitamins and enzymes. Through enzymes, vitamins stimulate metabolic processes, converting food to energy and accelerating biological functions. They are truly *vital* or 'life-giving' as the first part of their name implies. They create blood, skin and bone, detoxify the body, release energy, enable reproduction to take place and promote longevity.

Vitamins are not a part of the body's structure. They are just agents that help to regulate its maintenance and activity. Measured in milligrams (mg), most are water-soluble and, therefore, any surpluses are eliminated through urination. On the other hand, a small group of fat-soluble vitamins, which are not soluble in water and are measured in International Units (IU), are harder to eliminate and easier to accumulate. Prolonged overdosing with these can cause adverse effects.

Although each one of us basically needs the same vitamins and minerals, individual requirements vary with sex, age, occupation, lifestyle and metabolic rate. Up to now, science has not come up with a general formula to determine individual needs, which can vary tremendously from person to person. Vitamins A and C, for example, can vary at least twentyfold.[1] Calcium and protein requirements may vary by a factor of five.[2] This is the principle of 'biochemical individuality', a phrase coined by Nobel laureate Dr Roger Williams, the Texan biochemist who first isolated pantothenic acid (vitamin B5).

The principle of biochemical individuality was dramatically illustrated after World War II when prisoners of war were released. Most of them were obviously malnourished, but a few were merely underweight. These were individuals with low nutrient requirements and exceptionally efficient metabolic systems. Their bodies were able to absorb enough nutrients from their meagre diet to sustain reasonable health.

DAILY VITAMIN REQUIREMENTS

Although there is no general formula to determine individual vitamin requirements, there are a few tables of average nutrient needs. These tables, however, are very inadequate and often misleading, nor do they contain all known nutrients. The figures are revised from time to time and 'new' nutrients are added. The tables I am referring to are the RDA (Recommended Daily Allowances) and the US RDA (US Recommended Daily Allowances). The former were drawn up by the Food and Nutrition Board of the National Research Council of the Academy of Sciences, established by the U.S. government to protect public health. The latter were formulated by the U.S. Food and Drug Administration (FDA), mainly as a standard for food labelings.

How were RDA levels determined? Simply by observing statistically the average food intake of healthy Americans, calculating the vitamin content and adding a margin of safety. RDAs do not and cannot take into consideration specific individual needs, nor special requirements due to metabolic defects, allergies or stress. No wonder they cannot serve as a reliable general guide for nutrient intake. The low amounts of nutrients they recommend are just enough to keep us on our feet! By no means should these low amounts be expected to promote radiant health, sustain a feeling of energetic well-being, or prevent deficiency disorders.

These tables mislead many people. I often hear the remark: 'I just ate an orange. I've had my daily quota of vitamin C.' Instead of relying on daily quotas, we should adopt the approach of optimum nutrition, which seeks to supply an abundance of balanced nutrients. Biological processes can then achieve their peak efficiency, promoting physical and mental fitness. Only then can we live our lives to the fullest.

In the list of vitamins on pp.54-91, the RDA values quoted are those compiled by the Food and Nutrition Board of the National Research Council. They should, however, be considered as only the barest, minimal requirement to sustain life, not to promote health. Nutritional needs can increase dramatically during periods of illness, stress, crisis, after operations, and during convalescence, pregnancy and lactation. For the best results, each person should experiment with dosages to find out his or her own individual requirement for specific nutrients. This can be done by starting supplementation with the lowest doses available and then slowly increasing the dose. Watch out for allergic reactions. Note how you feel with the initial dose for a few days, then increase it by about 50 per cent at a time for as long as you feel comfortable. Keep a record of your supplement intake. Have a thorough medical check-up to determine your state of health and reveal possible weak spots in your body. Consult a qualified nutritionist or a physician in case of doubt, and have the results of your check-up evaluated professionally.

CAUTION: Beware of excessive supplementation. Each person must learn his or her tolerances – what is excessive in one person may be well tolerated in another. People with specific conditions must get clearance from their doctors before taking supplements.

We must remember that everything can become toxic in excessive amounts, even water, our safest nutrient. If we were to drink four times our usual daily intake of water, we would die of uremia in a few days.[3] Excessive intake of vitamin D, for example, can elevate calcium level dangerously; too much vitamin C may cause kidney stones in susceptible people unless balanced with magnesium; excess choline can cause vitamin B6 deficiency. Massive doses of nutrients intended to treat special conditions should always be taken under the guidance of a nutritionist or nutritionally-oriented physician.

Recently, however, self check-up kits have been developed to determine and monitor individual needs for vitamin C and calcium. These kits, now sold in health food shops at very reasonable prices, can tell you how much vitamin C and calcium supplements you should take at any given time. As we have seen, individual requirements for many nutrients fluctuate according to individual conditions. The need for vitamin C, for example, can vary drastically with stress, dieting or allergies, and in smokers, athletes, contact lens wearers and people living in areas where air pollution is bad. A 15-second, drop-on-the-tongue test indicates the level of vitamin C in the body and how to correct it if necessary. A 1-minute urine test determines calcium level – if it is low, you may be losing too much calcium and therefore be vulnerable to osteoporosis and hypertension, or if it is high, you run the risk of developing kidney stones. So self check-up kits are a most convenient way of monitoring calcium and vitamin C requirements, and cost very little compared to laboratory tests. Also available now are self check-up kits for stomach secretions, rate of absorption of nutrients and bowel performance. These give early warnings of conditions which may one day develop into ulcers, colitis and cancer. Domestic kits are a powerful health-preserving tool for those who truly want to take responsibility for their health.

VITAMIN A

Vitamin A is a fat-soluble vitamin which occurs in two forms in nature. It occurs in its true form (also called retinol) in animal foods such as fish oils and liver. In this form, it is readily used by the body. It is stored in and released by the liver. However, in order to be transported throughout the body, it needs a special protein carrier. Hence the importance of adequate protein intake when vitamin A intake is increased.[4]

Vitamin A also occurs in vegatables in the form of beta carotene, or provitamin A, which is the precursor of the actual vitamin. Beta carotene is abundant in root vegetables, such as carrots and yams, leafy vegetables such as spinach and kale and yellow fruits such as cantaloupe and mango. Beta carotene cannot be directly used by the body as actual vitamin A. It has to be converted into retinol in the presence of fats and bile before this can happen.[5] This is why it is advisable, when eating a salad, to sprinkle a little salad oil on it. In this respect, cooked carrots are better than raw ones, as the cooking of carotene helps the liver to convert it to the retinol form of Vitamin A.

Although it got most scientific attention in the past, beta carotene is now known to be only one of several hundred plant pigments known collectively as carotenoids. These plant pigments which can absorb dangerous sunlight wavelength rays, were also found to act as antioxidants. As such, they neutralize the destructive molecules known as free radicals. Carotenoids protect plants from the damage caused by the free radicals which are formed when plants are exposed to sunlight. Without the protective carotenoids, the plants would shrivel quickly. People can acquire these antioxidant effects by eating carotenoids. This is important because free radicals are now considered to be the underlying cause for the degenerative diseases of aging such as heart disease and cancer. Some of the dietary carotenoids include lycopene, alpha carotene, lutein and zeaxanthin. Tomatoes, which are the major source of lycopene, were found to be related to a lower risk of prostate cancer.[6] Alpha carotene was found to help prevent the growth of some forms of cancer,[7] and studies by Dr Joanne Curran-Celentano of the University of New Hampshire revealed that supplementation of lutein and zeaxanthin, two carotenoids found in the retina of the eye, may prevent macular degeneration (AMD), which is a leading cause of blindness in the elderly.[8]

Vitamin A can be stored in the liver until needed. Nevertheless, deficiencies can occur, especially among dieters on low fat regimes or vegetables. The beta carotene they consume can only partly be converted to retinol if their fat intake is insufficient. Normal healthy people convert only 25 per cent of their beta carotene to vitamin A, and diabetics even less,[9] so the importance of adequate vitamin A supplementation, especially in unbalanced diets, is obvious. Being a fatty acid, vitamin A is easily oxidized in the body. It is therefore advisable to take some vitamin E, which prevents oxidation, along with it.

BENEFICIAL EFFECTS
Vitamin A helps to fight colds and infections, particularly in

the mucous membranes of the eyes, ear, nose, throat, lungs and bladder. It increases the resistance of these tissues to bacterial infections. As for the eyes, vitamin A is necessary for the formation of the photosensitive pigment known as visual purple; this contains beta carotene, vitamin A and protein, and maintains good vision. Night vision depends entirely on vitamin A. This multi-role vitamin also helps to maintain a healthy skin, preventing acne and dermatitis. It is also known to prevent kidney stones.

Several studies conducted recently have shown some types of vitamin A to possess anti-cancer effects, protecting mainly soft tissues.[10] Retinoids and beta carotenes have been shown to prevent cancer of skin, lung, bladder and breast in experimental animals and to be involved in controlling cell differentiation.[11] As a result, a growing number of therapists are now using megadoses of vitamin A to prevent and treat certain types of malignancy, particularly lung cancer. A 19-year study of about 3,000 middle-aged men has provided evidence that beta carotene can protect smokers by reducing their risk of lung cancer.[12] Daily doses of about 10,000 IU of beta carotene were found effective. This, of course, does not mean that it is safe to smoke if you take beta carotene supplements. Smoking has deleterious effects on the cardiovascular system and these would not be minimized by taking beta carotene. Beta carotene capsules, by the way, are now available in most good health food shops.

DEFICIENCY SYMPTOMS
Red, itchy eyes are a common symptom of vitamin A deficiency. Other symptoms are night blindness, vision difficulties in dim light and sensitivity to bright light; dry or rough skin; a predisposition to colds and infections; broken tooth enamel; kidney stones; allergies.

BEST NATURAL SOURCES

Fish liver oil and animal liver; carrots, yams, sweet potatoes, pumpkin and other yellow vegetables; yellow fruits such as apricots, peaches, papaya (pawpaw) and cantaloupe melon; eggs; milk and dairy products.

DAILY DOSAGE

Adults 5,000 IU, children 3,000 IU. Requirements increase during illness, pregnancy and lactation, but decrease when using oral contraceptives. A more reasonable intake is: adults 10,000 IU, children 5,000 IU. In spite of well publicized concern about vitamin A toxicity, some people have taken up to 50,000 IU a day without experiencing any adverse symptoms. Our parents were given daily tablespoons of cod liver oil in childhood, each containing 33,000 IU, to promote growth and health, but that was before the RDAs labeled any dose over 5,000 IU as excessive and dangerous. However, toxic effects were noticed in people taking between 50,000 IU and 100,000 IU daily for extended periods, i.e. for three to six months.[13]

VITAMIN B COMPLEX

All of the B complex family are water-soluble. Up to now, some sixteen B vitamins have been isolated. These are referred to as the B group because they occur together in many vegetables and animal foods. Each will be discussed separately below.

B group vitamins are vital for converting carbohydrates to glucose and food into energy. When B vitamins are lacking in the body, carbohydrates do not burn fully but produce 'smoke', so to speak. This appears as nervousness, constipation, fatigue and indigestion, to name but a few disorders commonly associated with a lack of B vitamins. Most of the Bs are concerned with various processes in the liver, eyes, skin and hair. Their action includes a wide range of effects, from alleviating stress to preventing atherosclerosis.

Foods rich in the entire B complex are: organ meats (particularly liver), brewer's yeast, raw wheat germ and rice bran, the fibrous coating of the rice grains (available in most health food stores). This is one reason why biologic nutrition recommends eating whole unpolished brown rice.

Being water-soluble, the B vitamins in raw vegetables readily dissolve once they are cooked in water, as for soup, or even just soaked in cold water. The soup or cooking liquid is highly nutritious, which is why, if you boil rice, particularly brown rice, you should save and use the cooking water rather than throw it away; it is a concentrated source of natural B complex.

It is important to eat the whole B complex group as it occurs in the natural foods listed above.[14] Since the B vitamins are interrelated, excessive consumption of only one of them disrupts their balance and can cause depletion of the others through excretion. When a specific B vitamin is needed to treat a specific condition, it is therefore advisable to take it in conjunction with a whole B complex source, such as brewer's yeast or B complex tablets. People on reducing diets, who take massive doses of vitamin B6 to help them burn off fat, are particularly susceptible to vitamin B imbalance.

BENEFICIAL EFFECTS

The B group is helpful in strengthening the nervous system. People under conditions of stress, physical or emotional, can be helped by eating foods such as liver and brewer's yeast. The Bs can prove most beneficial for individuals with a weak digestion, poor appetite, constipation, fatigue, anaemia and migraines. Some B vitamins can even prevent hair greying.

DEFICIENCY SYMPTOMS
In processed foods a large part of the B complex is destroyed. If you eat large quantities of refined sugar and white flour, your intake of B vitamins is likely to be low. Alcohol consumption also drains certain B vitamins from the body. No wonder the B complex, as a whole, is deficient in vast numbers of people today. Typical deficiency symptoms are: fatigue, nervousness, depression, suicidal tendencies and low morale; senility; hair loss; high cholesterol levels; poor appetite; constipation.

DAILY DOSAGE
Although certain functions of many B vitamins overlap, each has its own characteristics and they cannot replace each other. As they are all water-soluble, it is hard to accumulate excesses, particularly when the diet is not massively supplemented. RDAs are given for each B vitamin separately.

VITAMIN B1
(THIAMINE)

Thiamine is vulnerable to heat and air as well as water. It plays an important role in converting carbohydrates to glucose, the only type of sugar the body can convert to energy. It also prevents excess formation of pyruvic acid, a by-product of carbohydrate metabolism, known to cause nervousness and irritation (particularly among alcoholics),[15] and ensures proper oxygen levels in the blood for optimal release of energy.

Thiamine is quickly absorbed from food, but the body

cannot store it in meaningful amounts. A consistent daily supply is therefore needed. Substances which block its absorption are: white sugar, white flour, alcohol, caffeine, antibiotic drugs and contraceptive pills. Alcoholics are particularly vulnerable to thiamine deficiency,[16] and should protect themselves with massive supplementation.

Prolonged thiamine deficiency causes beriberi, the symptoms of which are weakness, emaciation, hair loss, oedema, indigestion, nervousness, and finally heart attack. Beriberi occurred in its acute form in the Far East during the early years of this century, after people started eating white polished rice instead of whole brown rice as their main staple.

BENEFICIAL EFFECTS

Thiamine has been called the 'morale vitamin' due to its salutary effect on the central nervous system. It establishes a feeling of optimism; helps to overcome emotional stress and relieve depression and anxiety, confusion and poor memory; stabilizes appetite and stomach acid secretions; maintains normal heart function; is important to growth, lactation and fertility; and also helps to alleviate motion sickness.

DEFICIENCY SYMPTOMS

Nervous disorders such as neurosis, neurasthenia (nervous exhaustion), irritability, sensitivity to noise, loss of morale, fear, anxiety and confusion. Physical disorders such as low thyroid function, appetite loss and heart palpitations.

BEST NATURAL SOURCES

Brewer's yeast, rice bran, raw wheat germ, whole grains, peanuts, green and yellow vegetables, fruit, milk.

DAILY DOSAGE
Adults 1.2 to 1.4 mg, children 0.7 to 1.2 mg. Need increases
to 1.4 mg during lactation, stress, illness or after surgery. Many
people find a daily dosage of 10 to 50 mg much more
effective (and safe) for an improved feeling of well-being.

VITAMIN B2
(RIBOFLAVIN)

Riboflavin is another B vitamin which can't be stored in the
body. It can withstand heat and oxidation, but not light. That's
why milk, which is a good source of riboflavin, shouldn't be
kept in clear containers. Riboflavin functions as a part of the
enzyme system involved in the breakdown of carbohydrates,
fats and proteins. It also takes part in the synthesis of nucleic
acids and of enzymes which prevent certain aging processes.
It is considered highly deficient in the American diet.

BENEFICIAL EFFECTS
Contributes to good vision (along with vitamin A) and maintains healthy skin, hair and nails; promotes growth, fertility
and iron assimilation; helps to convert tryptophan (an important amino acid) to niacin (vitamin B3). Large doses have
been reported to increase resistance to athlete's foot and similar fungus infections, to bring relief to sufferers of certain
eczemas and allergies,[17] and to counteract a sweet tooth.

DEFICIENCY SYMPTOMS
Mouth and lip lesions, tongue inflammations; sensation of
sand in the eyes, red itchy eyes, cataracts; scaly skin on face;
impairment of red blood cell formation leading to anaemia
and heart disease; dental problems; congenital birth defects.

BEST NATURAL SOURCES
Milk, liver, brewer's yeast, dairy products, leafy green vegetables, fish, eggs.

DAILY DOSAGE
Adults 1.7 mg, children 1 mg. Some nutritionists advocate no less than 5 mg. Pregnancy and lactation require 1.5 and 1.7 mg respectively. Need increases in stress situations. Popular B complex tablets contain 50 mg of riboflavin.

VITAMIN B3
(NIACIN AND NIACINAMIDE)

There are two forms of vitamin B3, niacin and niacinamide. Sensitive people who become flushed as a reaction to one form can use the other. However, the form commonly found in plants is niacin. This can be produced in the body from the essential amino acid tryptophan, provided that the intestinal flora (bacteria) are healthy and that the diet contains sufficient B2, B6 and protein. Niacin is stable in heat. It assists enzymes in breaking down nutrients and is essential for the synthesis of sex hormones (oestrogen, progesterone and testosterone) and other hormones such as cortisone, insulin and thyroxine. Small quantities of niacin are present in most foods. Unlike some of the other Bs, it can be stored, in the liver. However, deficiencies can and do occur, especially when taking antibiotics or overindulging in sweets. People susceptible to depression may have high requirements for niacin and can be greatly helped by massive supplementation.

A vitamin B3 dependant coenzyme, NADH (Nicotinamide Adenine Dinucleotide), which occurs naturally in the body, but which declines with age, has been recently hailed as a nutritional breakthrough. NADH enhances cellular energy and helps produce energy from food. It has potent antioxidant and antiaging effects and is now used to relieve chronic fatigue (CFS), treat Parkinson's disease[18], reduce high cholesterol level[19]) and increase athletic performance[20]. It is available in health food stores as a supplement called 'Enada'.

BENEFICIAL EFFECTS

Vitamin B3 assists macronutrient metabolism; strengthens digestion; improves blood circulation by restoring electrical polarity to blood cells, preventing them from agglutinating and contributing to arteriosclerosis and heart attacks; lowers cholesterol level if taken in doses of 3 grams or more a day;[21] is vital to a healthy nervous system and normal mental function; releases histamine (a chemical which is released largely during allergic reactions but which is also, in small amounts, vital to such functions as growth, healing, orgasm and stomach acid secretion); raises levels of heparin (a blood anticoagulant); can be used to treat alcoholism, smoking and suicidal tendencies;[22] and decreases the effects of hallucinogens such as LSD and mescaline.[23]

DEFICIENCY SYMPTOMS

Clinical (severe) deficiencies can bring about pellagra, at one time a very widespread disease characterized by eczema, diarrhoea and delirium. Subclinical deficiencies, very common in modern life, manifest themselves as: indigestion; fatigue; mouth disorders such as bad breath; arthritis[24]; loss of sense of humour[25] and headaches. In susceptible people, deficiencies can cause depression, dementia and even schizophrenia. Niacin is often used as part of megavitamin therapy in the treatment of schizophrenia.

BEST NATURAL SOURCES
Liver, brewer's yeast, raw wheat germ, fish, eggs, peanut butter, avocados, dried fruits such as dates, figs, prunes.

DAILY DOSAGE
Adults 13 to 18 mg, children 9 to 16 mg. Requirements increase during illness, pregnancy and lactation. The National Research Council suggests that the RDA of niacin should be based on caloric intake: 6.6 mg for every 1,000 calories consumed. The essential amino acid tryptophan is transformed in the body to niacin and can provide part or all of the daily requirement – 60 mg of tryptophan yields 1 mg of niacin.

VITAMIN B5
(PANTOTHENIC ACID)

Pantothenic acid, or vitamin B5, occurs in most foods in small amounts. 'Pantothenic' is derived from the ancient Greek word *pantothen*, which means 'from all sides'. None the less, it is a widely deficient vitamin. Dr William Rogers, the research biochemist from the University of Texas at Austin who discovered it, writes in *Nutrition Against Disease*: 'While no one ever ate a meal without getting some pantothenic acid, it is wishful thinking to suppose that people always get enough.' Deficiency reduces blood sugar levels, which results in a feeling of exhaustion, and reduces the release of adrenalin,[26] the hormone we need to overcome sudden stress.

Pantothenic acid is often referred to as the 'stress vitamin'.

Pantothenic acid is an important ingredient of 'Royal Jelly', the special substance which transforms a worker bee into a queen who can lay eggs. Its high concentration in cod's roe also points up its importance in reproduction. It is essential to macronutrient metabolism, and to the synthesis of cholesterol, fats, antibodies and acetylcholine (a chemical which transmits nerve impulses). It has also been found to speed up food transit time in the digestive tract if taken in high daily doses of 1 to 3 grams – a boon to the constipated and to dieters.[27] B5 is especially concentrated in organs important to metabolic activities such as the liver, kidneys and adrenal glands. However, it is neutralized by antibiotics and sulpha drugs, most sleeping pills, contraceptive pills, stress and alcohol.

BENEFICIAL EFFECTS
Vitamin B5 stimulates adrenal function, prevents fatigue and reduces stress; increases antibody production and helps fight infections; is good for post–operative shock; reduces the toxic effects of antibiotics; and promotes fertility and longevity.

DEFICIENCY SYMPTOMS
Mental stress, often expressed as irritability or depression; hypoglycaemia; allergies; arthritis; gastric conditions such as indigestion, constipation and ulcers; fatigue; greying hair; skin disorders.

BEST NATURAL SOURCES
'Royal Jelly,' cod's roe, meat, raw wheat germ, organ meats (liver, kidneys), whole grains, beans, brewer's yeast, molasses, nuts.

DAILY DOSAGE
Adults 10 mg, children 5 mg. Paavo Airola and some other nutritionists recommend 30 to 50 mg a day.

VITAMIN B6
(PYRIDOXINE)

One of the busiest Bs, B6 or pyridoxine takes part in many metabolic functions, including release of glycogen from the liver whenever muscles need energy. It converts linoleic acid to arachidonic acid (a more active fatty acid),[28] and so helps to control obesity. It assists the metabolism of and even conserves protein. It also helps to balance sodium and potassium in the body, and therefore helps to regulate body fluids, acid-alkaline balance and the function of nerves and muscles. It helps to synthesize nucleic acids, antibodies and red blood cells. Combined with magnesium, it prevents the formation of oxalic acid salts (the precursors of kidney stones). B6 is not stored and is deficient in vast numbers of people, particularly dieters and people who fast often. It is depleted from milk by pasteurization, partially destroyed by cooking and mostly removed from grains by refining. Contraceptive pills are among its greatest enemies.[29] Any woman on oral contraceptives should take B6 supplements. B6 has also been reported to increase the level of dopamine in the brain – dopamine is a chemical which prevents tremors and motor disorders of the kind seen in Parkinson's disease.[30]

CAUTION: Too much B6 can cause a magnesium deficiency. Therefore, massive doses of B6 should be accompanied by magnesium or dolomite tablets.

BENEFICIAL EFFECTS

Due to its remarkable metabolic properties, B6 is beneficial during dieting. According to Dr Henry Schroeder of Dartmouth Medical School, Vermont, it also prevents hardening of the arteries, one of the major causes of heart attacks.

It inhibits the release of histamine, and is therefore beneficial to allergy sufferers; prevents nausea during pregnancy;[31] prevents eclampsia (toxaemia) during pregnancy,[32] particularly when combined with zinc; prevents certain anaemias;[33] dries oily skin and controls dandruff. In mega-doses of 200–250 mg daily, pyridoxine is reported to be effective in treating the carpal tunnel syndrome (pain or numbness in fingers or palms), which is more common in women, reducing the need for surgery.

DEFICIENCY SYMPTOMS
Skin striations, linear nail ridges, inability to tan and sensitivity to sun; tongue inflammations and cracks around the lips; numbness of hands and feet; convulsions in children;[31] depression; tremors and seizures, as in epilepsy and Parkinsonism;[32] hypoglycaemia, diabetes; appetite loss; high cholesterol levels; kidney stones; arthritis; allergies; anaemia; oedema (water retention); poor dream recollection.[33]

BEST NATURAL SOURCES
Brewer's yeast, raw wheat germ, liver and kidney, molasses, cabbage, milk, eggs.

DAILY DOSAGE
Adults 1.8 to 2.2 mg, children 1.3 to 1.6 mg. Many nutritionists recommend up to 25 mg. Supplements are available up to 100 mg. Requirements increase considerably during pregnancy and after surgery. Dieters and women on contraceptive pills need supplements.

VITAMIN B12
(CYANOCOBALAMIN)

Vitamin B12 was discovered in 1926 by Drs. George R. Minot and William P. Murphy as a cure for pernicious anaemia. It was isolated in 1948, but due to its complexity its molecular structure was not established until 1955.

Although vitamin B12 requirements are tiny and measured in micrograms (mcg or μg) it is one of the most important of the B group. It is water-soluble and is the only vitamin that contains cobalt, from which its technical name is derived. It occurs in two forms, cyanocobalamin and hydroxocobalamin (more active). People allergic to the first form, which is the more popular, can use the second. For strict vegetarians, B12 is a problem since it hardly occurs in non-animal foods. Anyone who abstains entirely from animal foods should emphasize such plant foods as pollen, spirulina and brewer's yeast, which all contain some B12, and also take B12 capsules. In a less strict vegetarian diet, eggs, milk and dairy products should be taken on an occasional basis.

B12 is required by the body for a great variety of functions. In fact, it is essential to the functioning of all cells, from bone marrow to nerves. Therapeutically, it is mainly used as an anti-fatigue and anti-anaemia vitamin.[34] However, for optimal absorption it should be given by injection (with folic acid) rather than taken orally.[35] Substances which deplete B12 are alcohol, contraceptive pills and sleeping pills.

BENEFICIAL EFFECTS
Vitamin B12, with folic acid (see p.73), forms red blood cells in the bone marrow and therefore helps to prevent anaemia;[36] promotes growth and appetite in children; increases energy;

improves brain functions such as memory, learning ability and balance; maintains a healthy nervous system; helps the action of iron, vitamin C, pantothenic acid, folic acid and choline; stabilizes menstruation and prevents postnatal depression.

DEFICIENCY SYMPTOMS
Although vitamin B12 requirements are small, deficiencies are widespread and serious, the most severe being pernicious anaemia. Mild deficiencies can result in a sore tongue, shortness of breath, heart palpitations, apathy and a feeling of weakness. As a deficiency builds up, more advanced symptoms may occur, such as degeneration of the brain and nervous system (with or without degeneration of spinal cord), loss of co-ordination (ataxia), impaired memory and concentration, and senile dementia.

Many people think that if they don't have anaemia, their B12 level is okay, but deficiency symptoms take years to develop and are hard to diagnose. Even doctors have difficulties correlating fatigue and mental conditions with B12 deficiency. One study revealed that people with B12 deficiency had suffered from apathy, sharp mood swings, impaired memory and paranoia for years before their B12-deficiency anaemia was diagnosed.[37] Other pre-anaemic disorders were also observed: weakness of limbs and reflexes, walking difficulties, and varied temperatures in different parts of the body.

A deficiency of B12 can also occur in people whose diets are balanced but who lack a certain stomach secretion, known as 'intrinsic factor', which is vital for B12 absorption. These people need constant supplementation of B12, preferably by injection.

BEST NATURAL SOURCES
Liver and kidneys, meat, eggs, dairy products and spirulina.

DAILY DOSAGE

Adults 3 mcg, children 2 to 3 mcg, pregnant and lactating women 4 mcg. Supplements are available in potencies between 60 mcg and 2,000 mcg.

VITAMIN B15
(PANGAMIC ACID)

This is a relatively 'young' vitamin. It is mostly used in Russia, to improve heart conditions and athletic performance. At the time of writing, it is still unrecognized by the FDA. Vitamin B15 is a potent antioxidant, as are vitamins C and E and therefore prevents the formation of destructive peroxides, a major cause of aging. Being a lipotropic substance, it also prevents fat accumulating in the liver.

BENEFICIAL EFFECTS

B15 is an anti-oxidant and anti-pollutant, eliminating environmental toxins from the body; it also extends cell life span; lowers cholesterol levels and protects the liver from cirrhosis; increases general immunity; and helps to reduce alcohol cravings and the effects of hangovers.

DEFICIENCY SYMPTOMS

Reduced oxygenation of cells, leading to fatigue, low levels of fitness, premature aging, heart disease, and glandular and nervous disorders.

BEST NATURAL SOURCES

Brewer's yeast, brown rice, whole grains, pumpkin, sesame seeds.

DAILY DOSAGE

Not given in RDA tables. However, the daily dosage most

often used is between 25 to 100 mg. It is sometimes available in health food stores as 'calcium pangamate'.

VITAMIN B17
(LAETRILE)

Laetrile, or amygdalin, is the most controversial 'vitamin' of recent years because of its use by some therapists as a cancer treatment.[38] It contains benzaldehyde and cyanide, is extracted from apricot kernels and is one B vitamin that does not occur in brewer's yeast.[39]

BENEFICIAL EFFECTS
Claimed to have cancer-preventive properties.[40]

DEFICIENCY SYMPTOMS
Fatigue, increased susceptibility to cancer.

BEST NATURAL SOURCES
Found in small amounts in apricot, cherry, peach and plum kernels, and in apple pips.

DAILY DOSAGE
No RDA has been established, but the usual dosage is between 250 and 1,000 mg. The FDA rejects laetrile on the grounds that it contains cyanide.

PABA
(PARA AMINO BENZOIC ACID)

PABA is related to folic acid (see p.73) and stimulates its synthesis in the intestines. PABA is water-soluble and a 'recent' member of the B group. It can be synthesized by the body and helps to utilize protein. With manganese, it stimulates pituitary gland function. It also has sunscreen properties and is therefore used in sunscreening ointments to prevent sunburn. PABA ointments are also reported to delay skin aging signs such as wrinkles and dark spots.[41] Along with pantothenic acid, PABA is known to restore grey hair to its natural colour in animals. It is also known to protect the lungs from ozone damage (ozone is found in smog and cigarette smoke), and is therefore very important for smokers and city dwellers. PABA is destroyed in the body by antibiotics and alcohol.

BENEFICIAL EFFECTS
Corrects loss of pigmentation in skin and hair (conditions such as vitiligo); protects against sunburn; aids fertility; fights senility; and increases synthesis of oestrogen and insulin.

DEFICIENCY SYMPTOMS
Skin conditions such as eczema, wrinkles and pigmentation loss; fatigue, irritability and depression; senility; arthritis and bursitis; gastric disorders.

BEST NATURAL SOURCES
Organ meats, brewer's yeast, whole grains, raw wheat germ, molasses.

DAILY DOSAGE
No RDA has been established, but 30 to 100 mg per day are reasonable. NOTE: PABA interferes with the action of sulpha drugs and neutralizes them. Supplementation should therefore be discontinued when sulpha drugs are taken.

FOLIC ACID

Folic acid, or folacin, is another water-soluble B vitamin, and its requirements are measured in micrograms. It is partially synthesized in the intestines by coliform bacteria. This important vitamin takes part, with B12, in the synthesis of nucleic acids and certain amino acids.[42] Our diets are very deficient in this vitamin. Easily destroyed, its antagonists are antibiotics, contraceptive pills and anti-convulsants such as Dilantin. Women taking oral contraceptives would do well to supplement their diet with folic acid. Pregnant and lactating women are particularly vulnerable to deficiencies and should increase their intake.[43] NOTE: Large amounts of vitamin C deplete folic acid, so when taking vitamin C in high doses, the diet should be supplemented accordingly.

BENEFICIAL EFFECTS
Stimulates stomach acid secretions, which prevent food poisoning and improve digestion and appetite; increases oestrogen levels; stimulates formation of red blood cells (with B12); improves lactation; promotes mental and emotional health; helps the body to synthesize brain neurotransmitters,[44] (chemicals which transmit nerve impulses in the brain); and raises blood histamine level, benefiting nervous disorders due to low levels of histamine.

DEFICIENCY SYMPTOMS
Megaloblastic anaemia; depression, psychosis and epileptic fits;[45] lack of appetite, sore tongue and digestive disturbances.

BEST NATURAL SOURCES
Green leafy vegetables, liver, egg yolk, Torula yeast, carrots, cantaloupe melons, pumpkin, avocados, beans.

DAILY DOSAGE
Adults 400 mcg, pregnant women 800 mcg, lactating women 600 mcg.

CAUTION: Excess folic acid supplementation may mask the anaemia caused by B12 deficiency. Since B12 and folic acid are so closely interrelated in their biochemical functions, these two vitamins are best taken simultaneously. Pregnant and lactating women who are on high folic acid supplementation should eat a well-balanced diet with adequate supplies of vitamin B12. Strict vegetarians are the most vulnerable. Subsisting for long periods on diets deficient in B12, they may absorb a lot of folic acid from a heavy consumption of green leafy vegetables, which may mask the development of a B12 deficiency, the devastating symptoms of which may take years to appear.

BIOTIN

Biotin is water-soluble and very stable when heated. It helps to utilize protein, folic acid and vitamin B12, and is synthesized by intestinal bacteria (flora). Deficiencies are not widespread. It is worth knowing, however, that raw egg white contains a substance called avidin, which prevents absorption of biotin. To prevent a deficiency, eggs should be eaten cooked.

BENEFICIAL EFFECTS
Maintains healthy skin and alleviates eczema and dermatitis; prevents grey hair and promotes healthy hair growth; and eases muscle aches and pains.

DEFICIENCY SYMPTOMS
Eczema and dermatitis; lack of appetite; fatigue; muscle aches
and pains.

BEST NATURAL SOURCES
Brewer's yeast, liver, brown rice, nuts, egg yolks, milk, fruits.

DAILY DOSAGE
Usually 150 to 300 mcg. Requirements increase during pregnancy and lactation.

CHOLINE

Choline is related to inositol as a constituent of lecithin. It is
lipotropic (emulsifies fat) and is involved in the utilization of
fats and cholesterol. Together with betaine and methionine,
choline helps the transportation of fat particles to cells. In the
body, choline is synthesized to acetylcholine, a neurotransmitter chemical vital for proper brain and nerve-muscle function. This action takes place in the presence of pantothenic
acid and manganese. Choline is one of the few substances that
can penetrate the blood-brain barrier (this barrier ensures
selective admission of nutrients to the brain, which requires
consistent nutrient levels regardless of daily variations in diet).

Choline can be formed in the body from the amino acid
methionine in the presence of B12 and folic acid.
Nevertheless, deficiencies do occur because of metabolic
defects or inadequate diet. Choline is also destroyed by alcohol, antibiotics, and food processing. In one study with rats,
severe deficiencies of choline for a period of eight months
were shown to impair liver function, causing a fatty liver, cirrhosis and, finally, cancerous tumours.[46] When taking supple-

mentary choline or lecithin, it is advisable to take calcium as well, since choline tends to raise phosphorus levels. Calcium restores a proper calcium-phosphorus balance.

BENEFICIAL EFFECTS
Reduces cholesterol; improves transmission of nerve-muscle impulses; improves memory and learning ability,[47] promotes sleep; maintains the health of the liver, kidneys and nerves; decreases oestrogen activity, easing menstrual cramps and lowering the risk of oestrogen-related breast lumps and breast cancer; and increases the synthesis of hormones such as adrenalin.

DEFICIENCY SYMPTOMS
Fatty degeneration of the liver; nephritis (kidney disease); intolerance of fats (gallbladder syndrome); gallstones; nerve-muscle diseases such as myasthenia gravis and tardive dyskinesia; high cholesterol; atherosclerosis; hypertension.

BEST NATURAL SOURCES
Egg yolk, brains, liver, brewer's yeast, raw wheat germ, green leafy vegetables.

DAILY DOSAGE
No RDA has been established. Average diets are thought to contain about 1 gram or more. For therapeutic effects, up to 6,000 mg are prescribed. NOTE: Massive and prolonged supplementation of choline depletes vitamin B6; in such cases, vitamin B6 should be used as an additional supplement.

INOSITOL

Inositol functions in cooperation with choline and biotin. Like choline, inositol is lipotropic and helps to metabolize fats and cholesterol. With choline, it is part of the structure of lecithin.

The brain and spinal cord contain large amounts of inositol. It was therefore assumed, and later established, that inositol supplements beneficially affect mental behaviour, producing a calming effect.[48]

In humans and animals, inositol (and choline) combines with phosphorus, fatty acids and nitrogen to form phospho-lipids. These form part of all cell membranes and are one of the means by which fats travel through the body. In cereals, seeds and legumes, inositol occurs as phytic acid, which binds with calcium, iron, zinc and other minerals, preventing their absorption into the bloodstream. To prevent mineral defi-ciencies, phytic acid must be deactivated. This is done by cooking, sprouting or leavening. Sprouted beans and grains such as soy and alfalfa can be eaten safely. In bread-making, leavening flour with yeast serves to deactivate phytates.

BENEFICIAL EFFECTS

Inositol helps to lower cholesterol in the liver,[49] maintains a healthy skin, and reduces undesirably high oestrogen levels in women (excess oestrogen can cause disorders such as breast lumps or breast cancer). Adelle Davis, the well-known author and nutritionist, found inositol very helpful, along with other B vitamins, in counteracting hair loss in men. Dr Carl Pfeiffer, head of the Brain-Bio Nutrition Research Institute in Princeton, New Jersey, considers inositol an effective treat-ment of high blood pressure when taken in daily doses of 2,000 mg. Dr Robert Atkins, physician and founder of the

Atkins Centre for Alternative Therapy in New York, finds that 2,000 mg a day helps to induce sleep when taken at bedtime, while 650 mg makes an effective daytime sedative. Dr Pfeiffer also finds that inositol has an anti-anxiety effect.

DEFICIENCY SYMPTOMS
Hypertension (high blood pressure); high cholesterol levels; atherosclerosis; dermatitis; constipation; hair loss. NOTE: Diabetics and alcohol and coffee drinkers over-excrete inositol and therefore need supplements to prevent deficiencies.

BEST NATURAL SOURCES
Organ meats, brains, brewer's yeast, wheat germ, cantaloupe melons, molasses, peanut butter.

DAILY DOSAGE
An RDA has not yet been established, but most nutritionists recommend the same intake as choline, about 1 gram (1,000 mg).

VITAMIN C

Vitamin C, also known by its chemical name ascorbic acid, is another water-soluble vitamin. It is very unstable and disintegrates not only in cooking but also when fruits and vegetables are peeled or stoned. Merely soaking unpeeled fruits in cold water causes depletion. Vitamin C, like other vitamins, does not occur in an isolated form but is always surrounded by various accompanying nutrients. These, in combination, are called the bioflavonoid complex (see p.89). They were discovered in Hungary in 1936 by Dr Albert Szent-Gyorgyi, the same biochemist who had isolated vitamin C three years earlier. The bioflavonoids, also collectively referred to as vitamin P, assist the function and increase the effects of vitamin C in the body.

Vitamin C influences several other nutrients. For example, it improves the body's ability to absorb calcium and iron,[50] and excrete poisonous copper,[51] lead and mercury. It lowers cholesterol by converting it into bile acids and is, in turn, helped to perform its duties by zinc. Vitamin C also assists the absorption of certain amino acids, and is needed in greater amounts in the high protein diets used by dieters and hypoglycaemics. It helps to neutralize nitrosamines, carcinogenic substances which are formed when smoked meats such as ham and bacon are cured with nitrites to prevent botulism and preserve an appetizing appearance.

The most famous vitamin C deficiency disease is of course scurvy, a fatal condition in its acute form. The symptoms of scurvy are bleeding gums, loss of teeth, opening of old wounds, anaemia, loss of appetite, fatigue, depression and hysteria. It was not until 1747, when Scottish physician Dr James Lind tested oranges, lemons and limes on British sailors, that a cure for scurvy was found. Scurvy still exists in populations ravaged by starvation and malnutrition. In the United States, subclinical (less acute) symptoms of scurvy are still found in many people, particularly those who subsist on junk foods.

Human beings are one of the very few mammals that cannot synthesize their own vitamin C. We therefore require a regular daily intake in our food. Vitamin C is not only water-soluble, but also easily perishable. If eaten at breakfast, it is gone from the bloodstream by noon.[52] So natural vitamin C foods such as fresh fruits and vegetables, or vitamin C tablets, should be taken throughout the day, every day. Smokers need more vitamin C than non-smokers, as each cigarette destroys 25 mg. Although vitamin C is non-toxic, it is known to increase urinary oxalic acid salts, so when taking high dosages of vitamin C (and calcium), magnesium intake should be increased to prevent the formation of calcium-oxalate kidney stones.

BENEFICIAL EFFECTS

Despite much controversy in recent years, the ability of vitamin C to fight the common cold is now well accepted among nutrition-oriented doctors and nutritionists. Although still not officially recognized by the conservative medical establishment, vitamin C attracted wide public attention when Dr Linus Pauling, the Nobel laureate biochemist, published a small pamphlet called Vitamin C and the Common Cold.[53] His investigations into the effects of massive vitamin C dosages continue at the research institute he headed at Menlo Park, California. Few people realize that vitamin C has many more uses than just preventing scurvy. For example, as an antioxidant, it delays aging; as an anti-histamine, it alleviates allergies; and as an anti-pollutant, it helps to eliminate toxic substances from the body, from poisonous lead to snake venom.

One of ascorbic acid's main biological functions is to help form collagen (a sub-skin 'cement'). Reduced collagen may be reflected in wrinkles, thought to be a sign of aging. They could, in fact, be a sign of lifelong vitamin C deficiency.

Vitamin C increases our immune response to infectious diseases by boosting leukocyte (antibody) function and raising production of interferon,[54] a type of protein secreted by the white cells of the immune system which prevents viruses from proliferating in the body. Recent studies confirm that vitamin C lowers the risk of cancers of the mouth, oesophagus, lung, stomach, colon, cervix and breast.[55] It was also found that breast cancer risk could be reduced if post-menopausal women took 380 mg vitamin C a day.[56] In the treatment of cancer, megadoses of vitamin C have been found to inhibit tumour development and prolong the survival of terminal cancer patients.[57] Vitamin C speeds up the healing of wounds and strengthens capillaries and blood vessels,[58] preventing strokes. It helps to prevent anaemia (with B12 and folic acid). It promotes healthy teeth, and relieves fatigue, anxiety and depression by assisting in the formation of nor-epinephrine, an important neurotransmitter.[59]

Several studies have established the ability of vitamin C to lower cholesterol levels – it does this by accelerating its transformation into bile acids.[60] A British study showed that cholesterol can be lowered with daily supplements of 1,000 mg of vitamin C.[61] Dr Constance Spittle, the research scientist who conducted this study, has also suggested that athero-sclerosis may be the result of long-term deficiency of vitamin C, which allows high cholesterol levels to build up in the arteries. Finally, vitamin C has been found to provide additional protection against the devastating effects of alcoholism and smoking – it does this by reducing the formation of acetaldehyde, a toxic by-product of alcohol and nicotine metabolism.[62]

DEFICIENCY SYMPTOMS
Susceptibility to colds, infections and allergies; bleeding or inflamed gums and defective teeth; broken capillaries and sub-skin haemorrhages; strokes; anaemia; skin wrinkles; loss of appetite and fatigue; nervousness, anxiety and depression; impaired healing of wounds.

BEST NATURAL SOURCES
Whole citrus fruits and juices, peppers, broccoli, tomatoes, cabbage, green leafy vegetables, melons, yams, potatoes.

DAILY DOSAGE
Adults 60 mg, children 45 mg, pregnant and lactating women 100 mg. In view of recent studies, these RDAs are ridiculously low, although they will prevent scurvy. They will not promote immunity and health. Nutritionists prescribe doses of several grams a day. Dr Linus Pauling concludes, from comparative studies of animals which synthesize their own vitamin C, that humans need 1.5 to 4.0 grams daily. NOTE: High doses of vitamin C should be supplemented with magnesium tablets to keep calcium soluble and prevent kidney stones. People with an over-acidic stomach, or those who suffer from heartburn, can use buffered vitamin C, calcium ascorbate or ester C which are less acidic. Ester C is a gentler form of vitamin C. It stays longer in the bloodstream and has less tendency to cause kidney stones in susceptible people.

VITAMIN D

Vitamin D is a fat-soluble vitamin and is supplied either by food or by exposure to the sun. It is known as the 'sunshine vitamin' since the sun's ultraviolet rays convert sub-skin cholesterol into vitamin D.

In food, vitamin D is absorbed, together with emulsified fats, through the intestinal wall. When produced by the sun, it is absorbed directly into the bloodstream. After absorption, it is stored in the liver. It is also stored, in smaller quantities, in the skin, brain, and bones. People who do not drink milk or who are strict vegetarians should be concerned about their vitamin D intake. Vitamin D is scarce in vegetables. City dwellers employed indoors should also take care to obtain proper amounts of vitamin D. It is worth noting that when a suntan is maintained, the skin ceases to manufacture vitamin D. NOTE: If you drink large quantities of vitamin D fortified milk you should be aware that synthetic vitamin D considerably increases excretion of magnesium from the body. It would therefore be wise to supplement your milk with magnesium or dolomite tablets.

BENEFICIAL EFFECTS
Promotes absorption of calcium and phosphorus,[63] both vital for strong teeth and bones, and for preventing rickets (bent legs in infants and children) – rickets has been treated since the Middle Ages with cod liver oil, a rich source of vitamin D; helps to assimilate vitamin A; maintains a healthy nervous system, normal heartbeat and efficient blood clotting.

DEFICIENCY SYMPTOMS
Soft and porous bones and teeth, leading to rickets and tooth decay; fatigue; arthritis. One report cites myopia (shortsightedness) as a consequence of vitamin D deficiency.

BEST NATURAL SOURCES
Fish liver oil, sardines, herring, salmon, tuna, fortified milk.

DAILY DOSAGE
Adults and children 400 IU, pregnant and lactating women 600 IU. NOTE: Daily overdoses of 1,800 IU or more may lead to overaccumulation of vitamin D and to toxicity symptoms such as diarrhoea, nausea, excessive urination, calcification of the arteries and kidney damage.

VITAMIN E

Vitamin E is another fat-soluble vitamin. It is composed of a group of substances called tocopherols, which are subdivided into alpha, beta, gamma, etc. Of all these, alpha tocopherol is the most chemically active; the others have anti-oxidation effects.

'Tocopherol' comes from a Greek word meaning 'child-birth'. Most early studies of vitamin E were connected with sterility problems and it was found that women with a history of miscarriage responded well to large doses of it.

Vitamin E is most important as a potent antioxidant. According to Dr Wilfrid Shute, director of the Shute Institute in Ontario, Canada, and a leading authority on vitamin E for 45 years, it is three times as potent in this respect as vitamin C.[64] Vitamin E unites with oxygen and prevents the formation of destructive peroxide products, and therefore has wide-ranging beneficial effects. For example, it prevents unsaturated body fats from oxidizing and forming damaging particles known as free radicals. Uncontrolled oxidation (peroxidation) of lipids (body fats) has many harmful effects. These include: damage to fatty brain cells, causing senility; rupture of red blood cells, causing haemolytic anaemia (which is not responsive to iron but to vitamin E); weakening of immune cell function, causing auto-immune diseases such as arthritis; damage to DNA (nucleic acids which carry the genetic code), leading to the kind of mutations which cause cancer. Vitamin E protects prostacyclin (PGI2), a hormone-like compound which protects blood vessels from undue blood-clotting and therefore prevents atherosclerosis and heart attacks. [65]

The ability of vitamin E to bind oxygen can benefit runners and joggers who inhale lots of oxygen during their aerobic activities. This extra oxygen can cause dangerous peroxidation unless counterbalanced by additional vitamin E. Moreover, vitamin E improves cell respiration, which enables muscles, including the heart muscle, to function with less oxygen and so increase their efficiency. No wonder vitamin E supplements are so popular among athletes.

Substances which render vitamin E ineffective are: oxygen, iron, oestrogen-containing pills, chlorine and mineral oil. Inorganic iron supplements such as ferrous sulphate destroy vitamin E, while organic iron preparations such as ferrous gluconate or succinate do not. Therefore, when using a supplement which contains ferrous sulphate, take vitamin E at least 8 hours before or after.

Vitamin E is essential to pituitary hormone production – the hormones produced by the pituitary gland control, among many other things, adrenal function and childhood-growth. Oestrogen can neutralize vitamin E, and it is thought that many of the side effects of oral contraceptives – weight gain, varicose veins, water retention (oedema) – are a result of vitamin E deficiency. People who live in highly polluted air, or whose water supply is rich in chlorine, should also take vitamin E supplements.

At a nutritional convention in 1979,[66] Dr Wilfrid Shute reported that vitamin E has a variable influence on blood pressure: in one third of his patients vitamin E raised blood pressure, in another third it lowered it, and in another third it had no effect. Nevertheless vitamin E was found to be of great help to the thousands of patients treated by Dr Shute. However, Dr Carlton Fredericks,[67] the well-known research nutritionist and author, advises cardiac patients to use vitamin E only under the supervision of a cardiologist. Minimal doses should be taken to begin with, and then increased very gradually, in order to give the weak heart and circulatory system a chance to adjust. Dr Shute's book, *Vitamin E for Ailing and*

Healthy Hearts, contains explicit instructions for the use of vitamin E in such cases.

Two recent studies from Harvard showed that nurses and other health professionals who took at least 100 IU of vitamin E for at least two years had a forty per cent lower risk of heart disease than non-users of vitamin E.[68] Finally, several studies have shown that people with low levels of vitamin E increase their risk of cancer.[69]

BENEFICIAL EFFECTS

Vitamin E acts as an antioxidant, and therefore assists cell regeneration and delays aging. It protects fat-soluble vitamins and hormones, and in high doses guards against the effects of pollutants in food, water and air. It also acts as an anticoagulant (an anti-clotting factor), lowering blood cholesterol and thinning the blood; this prevents the formation of arterial blood clots and conditions such as phlebitis (inflammation of the veins). Phlebitis often results in a blood clot (thrombophlebitis) which is liable to detach itself from the vein where it was formed and move to block a vital artery in the lungs or heart.

Vitamin E plays an important role in alleviating the primary causes of death in affluent Western societies: heart disease, cancer, diabetes and accidents, including burns.[70] Having treated more than 35,000 patients in the last 40 years, Dr Shute has conclusively shown the ability of vitamin E to improve blood circulation and prevent heart disease. He has also found that treating major burns and sunburn with vitamin E ointment helps to prevent blistering and scarring, accelerates healing, and often completely regenerates the skin.

Dr Shute has also treated diabetic gangrene of the leg with oral doses of vitamin E only. The gangrenous tissue fell off of its own accord, eliminating the need for surgery. It was found that the white cells of the immune system had engulfed and digested the gangrenous cells next to them, forming a line of cleavage along which detachment took place. Research biochemist Dr Raymond Shamberger and others have shown the ability of vitamin E (and other antioxidants such as vitamin C) to suppress cancer development by inhibiting the action of carcinogens.[71]

Vitamin E is well known to be beneficial for fertility and sexual potency. Women who take oestrogen to prevent hot flushes and nervousness during the menopause would do well to use vitamin E instead. Vitamin E is involved in the production of a substance which delivers nerve impulses to muscles, and is therefore beneficial in chronic debilitating diseases such as multiple sclerosis, myasthenia gravis and certain other paralytic conditions.

DEFICIENCY SYMPTOMS
Fatigue and premature aging; infertility, sterility and miscarriage; muscular dystrophy; haemolytic anaemia (not responsive to iron intake); circulatory disorders such as coronary heart disease, thrombosis, swollen and inflamed veins (thrombophlebitis); lameness due to poor circulation (claudication); kidney inflammation (nephritis); degeneration of sex glands (testes and prostate); poor healing of wounds and burns.

BEST NATURAL SOURCES
Raw wheat germ and wheat germ oil, vegetable oils, soya beans, leafy green vegetables, whole grains and cereals, eggs.

DAILY DOSAGE
Adults 12 to 15 IU, children 7 to 12 IU. However, most nutritionists recommend much higher doses, 100 IU and over.

Many people supplement their diets with 400 to 600 IU.

VITAMIN K

Vitamin K is another fat-soluble vitamin which occurs in three forms, called K1, K2 and K3. K1 and K2 are synthesized by the intestinal flora. Synthetic K3 is available for those who cannot absorb it from food.

To ensure adequate absorption of vitamin K, cultured milk products (yogurt for example), other dairy foods, and vegetable oils, must be included in the daily diet. Over-consumption of sugar and sugary foods should be avoided. Healthy intestinal flora can be maintained by regularly eating yogurt and buttermilk and supplementing the diet with lactobacillus-acidophilus capsules. Antibiotics, which indiscriminately kill hostile and friendly intestinal bacteria, are antagonistic to vitamin K and should be used as sparingly as possible. When they must be taken, their destructive action should be counteracted by eating additional yogurt and buttermilk.

BENEFICIAL EFFECTS
The liver needs vitamin K in order to produce prothrombin, one of many factors involved in blood clotting. Vitamin K therefore plays a part in preventing internal bleeding and reducing excessive menstrual flow. It also helps to prevent coronary thrombosis.

DEFICIENCY SYMPTOMS
Deficiencies of vitamin K are usually caused by a defect in metabolism or a malfunction of the liver, or by colitis or coeliac disease. Coeliac disease is caused by intestinal intoler-

ance to gluten, a protein found in wheat, rye and barley. Coeliac victims must emphasize vitamin K foods and supplement their diets not only with vitamin K but with the other fat-soluble vitamins – A, D and E – and also with calcium and B complex. A deficiency causes delayed blood-clotting, haemorrhages such as nose bleeds, and a lack of blood platelets (the small discs around which blood coagulates).

BEST NATURAL SOURCES
Alfalfa, green leafy vegetables, kelp, yogurt and buttermilk, egg yolks, fish liver oil, safflower and soybean oil.

DAILY DOSAGE
No official dosage has been established, but 300 mcg are generally considered adequate for an adult.

VITAMIN P
(BIOFLAVONOID COMPLEX)

Vitamin P is the collective name for a group of water-soluble substances called bioflavonoids, annexed in plants to vitamin C. Citrus pith is now known to be a rich source of bioflavonoids, which is why it is always preferable to eat whole, thinly peeled oranges rather than drink strained orange juice. Vitamin C complex, which includes the bioflavonoids, is better than plain vitamin C, which provides only ascorbic acid.

As a group, between 600 and 800 flavonoids have been identified in fruits, vegetables, nuts, seeds, leaves, flowers and barley. Many medicinal plants owe much of their activity to flavonoids such as quercetin and rutin. The typical Western diet contains 1 gram of mixed flavonoids of which 50 mg is quercetin.

BENEFICIAL EFFECTS

The bioflavonoid rutin increases absorption and utilization of vitamin C,[72] and therefore helps to maintain healthy collagen, the vital 'cement' between all body cells. It also strengthens the walls of capillaries, making them less likely to rupture and cause bleeding and bruising.

Rutin is well known, especially among herbalists, as an effective treatment for piles, varicose veins and high blood pressure. For these conditions, a tea made from buckwheat leaves, a fine source of rutin, is sometimes recommended. Rutin is mentioned by Dr Carlton Fredericks as a preventive against menopausal flushes.

Bioflavonoids have been successfully used in the treatment of stomach ulcers. This is not surprising since they make weak capillaries less vulnerable to attack and rupture by stomach acid. While bioflavonoids strengthen capillaries, vitamin C speeds up the healing of these which have broken. These combined effects are also beneficial against nose bleeds, bleeding gums, oedema, arthritis and various infections.

BEST NATURAL SOURCES

Citrus fruits (especially the pith and rind), grapes, plums, blackcurrants, apricots, buckwheat leaves, cherries, blackberries, rosehips.

DAILY DOSAGE

No official dosage has been established, but many nutritionists advise at least 50 mg for every 300mg of vitamin C.

QUERCETIN

Quercetin is the bioflavonoid that has drawn the special attention of science in recent years. Research studies have revealed that quercetin is the most active of all flavonoids, with remarkable beneficial effects on an array of health conditions.

Quercetin was found to be an excellent antioxidant and free radical scavenger.[73] This contributes to a reduced predisposition to diseases and increased lifespan. Quercetin was also reported to possess a strong and prolonged anti-inflammatory effect,[74] and wound-healing effect.[75] Quercetin was also found to be effective against human viruses, especially against *Herpes simplex* virus.[76]

Quercetin has also manifested a wide anticarcinogenic activity. Several studies have shown its ability to inhibit the growth of several types of cancer cells, such as breast cancer,[77] ovarian cancer [78] and leukaemia.[79] Quercetin was also shown to be an efficient inhibitor of histamine release,[80] and therefore, helpful in treating allergies. Additional studies reported quercetin's ability to delay the onset of cataract by decreasing the accumulation of sorbitol which crystallizes in the lens of diabetic animals.[81] It does so by inhibiting the enzyme, aldose reductase, which converts glucose to sorbitol. Quercetin is also useful in diabetes for its ability to enhance insulin secretion.[82]

The discoveries about the healthful effects of quercetin have made it very popular in the 1990s. It is now available as a food supplement in health food stores.

ENZYMES

Although much has been written about vitamins, minerals and other nutrients, very little has been published on the subject of enzymes. Yet these remarkable substances are the most important of all metabolic elements. They act as catalysts, that is, agents that speed up chemical reactions that otherwise would not take place, or would take place so slowly as to appear not to be occurring. Without digestive-enzymes in our digestive tract, vitamins, minerals and other nutrients have no value to the body.

Enzymes are complex proteins. Some of them contain metallic minerals, while others function in cooperation with vitamins, especially B vitamins, which act as co-enzymes. Digestive-enzymes stimulate metabolic processes without being chemically changed in the process. They can, for example, enable sugar and fat to burn at normal body temperature (98.4°F/37°C) in the presence of oxygen, releasing carbon dioxide and water. Copper-containing enzymes in the body combine oxygen and hydrogen to create water, a reaction which would otherwise be explosive.

Life on our planet began to evolve principally through the action of enzymes in the water and gases that covered the earth's surface. Enzyme reactions started fermentation, which formed plants, which in turn converted the carbon dioxide-rich atmosphere into an oxygen-rich one suitable for the evolution of animal life.

The human digestive system is a reflection of those first processes of evolution. The digestive tract supplies the water and the food, which are then metabolized through enzyme intermediaries. Enzymatic breakdown of foods (hydrolysis) begins in the mouth. Saliva contains ptyalin, a starch-reducing enzyme which acts on starch as food is chewed. The stomach then secretes pepsin, an enzyme which gets to work on proteins, provided it is in an acid environment. The intestines, which are an alkaline environment, contain various enzymes which dismantle all the remaining nutrients, converting them to simpler substances which the body can use – proteins into amino acids, fats into fatty acids, carbohydrates into glucose. Since each specific enzyme acts only on one specific substance (substrate) and brings about only one specific chemical reaction, the reader will readily appreciate that the mechanism of metabolism – the sum total of all the chemical reactions which take place in the body – is very complex and delicate. The liver alone produces over 1,000 different enzymes.[83] The lack of even one enzyme can break the chain of biochemical reactions, causing imbalances which manifest themselves as allergies, nutritional deficiencies and illness. For example, the lack of a stomach enzyme known as 'intrinsic factor' can lead to pernicious anaemia unless the diet is fortified with digestive-enzyme tablets and vitamin B12.

To properly digest foods, digestive-enzymes that break down all the main food groups must be present: protease for proteins, lipase for fats and carbohydrase for sugars and starches. Even to completely digest just protein, the other enzyme groups are helpful.

With aging however, the secretion of enzymes in the body is gradually reduced. It is a well-known fact that young people can digest food more efficiently than older people. Deficiencies of digestive-enzymes in older age can cause common symptoms of indigestion, poor absorption of nutrients, malnutrition, toxicity and allergies to by-products from poorly digested foods, headaches, fatigue and lower immunity to diseases. Dr Humbart Santillo has said that 'Enzyme deficiencies are America's number one nutritional problem, and are responsible for more disease than all other nutritional shortages combined.' In fact, enzymes may be a key factor in preventing disease and extending life-span. Enzyme supplementation from middle age and beyond, is therefore very desirable and can relieve many digestive discomforts.

Enzyme supplementation is available through health food shops in various forms. Some come from vegetarian origins, such as papain from papaya and bromelain from pineapple. Others are from animal origin like pancreatin, which is made from cattle or hog pancreas, handles more food groups and has a strong digestive activity. Pancreatin tablets usually contain protease, lipase and amylase for the digestion of protein, fat and starch. People who have digestive discomfort from low stomach acid secretion, can use betaine HCl tablets. Many marketed preparations combine enzymes of both animal and vegetable origin, and assist digestion in a balanced way. Enzymes are usually taken after a meal, except some detoxifying enzymes which are better taken between meals.

THE IMPORTANCE OF FRESH, RAW FOODS

Enzymes are found abundantly in fresh, unprocessed, natural foods. However, they are easily destroyed by heating to temperatures over 120°F (49°C), and are also sensitive to other food processing procedures. Peeling, cooking, pasteurizing, refining, preserving, smoking, grilling, frying and baking largely destroy enzymes. Nevertheless, as our civilization has 'progressed', we have gradually parted company with natural unprocessed foods. Until recently, the more complex the ingredients and the preparation of a recipe, the more 'gastronomic' it was considered to be. Fresh simple food, consumed à la nature, was regarded as unfit or unhygienic for intelligent civilized people.

Wild animals eat fresh uncooked food, but when zoo keepers tried to feed animals cooked food, they began to get 'human' diseases. The late Dr Francis F. Pottenger, Professor of Medicine at the University of Southern California, carried out a famous experiment using three generations of cats. The first generation was reared on a natural diet of raw milk and raw meat, and produced healthy kittens. The kittens ate processed foods, such as condensed milk and cooked meats, their health deteriorated and they displayed many human afflictions such as loss of teeth, irritability and heart trouble. Their offspring, suffering from a variety of ailments, were put back on a diet of fresh natural foods; gradually they were restored to the glowing health of the first generation. The 'rawness' of the foods they ate made the difference.

Quantities of fresh unprocessed foods can do the same for humans as well, restoring health even to weak, unhealthy people who have subsisted on junk food for many years. But the changeover should be gradual. After a lifetime of habituation to processed foods, it is hard to convert to an exclusively raw food diet. And it is true that some foods, such as legumes and fish, need cooking. But in general we over-cook and over-process our food.

Linda Clark the American nutritionist, in her book *Stay Young Longer*, tells the story of the Russian scientist Kouchakoff, who found that after cooked food is eaten, white blood cells increase in the intestines. Now white cells, which are part of the immune system, always increase in number when there is a need to eliminate hostile invaders. Their extra concentration indicates the start of an inflammation or disease. In other words, cooked foods place an added strain on the immune system. Eating raw foods, however, does not cause an increase in white cell numbers. In fact, Dr Bircher-

Benner, the famous Swiss nutritionist, discovered that eating raw vegetables before cooked food prevents the appearance of the extra white cells. That is why fresh raw salad is always the first course of a meal in his sanatorium.

There is no scientific dispute over the fact that, as the body ages, enzymes become less plentiful. In fact, a shortage of enzymes is the main cause of digestive disorders, which are so widespread that they are often accepted as normal. Let us, therefore, emphasize enzyme-rich foods – plenty of fresh raw vegetables, fruits and grain sprouts – in our diets and aim for optimum health and well-being for as long as we live.

CHAPTER 4

BULK MINERALS AND TRACE ELEMENTS

Since the first decades of this century, scientific and public interest has focused on vitamins. In recent years, however, research has revealed the crucial importance of minerals and trace elements as well. As constituents of various enzyme systems, minerals are vital factors in health and well-being. Different studies have shown that minerals and trace elements can prevent and treat various disorders, from diabetes to premature aging, and from low sexual potency to heart disease.

Minerals are elements found abundantly in the earth's crust. Calcium, phosphorus, potassium, sodium, magnesium, sulphur, silicone and chlorine are all necessary to the body in relatively large amounts and are therefore referred to as bulk minerals. They should be supplied by plant or animal foods. Among the many important processes they help to regulate are heartbeat, water balance, and the functioning of nerves and muscles.

Trace elements, which are also minerals and no less important than bulk minerals, are necessary in extremely small amounts. Iron, zinc, copper, manganese, chromium, iodine, selenium, fluorine, and molybdenum are all trace elements, and each forms less than one hundredth of one per cent of the human body. However, this should not mislead us as to their vital importance to health. Deficiencies of trace elements can result in many and varied ailments, including diabetes (high blood sugar), hypoglycaemia (low blood sugar), obesity, anaemia and nervousness.

However, although trace elements are indispensable to the body, excesses are not desirable. Essential trace elements such as zinc and chromium are non-toxic and occur in foods in such tiny amounts that excesses are improbable, unless heavily supplemented, but others, such as fluorine and copper, while beneficial in specific minute amounts, are hazardous in larger amounts. Some elements, such as lead, cadmium and mercury, are highly toxic even in minuscule amounts and should be avoided at all costs. Water from lead pipes can cause mental degeneration[1] and infertility.[2] Soft water from rivers or water-softeners dissolve cadmium from metal water pipes, inducing high blood pressure and heart attacks.[3] Soft water from copper pipes will cause an excess of copper in the body, leading to arthritis, insanity,[4] and schizophrenia.[5] Acid foods and drinks such as lemonade can absorb sufficient antimony from enamelware to cause vomiting.[6] Aluminium salts from foods cooked in aluminium utensils or foil are implicated in loss of memory and pre-senile dementia.[7] Other sources of aluminium in daily life are processed cheese, baking soda, table salt and antiperspirants, all of which should be used minimally.

POOR SOIL, POOR FOOD

Why is it even more important to be aware of minerals and

essential trace elements than of vitamins? First, because vitamins depend on minerals for their absorption, and second, because vitamins are usually supplied by a wide range of readily available plant foods. Some are even synthesized by the body. Minerals, on the other hand, are not always found in plants and must be present in the soil before plants and grazing animals can make use of them. Fortunately, bulk minerals are spread copiously and evenly throughout the soil, but this is not the case with essential trace elements. In some parts of the world important elements such as iodine and molybdenum are either entirely lacking in the soil or exist in such negligible amounts that they cannot be utilized. Large parts of the American Midwest, for example, are deficient in iodine, which results in high incidence of goitre. The best way of combating the deficiency is to use iodized salt.

Molybdenum, required by legume roots for the growth of the nitrogen-fixing bacteria which synthesize protein, is another element which is deficient in many soils. Foods grown on zinc-deficient soil can cause prostate trouble. Foods grown on iron-deficient soil may result in anaemia. In areas short of magnesium, plants grow poorly because photosynthesis is impaired (magnesium is an ingredient of chlorophyll, which catalyzes photosynthesis in plants).

Recent research has put the limelight on selenium and chromium. Dr Richard Passwater, nutrition researcher and gerontologist, found that selenium is a fine antioxidant capable of neutralizing dangerous peroxide compounds, fighting cancer, building a healthy heart and slowing down the aging process.[8] Dr Walter Mertz of the Human Nutrition Laboratory in Beltsville, Maryland, discovered that chromium is the major component of the glucose tolerance factor (GTF) and of great value in preventing diabetes and hypoglycaemia.[9] Chromium in cereals and raw cane or beet sugar is removed by refining. Dr Henry Schroeder, a medical researcher from Brattleboro, Vermont, and a renowned authority on minerals, claims that if chromium intake were increased, the incidence of heart attacks would fall to what it was 80 years ago.

It is important to remember that the nutritional value of plants and animals depends on the quality of the soil. A shortage of any element will be reflected in the health of plants, animals, and eventually humans.

City dwellers who buy their food in supermarkets have no way of knowing whether the produce they buy is nutritious, unless it bears an 'organic', 'nitrate-free' or 'Soil Association' label. We live in an era of agricultural sprays, insecticides and chemical fertilizers, all of which contribute to mineral deficiencies. Farmers think more about intensifying growth, saving water and increasing yields per acre than about rehabilitating soils with essential trace elements. Organic fertilizing with manure and compost (which restores vital minerals to the soil, and increases the vitamin B12 and protein content of the crops) is regarded as impractical.

It is therefore important that we become conscious of our mineral intake. We cannot blindly rely on our diet. Since the same foods can vary greatly in mineral content from one locale to another, we should safeguard our health by eating a great variety of mineral-rich foods *and* taking multi-mineral supplements. Domestic organic gardening should be encouraged.

There is no doubt now that mineral-rich soils promote radiant health and contribute to longevity. Several ethnic groups living in isolated regions of the world on soils rich in minerals have been found to enjoy excellent health and exceptional longevity. The Hunzas of the Himalayas in Pakistan, for example, have been repeatedly investigated over the past 40 years.[10] These people were disease-free because they subsisted on foods grown on unpolluted, mineral-rich soils. Moreover, the soils were not depleted by intensive agriculture. Ancient methods of organic farming ensured that all minerals and elements were returned to the soil.

TRACE ELEMENTS VERSUS AGE AND CANCER

The more we study the elements, the more we learn about the vital roles they play in biological functions. Elements such as zinc, copper and manganese are now known to form an antioxidant enzyme in the body called SOD (superoxide dismutase). SOD has been shown to be positively correlated to lifespan.[11] This is because it protects the body from peroxides and free radicals, which attack body cells, causing age-related diseases such as arthritis, cataracts, atherosclerosis and multiple sclerosis.[12] SOD can also help to counteract the destructive effects of X-rays, which damage the body by generating free radicals. Selenium is needed for the formation of another antioxidant enzyme, glutathione peroxidase. This has been found to strengthen the immune system[13] and increase resistance to cancer. [14]

The study of trace elements is still far from complete. As a matter of fact, Dr Schroeder states that essential elements are still being discovered at a rate of two per decade, and there are still many questions to be answered. Preventing deficiencies through sensible eating, that is by eating whole unrefined foods, supplemented by mineral-rich health foods or multimineral tablets, is therefore in everybody's best interest.

Naturally rich sources of minerals and elements are raw seeds and nuts, raw wheat germ, alfalfa sprouts, brewer's yeast, pollen, spirulina, kelp, dolomite, bonemeal and molasses. All are available at health food stores. Spices contain relatively enormous amounts of trace elements, but are a poor source since only small quantities of them are consumed. Black pepper, for example, contains high concentrations of copper, chromium and manganese. Cloves are rich in copper and chromium. Thyme is also a good source of copper.

Synthetic mineral tablets are of questionable benefit since the body has difficulty absorbing them. The intestinal walls retain inorganic minerals and prevent their absorption into the blood unless they are combined (chelated) with proteins, which serve as carriers.[15] Most supplements sold at health food stores today are chelated minerals.

White sugar is one of the strongest antagonists of mineral absorption. Antibiotics are another enemy of minerals. Adelle Davis notes in her book *Let's Get Well* that the antibiotic streptomycin prevents manganese absorption. A deficiency of manganese impairs enzyme production and can cause convulsions, dizziness and loss of hearing. Minerals, like vitamins, are also depleted by stress, alcohol, smoking, lack of sleep, injury and illness.

Mineral dosages are controversial and some are not even established. Therefore, as in Chapter 3, RDA values will be quoted when available, and only as a starting point for nutritional planning.

BULK MINERALS

CALCIUM (Ca)

Calcium is the most abundant mineral in the body. Almost all of it, 99 per cent in fact, is found in the bones and teeth. However, the remaining 1 per cent is of great importance to body chemistry, since it normalizes nerve and muscle function, regulates heartbeat, is essential to blood clotting, maintains a proper acid-base equilibrium, induces sleep and generates skin health. For proper absorption and functioning calcium needs stomach acid (hydrochloric acid), vitamin D, phosphorus, magnesium, protein (for chelation), and vitamins A and C.

Absorption of calcium is very inefficient. Enough stomach acid must be present to dissolve it, and enough magnesium to keep it soluble, or it will be deposited and lead to various disorders, from kidney stones to arteriosclerosis. Supplements of stomach acid are available in health food stores as 'betaine HCL'; these are recommended for people with low gastric secretions, particularly to people over age 40, to improve absorption.

Calcium, in a balance of 2.5 parts calcium to 1 part phosphorus, is essential for strong bones and teeth. However, adequate calcium intake alone is not always enough to ensure healthy bones and teeth. Too much bedrest or a sedentary lifestyle causes calcium to dissolve out of bones and into the blood (due to the action of parathyroid hormone); this softens the bones and predisposes them to fractures. On the other hand, regular exercise strengthens the bones by encouraging bone calcification, or the deposition of calcium in bones. No wonder calcium deficiencies are so prevalent among older people. Not only do most of them lead a sedentary life, but their calcium absorption is also impaired due to diminution of gastric juices. Elderly women are particularly vulnerable since their average calcium consumption is less than that of men. More than 10 per cent of women over 50 suffer from bone loss leading to fractures. Every year, in the United States alone, 100,000 women over the age of 60 fracture their hips.[16]

Calcium also neutralizes excess lactic acid in the body.

Since lactic acid accumulates as a result of strenuous physical activity or mental stress, calcium is beneficial both to athletes in relieving fatigue and to people suffering from anxiety or depression.[17] Dr Lendon Smith, professor of pediatrics at the University of Oregon, has found calcium beneficial in calming hyperactive children.[18]

Phytic acid, found in raw cereals and legumes, can inhibit the absorption of calcium. Oxalic acid, another constituent of foods such as chocolate, spinach and rhubarb, combines with calcium to form insoluble compounds which cause kidney stones of the calcium oxalate type. Sugar disturbs the calcium–phosphorus balance. Strontium-90, from radioactive fallout, has an affinity with calcium – it can replace calcium in bones and eventually cause bone and blood cancer. Supplements of calcium can bind with strontium-90 and eliminate it through the faeces,[19] thus protecting us from radioactive pollution.

BENEFICIAL EFFECTS
Builds and maintains bones and teeth; facilitates transmission of nerve impulses and maintains a healthy nervous system; calms nervousness and helps insomnia if taken at bedtime; soothes menopausal emotional crises; promotes blood clotting; maintains a healthy complexion; reduces toxic effects of lead and cadmium; can neutralize some of the harmful effects of radioactive fallout.

DEFICIENCY SYMPTOMS
Porous and brittle bones, fractures, tooth decay (caries), rickets; nervousness, muscle aches, leg cramps, teeth grinding (bruxism); skin disorders such as loss of pigmentation, cold sores and mouth blisters; excessive menstrual flow; impaired growth.

BEST NATURAL SOURCES

Milk and dairy products, sesame seeds and sesame paste (tahini), soybeans, peanuts, green vegetables, walnuts, sunflower seeds, soups made with beef bones.

DAILY DOSAGE

Adults 800 mg, pregnant and lactating women 1,200 mg. Absorption of calcium becomes less efficient with age, so people over 40 should emphasize milk products in their diet, or if allergic, take calcium-rich supplements such as dolomite, bonemeal or oyster shell calcium tablets.

PHOSPHORUS (P)

Phosphorus is the second most abundant mineral in the body. It cooperates with calcium and functions best when in a balance of 1 part phosphorus to 2.5 parts calcium. Proper calcium-phosphorus balance ensures optimum bone mineralization.

Phosphorus is present in every cell of the body and is involved in most biological reactions. It is vital to the release of energy in every muscle cell and is needed for the conversion of glucose to glycogen, the form in which glucose is stored in the liver and muscles. Phosphorus is required for the synthesis of phospholipids such as lecithin, which transports fats throughout the body, for the transmission of nerve impulses, and for maintaining a proper acid-alkaline balance.

Phosphorus is a constituent of the nucleoproteins which carry our genetic code, and also of myelin, the fatty sheath which covers and insulates nerves, without which the nervous system would malfunction. Unlike calcium, it is very efficiently absorbed in the presence of vitamin D and calcium. Most of it is stored in the bones and teeth. Its enemies are sugar, which disturbs the calcium-phosphorus balance, and antacid preparations containing calcium carbonate. With age, the kidneys become less efficient at excreting phosphorus, and so it tends to build up, causing the calcium level to drop in order to maintain a proper calcium-phosphorus balance. A calcium deficiency is thus created, which explains why some nutritionists recommend decreasing phosphorus intake after the age of 40 by eating fewer phosphorus-rich foods.

BENEFICIAL EFFECTS
Maintains strong bones and teeth; promotes growth and body repair; provides energy by helping to metabolize carbohydrates and fats; maintains acid-alkaline balance and the proper functioning of nerves.

DEFICIENCY SYMPTOMS
Weak bones and teeth; rickets; gum infection and bleeding; arthritis; loss of appetite; muscle weakness.

BEST NATURAL SOURCES
Meat, eggs, fish, whole grains, raw wheat germ, nuts and seeds.

DAILY DOSAGE
Adults 800mg, pregnant and lactating women 1,200 mg. Deficiencies are very rare in people who eat balanced diets. NOTE: as phosphorus intake is increased (as in high protein diets), additional calcium should be taken to maintain proper calcium-phosphorus ratio.

POTASSIUM (K)

Potassium constitutes 5 per cent of the total mineral content of the body, and is found mainly in intracellular fluids (fluids inside cells). It has a multitude of functions: with sodium, it regulates sodium-potassium balance in the body and also stimulates kidney function; it maintains proper acid-alkaline balance; it stimulates insulin secretion; it helps to convert glucose to glycogen; it takes part in the transmission of nerve impulses, enabling muscle contraction to take place. A deficiency can be created by excessive vomiting or diarrhoea, or, more commonly, by using diuretics [20] – in such cases immediate potassium supplementation is necessary. Severe reducing diets (less than a 1,000 calories a day) also deplete potassium, and so do diets high in fat, salt and refined sugar. Patients with diabetes, high blood pressure or liver disease require additional potassium, which should be taken in the dosage and frequency recommended by their physicians.

BENEFICIAL EFFECTS
Promotes efficient disposal of body wastes; stimulates mental processes by increasing the supply of oxygen to brain; reduces blood pressure; helps diabetics by stimulating insulin secretion; stimulates stomach secretions through the vagus nerve (the cranial nerve which controls digestion).

DEFICIENCY SYMPTOMS
Oedema; hypertension; irregular heartbeat; nervousness and fatigue; arthritis.

BEST NATURAL SOURCES
Citrus fruits, green leafy vegetables, bananas, potatoes, tomatoes, pineapple.

DAILY DOSAGE

No RDA available. Normal average requirements are: adults 1,875–5,625 mg, children 550–1,650mg.

SODIUM (Na)

Most sodium is found in extracellular fluids, (the fluids which surround all body cells). With potassium, it maintains a pro-per acid-alkaline balance in the blood, and is highly important in maintaining osmotic pressure in tissues (osmotic pressure is created by the movement of fluids through cell membranes, from more concentrated to less concentrated solutions, enabling oxygen and digested nutrients to pass in and out of cells). With potassium, sodium also takes part in the transmission of nerve impulses.

The retention of sodium in the body is regulated by aldosterone, an adrenal hormone. People with Addison's disease, a condition of low aldosterone secretion, should be specially alert for sodium deficiency. Sodium tends to elevate blood pressure and constrict blood vessels, and should therefore be avoided by anyone who has hypertension or heart disease.

CAUTION: Excessive sodium can also cause oedema and hypertension. Anyone on a sodium-restricted diet should use salt substitutes based on potassium instead of sodium, or, even better, dried herb powders such as celery, allspice, basil, caraway, ginger, mustard, parsley, sesame, savory or tarragon.

BENEFICIAL EFFECTS

Stimulates the kidneys and keeps minerals soluble, preventing kidney stones; keeps calcium in solution and therefore assists efficient transmission of nerve impulses;[21] stimulates the secretion of gastric juices, helping digestion; promotes sweating, and therefore helps to prevent heat stroke; improves feelings of lassitude suffered by people with low blood pressure.

DEFICIENCY SYMPTOMS
Intestinal gas; weight loss; muscle wasting; fatigue; dehydration. NOTE: Deficiencies are very uncommon but can be caused by excessive perspiration.

BEST NATURAL SOURCES
Table salt, shellfish, kelp, meat, beets, carrots, chard and dandelion greens.

DAILY DOSAGE
No RDA available, however nutritionists estimate the following: adults 1,000 to 3,300 mg, children 325 to 975 mg. The Food and Nutrition Board of the National Research Council recommends no more than $1/2$ to 1 teaspoon of salt a day for adults, yet the average American consumes 2 to 2 $1/2$ teaspoons a day, which amounts to 4–5,000 mg of sodium, much more than the body needs. However, cutting out salt entirely does not necessarily solve the problem, since virtually all processed foods contain salt. If a reduction in salt intake is advised, a sodium counter should be used.
CAUTION: Excessive sodium intake should be balanced by increased potassium, since too much sodium causes loss of potassium in the urine.

MAGNESIUM (Mg)

Most of the body's magnesium is found in the bones, along with calcium and phosphorus. It is magnesium, not calcium, which helps to keep tooth enamel hard and resistant to decay. A smaller part of the body's magnesium is found in tissues and blood, where it plays an important role by activating many metabolic enzymes. Magnesium regulates heartbeat and muscle contraction, protects nerves, and helps the body to utilize vitamins E and C and convert glucose to energy. It also improves urine retention and keeps calcium soluble.

Magnesium is depleted by alcohol and excessive consumption of milk fortified with vitamin D; this is because synthetic vitamin D tends to bind magnesium and excrete it. People who eat white flour and white sugar products may have a magnesium deficiency because their bodies use stored magnesium to metabolize these refined carbohydrates. Magnesium and calcium are present in the body in a ratio of 1:2, so if consumption of calcium increases, so should magnesium consumption.

BENEFICIAL EFFECTS
Maintains strong bones and tooth enamel; calms the nervous system; regulates heartbeat; helps metabolism and weak digestion; maintains healthy prostate function in men;[22] improves urine retention and is therefore helpful for bed-wetting children; prevents kidney stones; regulates thyroid function.

DEFICIENCY SYMPTOMS
Irregular heartbeat and heart attacks; jumpy nerves and weak muscles; convulsions and seizures; prostate enlargement; fatigue; bed-wetting; kidney stones.

BEST NATURAL SOURCES
Figs, lemons, grapefruit, yellow corn, nuts, apples, raw wheat germ, green vegetables. Natural supplement: dolomite.

DAILY DOSAGE
Adults 350 mg, children 250 mg, pregnant and lactating women 450 mg. Magnesium deficiency can be a consequence of high alcohol consumption.

SULPHUR (S)

Known as the 'beauty mineral', sulphur is important for glossy, smooth hair, as well as healthy skin and nails. It is a non-metallic mineral, abundant in nature and present in every animal and plant cell.

Sulphur is important for the formation of collagen, the most abundant protein in our bodies. It also has a laxative effect because it absorbs water in the intestines (Epsom salts are, in fact, sulfate of magnesium).

Sulphur is linked with protein in the sulphur-containing amino acids cysteine, taurine and methionine. Cysteine, for example, is an important ingredient of reduced glutathione, an antioxidant enzyme which neutralizes dangerous peroxides and is therefore used in the treatment of auto-immune diseases such as arthritis. In fact, sulphur is an old-time remedy for arthritis and eggs, high in cysteine, are one of the best sources. Dr Carlton Fredericks has pointed out that children with rheumatic fever more often than not have a history of not eating eggs. In some cases, eggs have been more beneficial than penicillin in treating the disease.[23] Taurine, another sulphur-containing amino acid, is known to help control epileptic seizures by rectifying the unbalanced electrical activity of the brain.[24]

Recently a new form of organic sulphur, methylsulphonylmethane, or MSM, has become very popular in health food stores. MSM is a white, odourless powder which does not produce the intestinal gas or body odour that may occur with other forms of sulphur. MSM was found to be a safe, natural and highly assimilable nutrient.

BENEFICIAL EFFECTS
Helps the liver to secrete bile; improves mental functioning; maintains healthy hair and nails; prevents arthritis; treats skin conditions such as psoriasis, eczema and dermatitis when used in ointment form.

DEFICIENCY SYMPTOMS
Arthritis; dry hair, brittle nails and rough skin.

DAILY DOSAGE
No RDA available. Experienced nutritionists such as Dr Carlton Fredericks put daily requirements at 1 gram.

TRACE ELEMENTS

IRON (Fe)

Iron is the most abundant metallic trace element in the body. The average adult contains about 5 grams of iron, all of it combined with protein. Iron is absolutely indispensable to the formation of haemoglobin, the red pigment in red blood cells. It is this pigment which transports life-giving oxygen from the lungs to every cell in the body. Without iron, body cells, especially brain cells, starve to death from lack of oxygen. To be absorbed and utilized properly, iron needs copper, protein, calcium and vitamins B12, B6 and E.

A small daily loss of iron is normal and nothing to worry about as long as it is restored through a balanced diet. Men lose about 1 mg a day. Women, due to menstruation or pregnancy, lose more. During normal menstruation, women lose between 10 and 15 mg of iron, which is a large amount to compensate for. During pregnancy, 600 to 1,000 mg are lost, again creating a great deficiency unless counteracted by iron-rich foods and iron supplements. Today, iron supplementation is considered a must for pregnant women. It is estimated that one in two premenopausal women suffers from a degree of iron deficiency.

Babies are born with a store of 36 mg of iron. This is quickly spent because new cells are constantly being formed. Mother's milk is low in iron. Cow's milk is even lower. No wonder babies often develop anaemia toward the end of their first year, unless fed iron-enriched formulae. Children and adolescents can need extra iron for growth. Senior citizens may also need supplements due to inefficient absorption.

Iron absorption is problematic. Only about 8 per cent of naturally ingested iron is absorbed from the gut. It is therefore important to know that vitamin C, vitamin E and calcium help iron absorption when consumed simultaneously with foods containing iron. The most easily assimilated forms of iron are chelated organic iron supplements such as ferrous gluconate, but inorganic iron – ferrous sulphate, for example, which is included in certain multi-mineral supplements – actually destroys vitamin E. That is why inorganic iron should be taken 8 hours before or after vitamin E, never with it. Many health food shops now stock herb syrups which are naturally rich in iron (not fortified). Iron-fed yeast is also well absorbed.

Iron can be excessively accumulated by people who mistakenly equate 'anaemia' with 'iron deficiency anaemia'. Anemia is not always caused by iron deficiency, and anaemia due to other kinds of deficiency will not be solved by taking iron supplements. In fact, excess iron can have serious consequences, such as haemachromatosis or siderosis, liver damage and arthritis.[25] Before you start on an intensive course of iron supplementation, have your iron blood level measured.

BENEFICIAL EFFECTS
Relieves fatigue; prevents anaemia in women with heavy periods and in people suffering from internal bleeding (ulcers, colitis, haemorrhoids); promotes resistance to disease; aids growth.

DEFICIENCY SYMPTOMS
Iron-deficiency anaemia; pallor, weakness and shortness of breath; brittle nails.

BEST NATURAL SOURCES
Liver, kidneys, farina and oatmeal, raw clams and oysters, dried peaches, raisins, prunes, egg yolks, molasses, dried beans and green leafy vegetables.

DAILY DOSAGE
Men 10 mg, women 18 mg. Requirements increase during pregnancy, lactation, menstruation and haemorrhagic conditions.

ZINC (Zn)

Zinc is the most abundant trace element in the body next to iron; its weight in the body is estimated at about 1.8 grams. Zinc has numerous functions. It is found in at least 25 different enzymes and is an important constituent of insulin. It takes part in carbohydrate metabolism and in the breakdown of alcohol, and also in the synthesis of nucleic acids. It is vital to fertility and for the prevention of congenital birth defects, hence its importance during pregnancy. Zinc is necessary for proper growth and cooperates with vitamins B6, A and B12. It destroys toxic cadmium (found in cigarette smoke, for example) neutralizes excess copper, and is depleted by alcohol and perspiration.

Zinc is important to the function of the reproductive glands, especially the prostate in men, an important sex gland situated at the neck of the bladder. Human sperm and the prostate contain large amounts of zinc.[26] Various studies have confirmed the connection between adequate zinc levels and the health of the prostate. In one study, when the zinc level was reduced by 35 per cent, the prostate gland became enlarged, blocking the urethra and urine flow; with a 48 per cent zinc decrease, the prostate became inflamed (prostatitis); and with a 66 per cent decrease, prostate cancer was observed.[27]

Prostate trouble is very common in men over 45. In fact, it has been estimated that one out of every four men over the age of 55 suffers from a prostate condition. According to the statistics of the Metropolitan Life Insurance Company, some 20,000 men in the United States die every year of prostate difficulties.[28] Because of the delicacy of the problem, there has been a conspiracy of silence, with the result that the younger generation is largely unaware of possible prostate problems. This is a pity because the price of years of malnutrition is paid for with much suffering in later years. Smoking, coffee and alcohol,[29] all of which deplete zinc, are the main culprits.

BENEFICIAL EFFECTS
Zinc (with vitamin B6) lowers histamine production and is therefore very helpful in counteracting allergies. It is also beneficial in soothing nerves and depression, and even in

treating some types of schizophrenia.[30] Zinc also speeds up the healing of wounds and cures ulcers which arise as a side effect of cortisone treatment.[31] It stimulates growth, and plays a role in sexual maturation.

Zinc also helps diabetics because of its role in the formation of insulin; it also prolongs the effects of insulin. That is why zinc-rich brewer's yeast is used in the treatment of diabetes. Zinc neutralizes the bad effects of excess copper (one of the causes of arthritis) and the toxic effects of cadmium (a contributory factor in hypertension – smokers accumulate cadmium in their systems and are particularly vulnerable to hypertension). Zinc has also been shown to increase natural immunity against bacterial invasion,[32] and to promote skin health and alleviate psoriasis.[33] It can also help to reduce cholesterol levels.

DEFICIENCY SYMPTOMS
Prostate trouble; sterility, delayed sexual maturation, menstrual irregularities; retarded growth and dwarfism; birth defects such as mental retardation and slow learning;[34] susceptibility to infections and poor wound healing; joint pains; atherosclerosis and poor circulation; fatigue and lack of appetite; loss of sense of taste and smell;[35] susceptibility to diabetes; allergies; acne; stretch marks in pregnant women and obese individuals; depigmentation (white spots) of nails; offensive perspiration.

BEST NATURAL SOURCES
Raw oysters, meat, fish, raw wheat germ, mushrooms, brewer's yeast, pumpkin seeds, egg yolks, dried legumes, milk, ground mustard seeds

DAILY DOSAGE

Adults 15 mg, pregnant women 30 mg, lactating women 40 mg. Dr Schroeder recommends a daily intake of 200 mg during pregnancy.[36] Excessive sweating can cause a loss of 3 mg day.

COPPER (Cu)

Copper is an abundant trace element which helps in the absorption of iron; indirectly, therefore, it is responsible for the formation of haemoglobin. It takes part in many enzyme activities, in synthesizing phospholipids and utilizing vitamin C for example. It converts the amino acid tyrosine into a dark skin pigment which acts as a pigmentation factor for skin and hair, and reduces histamine levels, alleviating allergies.

Copper is an essential element, but needed in very small amounts. Accumulation of even small excesses can be damaging, causing disorders such as depression, arthritis, hypertension and heart attack.[37] Excesses are also suspected of causing one type of schizophrenia.[38] The most vulnerable people are those who drink water from copper pipes, smokers and city dwellers who inhale car exhaust fumes, and women who take contraceptive pills. Anyone who receives their water from copper pipes would do well to let the tap run for a minute or two, particularly in the morning, before using it. Zinc supplements can help to reduce high copper levels.

BENEFICIAL EFFECTS

Helps iron to form haemoglobin; prevents anaemia; lowers histamine level; helps to utilize vitamen C; convert tyrosine-to a skin and hair pigment.

DEFICIENCY SYMPTOMS
Anaemia; fatigue; shortness of breath; skin depigmentation.

BEST NATURAL SOURCES
Soybeans, legumes, whole wheat, prunes, liver, seafood, molasses.

DAILY DOSAGE
No RDA available, but a normal daily requirement for adults is considered to be 2mg.

MANGANESE (Mn)

Manganese is a trace element which takes part in the synthesis of cholesterol and fatty acids. It also activates many of the enzymes involved in carbohydrate metabolism. Manganese is important for the production of breast milk and sex hormones. It also helps to form thyroxine, the major hormone of the thyroid gland. With PABA (see p.71) it also stimulates the function of the pituitary gland. It forms part of the enzymes which manufacture acetylcholine, the neurotransmitter substance which is known to be deficient in muscle-nerve disorders such as myasthenia gravis. Manganese deficiency has also been found to lower glucose tolerance (the ability to remove excess glucose from the blood) and impair insulin secretion, promoting a diabetes-like condition.[39] A high intake of calcium and phosphorus increases the need for manganese.

BENEFICIAL EFFECTS
Has been found to help prevent diabetes; prevents muscle-nerve disorders and promotes muscle strength; promotes fer-

tility and male potency; stimulates production of breast milk.

DEFICIENCY SYMPTOMS
Low tolerance of carbohydrates; skeletal abnormalities (legs too short or too long in proportion to overall body length);[40] loss of muscle condition; convulsions.

BEST NATURAL SOURCES
Nuts, whole grains, green leafy vegetables, peas, cloves, ginger and tea leaves. In tea-drinking countries, a third of the daily manganese requirement comes from tea.[41]

DAILY DOSAGE
No official RDA has been set, but the estimated daily requirement is 2.5 to 5 mg. Lactating women may need more, up to 9 mg.

CHROMIUM (Cr)

Chromium is an essential micronutrient, which is mostly removed from common foods like sugar and flour by refining. It is involved principally in the metabolism of glucose and in the synthesis of fatty acids and cholesterol. Chromium-rich diets are a *must* for diabetics, hypoglycaemics and for anyone who has a high cholesterol level or hypertension.

Chromium was recently discovered to be the central component of the glucose tolerance factor (GTF), essential in carbohydrate metabolism because it enhances the function of insulin. It was found that chromium only binds with insulin if it is in the form of GTF. Normally, a healthy body produces its own GTF, from chromium, niacin (vitamin B3) and certain amino acids.

However, there are many people with a diminished ability to synthesize GTF who should supplement their diet with GTF instead of regular chromium. They will benefit from increased energy, improved mental function, better glycogen storage, reduced blood fats, and increased immune response.

The main causes of chromium deficiency are the overuse of refined sugar and flour products and depleted agricultural soils. Whole wheat, for example, contains an average of 175 micrograms of chromium per 100 grams while white flour contains only 23 micrograms.[42] Refining raw cane sugar into white sugar removes 93 per cent of its chromium.[43] If the use of white sugar and flour have long been a way of life, then Dr Schroeder's claim that chromium deficiency increases with age is hardly surprising. By middle age, accumulated deficiencies are severe enough to promote adult-onset diabetes, hypoglycaemia or heart attacks. What is more, only 3 per cent of the chromium in food is absorbed and absorption decreases with age.

Chromium on its own (as well as other minerals like zinc, iron and magnesium) is poorly absorbed into the cells. The cell membranes block the penetration of minerals because minerals have an electric charge (electric ion) that cannot be carried into the cells. To overcome that, minerals have to be chelated. The word 'chelate' comes from Greek, meaning 'claw'. That is, minerals have to be held by another chemical which neutralizes the mineral's ion. The mineral has then no charge, and can easily cross the cell membrane into the cell.

Picolinic acid was found to be the best natural chelator. It is produced by the body as the amino acid tryptophan is broken down to niacin (vitamin B3). And chromium picolinate, with its much better absorption in the body, or higher bioavailability, was   reported to lower glucose levels in diabetics, reduce cholesterol levels, and to speed up the development of muscles in athletes.[44]

Various studies confirmed the ability of chromium picolinate to help lose weight.[45] The results suggested that chromium picolinate on its own, even without exercise, could increase fat loss. And indeed in 1991, several new studies actually supported this suggestion that chromium picolinate does reduce body fat and builds muscle without additional dieting or increased exercise.[46] It was found to do it in two ways:

  a) by increasing the metabolic rate, i.e., increasing the rate by which fat is burned.[47]

  b) by helping the entrance of tryptophan into the cells.

Tryptophan increases production of serotonin, a calming neurotransmitter (nerve cell messenger), which is used by the appetite control centre to send a message of satiety.[48] This is a pleasant feeling of being well-fed. And the sooner the feeling of fullness the sooner one stops eating.

No wonder that chromium picolinate is now the chromium of choice in the health food market. As such it is also incorporated in many dieting formulas.

BENEFICIAL EFFECTS
Helps to metabolize sugar; regulates blood sugar level; prevents adult-onset diabetes and hypoglycaemia; may help to reverse atherosclerosis;[49] helps to lower high blood pressure and reduce weight.

DEFICIENCY SYMPTOMS
Fatigue; slow growth; obesity; hypertension; high cholesterol levels; impaired glucose metabolism.

BEST NATURAL SOURCES

Brewer's yeast (not Torula yeast, which is low in chromium), molasses, raw wheat germ, rice bran (husks), meat, shellfish and clams.

DAILY DOSAGE

No RDA available. Estimated daily requirements are: adults 50-200 mcg, children 20-80 mcg. Pregnant women are advised to take 1,500 mcg a day.[50] Chromium-GTF tablets are particularly recommended.

IODINE (I)

Iodine, in its iodide or salt form, is concentrated in the thyroid gland and is a constituent of the hormone thyroxine. As with all essential trace elements, a tiny amount has an enormous effect. The 25 mg in the average human body makes the difference between health and disease.

The influence of iodine, via thyroxine, is felt everywhere in the body. It raises the rate of metabolism, helping the body to burn excess fat and preventing the accumulation of cholesterol. Iodine calms nerves and improves the quality of hair, nails, skin and teeth. It also helps to convert carotene into vitamin A and aids the synthesis of cholesterol.

Iodine regulates the rate at which the body cells use oxygen, promoting growth and energy, and improving mental functions. It does this by stimulating the thyroid gland to produce thyroxine. There is a simple method of checking whether your thyroid is underactive. Upon awakening, place a thermometer in the armpit and keep it there for 10 minutes. A temperature of less than 97.8°F (36.7°C) indicates an underactive thyroid and a possible need for extra iodine.

People who constantly feel cold due to an underactive thyroid can also be helped by iodine supplementation. However, if low thyroid function is suspected, a doctor should be consulted first.

Raw vegetables of the *Brassica* family (broccoli, brussels sprouts, cabbage, kale) and also mustard seed oil contain factors which prevent uptake of iodine by the thyroid,[51] so should be avoided if thyroid function is low or if iodine is being supplemented. Peanuts, soy flour and foods rich in carotene are also claimed to inhibit iodine absorption. Produce grown on low-iodine soils is naturally poor in iodine. People living in such areas should use iodized salt or take kelp, other seaweeds or desiccated thyroid tablets.

BENEFICIAL EFFECTS
Reduces body fats and aids weight loss; calms nervousness; increases energy; promotes healthy skin and hair; reduces incidence of tooth cavities; increases resistance to colds.

DEFICIENCY SYMPTOMS
Deficiency of iodine results in goitre, characterized by swelling of the thyroid gland in the lower neck, and in hypothyroidism, decreased secretion of thyroid hormones. Symptoms of hypothyroidism include obesity, dry hair, rapid pulse, heart palpitations, a cold body, constipation, weakness, excessive menstruation, low resistance to colds and infections, nervousness and irritability.

BEST NATURAL SOURCES
Kelp, seaweeds, shellfish, onions. Supplements: iodized salt and desiccated thyroid tablets.

DAILY DOSAGE
Adults 150 mcg, children 120 mcg.

SELENIUM (Se)

Selenium is a trace element that works best in the presence of vitamin E. Like vitamin E, selenium is an antioxidant which protects the body from premature aging and keeps tissues youthfully elastic.

Studied intensively in recent years, selenium has been found to be needed by the body to form glutathione peroxidase, an important antioxidant and anti-aging enzyme which protects the body from the oxidative damage wrought by superoxides and hydrogen peroxide.[52] With vitamin E, selenium is reported to minimize the effects of lead,[53] cadmium[54] and mercury.[55] In fact, when mercury is present in sea water, tuna fish accumulate additional selenium in their bodies.[56] Selenium reduces the risk of cancer,[57] builds a healthy heart and can reduce some of the effects of arthritis[58] and cystic fibrosis.[59] Selenium is concentrated in the male sex glands and is lost in ejaculated semen. An ample supply can promote sexual function.

Selenium deficiency is known to be a factor in premature aging, heart attacks and cancer. In fact, the U.S. National Cancer Institute is now recommending a daily dose of 200 mcg as a prophylactic against cancer. According to certain epidemiological studies, it is estimated that if people took this much selenium daily, the incidence of cancer might eventually decrease by up to 70 per cent![60]

The availability of selenium from food is problematic as plants do not require selenium for growth. Wheat grown in selenium-rich soils can contain up to 100 parts per million (ppm) of selenium, while wheat grown in selenium-deficient soils may contain less than 0.1 ppm.[61] If you rely on plant foods grown in soil which has a low selenium or a high sulphur content (sulphur inhibits selenium), you run a risk of selenium deficiency, unless you supplement your diet. A deficiency of selenium can be partly relieved by vitamin E.[62]

BENEFICIAL EFFECTS
Increases immunity to diseases; slows down aging; alleviates menopausal discomfort; promotes energy and sexual potency; prevents auto-immune diseases such as rheumatoid arthritis and multiple sclerosis; prevents degenerative diseases such as atherosclerosis and cancer.

DEFICIENCY SYMPTOMS
Fatigue; susceptibility to infections and diseases; premature aging; predisposition to cancer; low sexual potency.

BEST NATURAL SOURCES
Raw wheat germ, tuna, onions, nuts and seeds, brewer's yeast (especially selenium-fed yeast).

DAILY DOSAGE
No RDA available. Average estimated requirements are: adults 50 to 200 mcg, children 50 to 80 mcg.

FLUORINE (Fl)

Fluorine is a non-metallic essential trace element which is concentrated in bones and teeth. It occurs as calcium fluoride in its natural form, and as sodium fluoride (used for fluoridating drinking water).

Fluorine is necessary for the formation of strong, hard bones and teeth. It increases resistance to tooth decay and bone fractures. Studies have shown that fluorine combines with the inorganic component of teeth (apatite) and converts it to a harder substance (fluoroapatite). Fluorine is also reported to reduce mouth acids which prosper in the presence of sugar and form dental plaque. It therefore helps to prevent tooth decay. In fact, fluorine deficiency is considered by some doctors to account for a large part of the tooth decay that plagues our population, and for the large number of fractured hips in older people.[63]

Although small amounts of fluorine are important to the body, even slight excesses can be harmful. Fluorine excess can destroy alkaline phosphatase, an enzyme which is believed to promote deposition of calcium salts in bones and teeth.[64] Excess fluorine can also neutralize other enzymes, mottle teeth and damage the brain.

Fluoridation of toothpaste and drinking water has had its enthusiastic proponents and opponents. Technically, it is difficult to keep the accepted concentration level of 1 part per million (ppm) in the water supply constant. This is very important, since concentrations over 2 ppm convert fluorine from friend to foe.

Recently, opponents of fluoridation have been on the increase. It has been found that, in the long run, fluorine protection for teeth is counteracted by excessive consumption of sweets. While fluorine guards against tooth decay, sugar destroys teeth.[65] Moreover, children using fluoridated toothpaste may ingest excessive fluorine because of insufficient rinsing.

One of fluorine's disadvantages is that it prevents the absorption of calcium. Overdoses can therefore deplete calcium and cause soft or porous bones, leg cramps and nervousness. In fact, excess fluorine has definitely been shown to cause brittle bones and fractures in some elderly people.[66] In this sense, calcium is an antidote for fluorine poisoning. It has also been suggested that there may be a direct relationship between the incidence of Down's syndrome and fluoridated drinking water.[67]

BENEFICIAL EFFECTS
Promotes formation of strong teeth and bones; helps to prevent tooth decay; prevents brittle bones in the elderly.
DEFICIENCY SYMPTOMS
Poor tooth development in children; tooth decay.

BEST NATURAL SOURCES
Kelp and seafoods, fluoridated drinking water, tea.

DAILY DOSAGE
No RDA available. Estimated adequate daily intakes are: adults 1.5-4mg, children 1.5-2.mg.
CAUTION: 20 mg and over are toxic.

SILICA (Si)

Silicon is the most abundant element in the earth's crust as a constituent of sand and rocks. Yet, it is present in the body only in trace amounts, no more than 15 micrograms per 100 ml of body fluid. Silicone oxidizes easily to form silica (silicon dioxide). Quartz crystals are pure silica.

Silica has been touted in the last decade as beneficial for hair, skin and nails. As such, it is incorporated in many nutritional formulas. No wonder it was dubbed 'the beauty mineral'. Biochemically, silicates have a diversified activity, since they can combine with other elements.

Silica appears in three forms in the body: protein-bound silica, fat-bound silica and water-soluble silica. In spite of its small total amount in the body, silica is present in almost every tissue and is essential for cell growth. Rich concentrations of silica are stored in the hair, nails and connective tissues. It helps store moisture in connective tissues like skin, keeping it smooth and supple. Silicone levels can be measured by hair tests. Silica gel can be used either orally or externally.

A distinction should be made between water-soluble silica and the controversial silicone breast implants. Natural silicone differs from breast implant silicone despite the similarity in the name. Silicone is an industrial polymer which contains a controversial hydrocarbon which is suspected of being carcinogenic.

BENEFICIAL EFFECTS

Silica gel as a mouth rinse is claimed to harden tooth enamel and prevent cavities. It also helps other mouth conditions such as bleeding or inflamed gums (gingivitis). Silicon helps strengthen bones and maintain bone density by assisting the process of bone mineralization. Silica has a definite beneficial effect on hair, skin and nails. It has been reported to halt hair greying; to add elasticity to skin and prevent wrinkles; and to beautify cracked, brittle nails. Indeed, several types of cosmetic silica creams, lotions and gels are marketed for these purposes.

In test cases with patients, reported in Dr Klaus Kaufman's book, *Silica the Amazing Gel,* silica was found to be beneficial in treating many and varied disorders such as: heartburn, ulcers, gastritis, varicose veins, colitis, bronchitis, arteriosclerosis, gum recession, allergic rashes and more.

DEFICIENCY SYMPTOMS
Demineralization of bones and teeth; wrinkled skin; lowered resistance to colds and infections; low energy levels.

BEST NATURAL SOURCES
Horsetail herb, oats, millet, barley, onions, whole wheat, red beet.

DAILY DOSAGE
No RDA available. Silica is included in many nutritional formulas. It is also sold on its own, as effervescent tablets, chewable tablets, capsules, powders and silica gel. The labels of the various products contain directions for use which must be adhered to.

MOLYBDENUM (Mo)

Molybdenum is a trace element widely distributed in raw foods and an essential part of several important enzymes. One such enzyme, xanthine oxidase, forms uric acid (by oxidizing RNA), stimulates the production of superoxides and hydrogen peroxide and is also involved in mobilizing iron from the liver. Another molybdenum-containing enzyme, aldehyde oxidase, oxidizes fats.

Like fluorine, molybdenum prevents tooth decay. It is also thought to prevent oesophageal cancer [68] and increase sexual potency in older men.

Molybdenum is mostly removed in the course of milling whole grains and refining raw cane sugar. As a result, the waste products of these milling and refining processes – bran, wheat germ, molasses – are a rich source. As with all essential trace elements, the best way to ensure an adequate intake of molybdenum is to see that whole, unrefined foods make up the major part of the diet. Excessive sweating depletes molybdenum. Toxicity resulting from excess molybdenum intake is unusual.

BENEFICIAL EFFECTS
Prevents tooth decay and aneamia.

DEFICIENCY SYMPTOMS
Predisposition to tooth decay; anaemia; oesophageal cancer; lowered sexual potency (men).

BEST NATURAL SOURCES
Legumes, whole grain cereals, dark green leafy vegetables.

DAILY DOSAGE
No RDA available. Estimated adequate daily intakes are: adults 150–6,500 mcg, children 60–150 mcg. A balanced diet usually supplies adequate amounts of molybdenum.

GERMANIUM (Ge)

Germanium is the most scientifically acclaimed trace element of recent times. It has been extensively studied medically, nutritionally and holistically during the last decade, and not without reason. It has been found to be non-toxic, immunity-enhancing, oxygen-enriching, radiation-protecting, detoxifying and potently analgesic. And these are but a few of its attributes.

Germanium was discovered by German scientist Clemens Winkler, who accidentally isolated it from a silver ore. It is a semi-metal and a semi-conductor, and was once widely used by the electronics industry to produce transistors before silicone technology developed.

In nutrition, only organic germanium (such as Ge-132) is used. This was first synthesized from the inorganic form in 1967 by the Japanese scientist Dr Kazuhiko Asai. Dr Asai now runs the Asai Germanium Clinic in Japan, in which germanium is used to treat people for a multitude of diseases.

The metabolic functions of germanium are not understood in detail yet, and there is still controversy as to whether it is essential to human nutrition. Much research is still needed, but it can be safely said, on the basis of the exciting effects discovered so far, that germanium is a small trace element with a great future.

BENEFICIAL EFFECTS

Because germanium is a semi-conductor, it enables plants to convert sunlight into tiny electrical currents, which in turn split water into oxygen and hydrogen. Oxygen is vital to life. Cells deprived of oxygen cannot perform their metabolic functions. So some of the beneficial effects of germanium are attributed to its ability to enrich the body's oxygen supply.[69] Organic germanium lowers the oxygen requirements of body organs, and protects them against oxygen-deficiency conditions such as carbon monoxide poisoning, the type of poisoning we are all exposed to in car exhaust fumes and cigarette smoke.

Oxygen, however, has its destructive side. When uncontrolled oxygenation takes place during certain metabolic processes, or due to radiation, extremely reactive superoxide particles called free radicals are formed. These are thought to be the primary cause of aging (see Chapter 15). The body therefore needs antioxidants, the most potent of which are vitamin E, vitamin C and germanium.[70] Germanium protects the body from many degenerative diseases, including cancer, leukaemia, asthma, diabetes, senility, digestive disorders, cardiac disorders such as angina, arteriosclerosis and hypertension, Parkinson's disease, epilepsy and eye diseases such as glaucoma and cataract.

GERMANIUM AND THE IMMUNE SYSTEM

Interferon is a potent antiviral substance produced, like antibodies, by immune cells. The more interferon there is in the body, the greater the resistance to viral diseases, including cancer. Germanium has been found to be an efficient booster of interferon production in the body.[71] It also activates macrophages, the large immune cells that destroy and engulf cancer cells,[72] stimulates production of T-suppressor cells which monitor antibodies,[73] and increases general immunity to disease.[74]

GERMANIUM AND CANCER

Organic germanium has been extensively studied for its effect on various types of cancer.[75] Germanium (type Ge-132) has improved cases of lung cancer.[76] It has also proved effective against ovarian malignancies.[77] In a clinical experiment with 17 patients afflicted with Hodgkin's disease (a disease in which the lymph glands and spleen become enlarged), germanium caused remission in five patients, two of whom were completely cured.[78] In the first international conference on germanium, which took place in Hanover, Germany, in October 1984, reports were submitted on the beneficial effects of germanium on colon cancer and other types of cancer. The reason for germanium's effects on cancer is thought to be its oxygen-enriching property, since cancer cells grow in the absence of oxygen.

GERMANIUM AND ARTHRITIS

Arthritis is a common debilitating disease. Medicine cannot actually cope with it. Now that the severe side effects of steroids are known, cortisone is no longer a miracle cure. Rheumatoid arthritis is sometimes referred to as an 'auto-immune disease' because some forms of it are the result of a faulty immune response. In such cases, due to a shortage of T-suppressor cells, antibodies cannot distinguish between friend and foe and therefore attack joint tissues as if they were foreign. The membranes around the joints become painful, swollen and inflamed, resulting in degeneration of cartilage, bones and ligaments. Studies conducted by Smith and Kline Laboratories have shown that germanium has anti-arthritic properties.[79] Its ability to promote the manufacture of T-suppressor cells is considered to be the reason.[80] This very same ability can also improve other auto-immune diseases such as multiple sclerosis. Germanium may also have a role in fighting AIDS, which is associated with HIV (Human Immunodeficiency Virus).[81]

DEFICIENCY SYMPTOMS

Increased susceptibility to the degenerative diseases associated with aging.

BEST NATURAL SOURCES

Trace amounts of germanium are present in most foods,[82] but richer amounts are found in ginseng, garlic, aloe vera and comfrey,[83] which may partially explain the great health-promoting effects of these foods. The amount of germanium in plants varies, depending on the soils they grow in. No official RDA has been established yet. Average daily intake varies greatly according to diet. The estimated intake of ovo-vegetarians (vegetarians who eat eggs) is over 3 mg, while high protein diets provide a daily average of only 0.8 mg.

Although germanium is a ubiquitous element, present in tiny amounts in many foods (usually in parts per million), it is impossible to derive a therapeutic dose from a normal diet, so supplementation is necessary. Germanium is non-toxic and is now sold as a supplement.

BORON (B)

Boron has been an overlooked element since the early 1900s. It was generally accepted as being essential for plants, but not for animals. However, since 1981, mounting evidence indicates that boron is also essential for humans.

Boron, a non-metal element, is very biologically active, and can easily interact with other compounds and vitamins. In 1981, it was reported that boron deficiency can depress growth in vitamin D deficient animals,[84] and that its beneficial action is increased by interacting with other elements in the body such as, calcium, magnesium, potassium, vitamin D and methionine.

In a 1987 study, a daily dose of 3 mg boron given to women reduced losses of calcium and magnesium. Boron also managed to elevate blood levels of estradiol, the most active type of oestrogen.[85] This has a special meaning to post-menopausal women: since lower estrogen levels in menopause reduces calcium absorption, increased estradiol in menopause, improves calcium absorption. This also means, that boron may be an important factor in the prevention of osteoporosis.

Boron supplementation was also effective in alleviating

symptoms of arthritis, including rheumatoid arthritis.[86] It was especially effective with cases of juvenile arthritis. Patients took a daily dose of 6-9 mg boron to achieve symptom relief followed by maintenance dose of 3 mg a day.[87]

BENEFICAL EFFECTS
Promotes absorption of calcium, magnesium; elevates estradiol levels in post-menopausal woman; helps prevent osteoporosis; alleviates arthritis. Stimulates growth.

DEFICIENCY SYMPTOMS
Calcium loss and bone demineralization; arthritis; low oestrogen levels in menopause; reduced growth.

BEST NATURAL SOURCES
Fruits, vegetables and nutritional supplements.

DAILY DOSAGE
No RDA available. Estimated daily intake is between 0.25 mg and 3 mg.

TOXIC ELEMENTS

The modern world is increasingly contaminated by toxic trace elements in the air, in food and in the water supply, and there is no longer any doubt whatsoever that such contaminants gradually accumulate in the body and produce mild to severe cases of poisoning – from headaches, nervousness and exhaustion to brain damage, cancer and heart attacks.

Intelligent nutrition is one way of minimizing the insidious and harmful effects of environmental pollutants. Certain minerals and vitamins have the ability to neutralize or inhibit absorption of known pollutants. Up to now, some sixteen toxic elements in our environment have been identified, of which lead, cadmium and mercury are the most prevalent. These three are cumulative and contribute in a major way to disorders often attributed to age rather than slow poisoning, that is to high blood pressure, arteriosclerosis and senility.

LEAD (Pb)

Lead is a highly toxic element, even in amounts of less than 1 mg a day. In larger amounts it can be fatal. Dr H. Schroeder, in his excellent book *The Poisons Around Us*, states that the inhabitants of industrialized countries are accumulating more lead daily (mostly in their bones) than they can excrete. He also claims that lead represents a far greater threat to human health than nuclear reactors.

The main sources of lead in the environment are: lead emission in car exhausts (the average car burning leaded gasoline emits 4 pounds of lead annually); industrial emissions; and cigarette smoke (1 mcg of lead per cigarette). Locally, lead poisoning can be caused by drinking from glazed pottery or from lead water pipes, ingestion of lead paint peelings by children or consumption of certain processed organ meats.[88] However, inhaled lead is much more dangerous than ingested lead. Forty per cent of inhaled lead is absorbed compared with only 5 per cent of ingested lead.[89]

Lead primarily attacks the brain and nervous system, causing symptoms such as feeling run-down, nervousness, depression, apathy, hyperactivity in children,[90] and also mental retardation.[91] In Dr Carl Pfeiffer's opinion, lead is such an important cause of hyperactivity that tests should be run on all children diagnosed as hyperactive in order to determine their lead level. Lead also weakens the immune system, causing frequent colds and infections. Higher levels of lead poisoning can cause sterility, damage to the kidneys and liver, hypertension, paralysis and even death. Lead neutralizes essential minerals such as iron, zinc and copper, so that even if these are taken in adequate amounts, the body does not get the benefit of them. Those most at risk of lead poisoning are smelters and garage workers, painters, plasterers and solderers, typesetters and printers, and people who work in battery-making plants.

Cases of lead poisoning have been found to respond to penicillamine, a chelating agent which binds with lead, increasing its elimination in the urine.[92]

NUTRITIONAL PROTECTION

Adequate dietary calcium prevents the accumulation of lead in the body.[93] Good calcium sources are bonemeal, dolomite, calcium lactate and oyster shell calcium tablets, milk and dairy products, and sesame paste. Vitamin C neutralizes lead. Take tablets of vitamin C, rosehips, or acerola, and eat a diet rich in fresh fruits and vegetables. Vitamin A activates the enzymes which prevent lead absorption. Fish liver oil capsules are convenient. Lecithin neutralizes poisons and protects the fatty sheath surrounding nerves. Take 1 to 3 teaspoons of pure lecithin granules daily. Kelp contains sodium alginate, which combines with lead so that it can be excreted through the bowels.[94] Take kelp tablets or sprinkle kelp powder on salads and stews. Use dried seaweeds in cooking, or add powdered algin, derived from kelp, to food and drinks.

MERCURY (Hg)

Mercury is about five times more toxic than lead.[95] Its main sources are fish, pesticides, fungistats (which prevent mould in seeds) and emissions from coal burning. Mercury accumulates in fish, so larger, older fish have a higher concentration than smaller, younger ones. That is why a large tuna can be many times more toxic than a sardine. The mercury which pollutes lakes and oceans is in the form of methyl mercury, a compound fifty times more toxic than pure mercury. Fish can become a highly concentrated source of mercury even if concentrations in sea or fresh water are comparatively low. Methyl mercury is dumped into rivers and lakes by industrial plants, especially chlorine plants, which use mercury for electrodes; by paper-making plants, which use mercury to protect paper from mould; and by plastics factories. Irreversible pollution has occurred in Lake Erie, where mercury levels are so high that fishing has been prohibited.

Mercury is more readily excreted than lead and lower amounts accumulate in the body. However, it is capable of causing damage to the brain and nervous system (paralysis and blindness, for example) and to the kidneys. The commonest sources of mercury are batteries, mercury vapour lamps, dental fillings, and mercury thermometers (if a thermometer breaks in the mouth, some of the mercury in it is almost certain to be ingested). According to Dr Pfeiffer, mercury poisoning should be treated promptly with penicillamine.

NUTRITIONAL PROTECTION
Selenium, an element which counteracts mercury, is available in tablets or from selenium-grown yeast. Other sources of

protection are calcium, vitamins A, C, E and B complex, stomach acid in the form of betaine HCL tablets, and lecithin.

CADMIUM (Cd)

Cadmium is an environmental pollutant that occurs naturally in zinc ores. It is a highly toxic metal – 1/2 to 1 ppm in water is thought to be toxic to most organisms. It accumulates in the body, mostly as the result of inhaling contaminated air.

Cadmium is present in car exhaust fumes because it is added to gasoline and engine oils. It is contained in phosphate fertilizers, through which it contaminates vegetation. Drinking water passing through old galvanized pipes may be high in cadmium. This is because the zinc that used to be used for galvanizing was poorly refined and contained many impurities, including cadmium. As a precaution, many nutritionists advise against drinking the first water that flows from a tap. It is better to let the water run a little first.

Cadmium is also found in cigarette smoke. A 20-pack of cigarettes contains 20 micrograms of cadmium, half of which are absorbed during smoking.[96] Nickel-cadmium battery plants are well-known sources of pollution, as are incinerators of discarded cars and zinc or copper smelting plants. Every year more than 2 million pounds of cadmium are released into the air from smelting plants alone.

Recently, cadmium has been used more often than zinc for metal-plating. Another source of slow cadmium poisoning is therefore enamelled kitchen utensils. Cadmium is used to paint enamel, just as lead is used to glaze pottery and ceramics.

Cadmium is deposited in the kidneys and arteries. It neutralizes antioxidant nutrients such as zinc and vitamin C, and is known to cause high blood pressure, atherosclerosis, cerebral haemorrhage, strokes and heart attacks. Emphysema is a nasty lung disease prevalent in long-time smokers. It is characterized by a loss of elasticity in the lung tissues, labored breathing and high blood pressure. Emphysema patients have been found to have more cadmium in their kidneys and liver than healthy people.[97] Since cigarette smoke contains cadmium, cadmium in cigarettes may be one of the causes of emphysema – another reason to quit smoking.

NUTRITIONAL PROTECTION
Vitamin C is effective in high doses of several grams a day. Zinc, which replaces cadmium in body tissues, is available from zinc-grown brewer's yeast or from chelated zinc tablets. Foods containing refined white flour should be avoided as they can increase zinc deficiencies. During flour milling, the wheat germ which contains the zinc is removed.

CHAPTER 5

SPECIAL HEALTH FOODS AND NUTRIENTS

Exactly what is meant by the term 'health foods'? Natural foods, much richer in specific nutrients than ordinary foods. A health food is a natural food which has been grown organically and prepared as simply as possible, without destructive processing or chemical additives. A food which has been grown and treated in this way contains nutrients in their natural proportions. It therefore stands the best possible chance of being absorbed and used by the body. This is why relatively small amounts of health foods go a long way towards supplying daily nutritional requirements and remedying deficiencies.

A distinction should be made between health foods and functional foods, which have recently been promoted as super foods by interested commercial companies. Functional foods are normal mass market foods to which nutrients have been added. This can enable manufacturers to make health claims on the labels. But these are ambiguous health claims, because many functional foods are high in fat, sugar or salt which counteract the other nutritional claims. There are many examples: a malted drink powder, which is nearly two thirds sugar, claiming to 'protect the body from some of the harmful effects of today's stressful lifestyles, because of its added vitamins,' disregards that sugar itself is a stress-inducing food; margarine with added omega-3 recommends itself 'for healthy hearts and minds' while it is 60 per cent fat, of which 28 per cent are saturated, definitely not the healthy type. Fibre in itself is not so palatable when eaten in large quantities. But fibre-rich cereals which are very common and tastier, and can cause more harm than good if eaten in excess. Dietary fibre is high in phytates, which inhibit the absorption of key minerals like calcium, iron and zinc. Several lavish serving-sizes a day, over a period of time, can cause a deficiency in these important minerals.

Functional foods are definitely convenience foods, which can mislead the unsuspecting health-seeking consumer. They are clearly no substitute for a natural diet supplemented with health foods and nutrients. The whole issue is still controversial and pending legislation.

In this chapter we will make the acquaintance of the commonest health foods. They are all available in health food stores and they work wonders for some people. Health foods are best bought from reputable companies, companies who have a reputation to lose. Better products cost more, but they will almost certainly be more effective. Always read the labels carefully, especially the information about ingredients and potencies. NOTE: Some preparations contain allergy-causing substances, included as fillers or binders.

MOLASSES

Molasses is a concentrated syrup, a by-product of cane sugar refining. After harvesting, the sugar cane is shredded, then the juice is squeezed out of it and boiled and thickened by evaporation. Tiny sugar crystals start to appear, which are later separated, by centrifuge machines, from the residual 'mother' syrup. This process is repeated until most of the crystals are extracted from the syrup. The residue is molasses, rich in nutrients and low in sucrose compared with ordinary sugar. In fact, those nutrients which are unharmed by heat are thirty times more concentrated in molasses than in the original cane juice.

Average molasses composition[1]	Per cent
Sucrose	33.5
Levulose and dextrose	17.5
Ash	9.0
Water	22.5
Organic matter	17.5

The table above shows that molasses is a fine source of natural sugars, only a third of which is sucrose. The 'ash' in molasses represents an abundance of minerals and trace elements, including iron, calcium, potassium, magnesium, copper, chromium, manganese, molybdenum and zinc.[2] Refined sugar contains none of these. In fact, one tablespoon of molasses supplies as much calcium as a glass of milk and as much iron as nine eggs! The 'organic matter' contains high levels of B vitamins. Moreover, molasses is an alkali-forming food, beneficial for maintaining a proper acid-alkaline balance in the body.[3] Molasses is one of the two natural foods which contain a special ingredient (wulzen factor) that has been shown to prevent and cure wrist-stiffness, muscular dystrophy and arthritis.[4] The other food is fresh unpasteurized cream. If nutritionists had their way, a jar of molasses would stand on every table, to be used regularly as a spread or sweetener.

The composition of molasses depends on the soil where the sugar cane was grown and on the milling processes used. However, it is generally accepted that molasses derived from sugar cane grown in the West Indies is the richest in iron and minerals, which is why it is the most sought after. From a nutritional point of view, crude or black-strap molasses, which is only mildly sweet, is preferable to sweeter varieties. Also, many types of molasses are preserved with sulphur and should be avoided. Insist on unsulphured molasses. High doses of sulphur can be toxic and will also undermine the nutritional value of molasses.

EFFECTS

In recent decades, testimonials have accumulated as to the beneficial, even miraculous effects of molasses on various disorders. In his book about molasses the British nutritionist Cyril Scott describes his own and other healers' successes in treating anaemia, rheumatism, arthritis, ulcers, colitis, varicose veins and benign tumours with molasses. Gayelord Hauser, the well-known nutritionist and author, particularly praises molasses as a natural laxative.[5] Scott testifies to the success of molasses in reversing hair greying and even in the external treatment of wounds. Molasses is high in iron and is therefore recommended to pregnant and lactating women.

The greatest advantage of molasses is its ability to conveniently supplement the diet of the busy twentieth-century citizen with easily assimilated natural nutrients. However, its effects are slow and cumulative, and it must be used regularly. It should also be understood that, in spite of its many testimonials, molasses is not an all-purpose cure.

USAGE

Molasses can be eaten right from the jar – 1 to 3 teaspoons a day is normally sufficient (half this quantity for children) – but it is more palatable stirred into a glass of water. Molasses should not be over-used because of is laxative effect. A delicious spread can be made from equal parts of molasses and honey (or maple syrup). Naturally, molasses can also be used in cakes, pies and cookies to improve their nutritional value. People who suffer from constipation should take 1 or 2 teaspoons at bedtime. NOTE: Like sugar, molasses can cause tooth decay, so either clean your teeth afterwards or at least rinse your mouth thoroughly, especially if you take it straight from a spoon. For convenience, molasses is also available in capsules.

CAUTION: Diabetics must not use molasses.

CIDER VINEGAR

Genuine cider vinegar is made by fermenting the juice of whole, fresh apples. Its beneficial effects come from the high mineral content of apples. Cider vinegar is considered to be both a food and a medicine, and is used by naturopaths as well as chefs.

The active factor in cider vinegar is in fact a combination

of minerals, organic matter and acetic acid, the latter giving it its characteristic taste and smell. Cider vinegar has an average acetic acid content of 5 per cent, and is high in minerals and low in natural sugars and vitamins. It is unusually high in potassium, calcium, phosphorus, sodium and trace elements. Dr D. C. Jarvis of Vermont claims that cider vinegar's ability to associate its potassium with other minerals is one reason for its versatile remedial effects.[6]

EFFECTS

Observations and case histories collected from medicine by Dr Jarvis and by the British nutritionist and author Maurice Hanssen, demonstrate cider vinegar's varied beneficial effects.[7] It has an astringent property which helps to inhibit diarrhoea. It increases blood oxygenation, improves metabolism, strengthens digestion, prevents tooth decay, acts as an antiseptic against intestinal parasites, and strengthens heart function. It can also be used to improve digestion in people who lack stomach acid. In such cases 1 to 2 teaspoons should be taken in a glass of water before main meals.

Cider vinegar is not a drug, so it can be taken with other medications. It is suitable for diabetics and for those on low sodium diets, and is equally suitable for children and the elderly.

In his book *Cider Vinegar,* Cyril Scott describes its 'miraculous' effects on so many disorders that he feels compelled to warn readers that it is not a universal panacea.[8] He emphasizes that cider vinegar only improves biological processes, but in so doing it helps to prevent or cure such disorders as obesity, excessive menstrual bleeding, infections of the ear, nose and throat, allergies, swollen veins and circulatory disorders. The effects of cider vinegar on a few of these typical disorders are worth describing in a little more detail.

WEIGHT CONTROL

Obesity is caused in most cases by overeating, lack of exercise and overindulgence. Cider vinegar was claimed to assist in reducing excess weight when combined with a calorie-controlled diet. It is thought to improve the rate at which food is converted to energy. Take 2 teaspoons of cider vinegar in a glass of water before each meal, preferably with two drops of iodine from seaweeds. Avoid salty and sugary foods. Being high in enzymes, cider vinegar was also claimed to help the underweight who are normally deficient in enzymes and therefore cannot use their food properly. To help normalise body weight take one tablespoon of cider vinegar and one teaspoon of honey in a glass of water first thing in the morning.

DIARRHOEA

In many cases mild diarrhoea represents the body's attempt to rid itself of toxins. However, in prolonged and serious cases, when the body becomes weak and stores of minerals are lost, cider vinegar can provide quick relief. Take 1 to 2 teaspoons in a glass of boiled or mineral water, several times during the day. For children over the age of three, halve the dose.

ANTISEPTIC EFFECTS

The antiseptic effects of taking cider vinegar are noticeable even after a few days – stools lose their pungent odour and even the breath smells better. This is because cider vinegar increases acidity and destroys putrefactive bacteria in the intestines. The poisonous by-products of putrefaction are partially absorbed through the intestinal walls into the blood, causing auto-intoxication of the body. Intestinal cleanliness is becoming increasingly popular as doctors realize that it is a basic requirement for a healthy life.

Some people also advocate using cider vinegar as a

mouthwash and throat gargle, as a general antiseptic against mouth or throat inflammations. Take 1 to 3 teaspoons in a glass of water, morning and evening.

ENERGY AND HEALTH, FATIGUE AND DISEASE

By observing the eating habits of animals given a free choice of food, Dr Jarvis also found a correlation between urine acidity and energy level and health.[9] He also discovered that fluctuations in urine acidity correspond to fluctuations in feelings of well-being in humans. Alkaline urine was found to be associated with fatigue, childhood diseases, hay fever, arthritis and other clinical conditions. However, when urine acidity was increased through the use of cider vinegar, the body regained its energy and health. Indeed, I have used cider vinegar for years to treat patients with fatigue caused by warm weather. In most cases, 2 to 3 teaspoons morning and noon are sufficient to relieve that run-down feeling. I have also found that, for many patients, a few tablespoons a day of cider vinegar help to dissolve certain types of kidney stones.

THINNING HAIR

Hair loss is sometimes a result of poor metabolism. Many case histories show that as a result of a few teaspoonfuls of cider vinegar each day for several months hair loss has stopped and the remaining hair become healthier and thicker. One reason for thinning hair is a deficiency of mineral salts, so it is easy to understand why mineral-rich cider vinegar can help.

To conclude this discussion, it is well to remember that cider vinegar will not work in the same way for everyone. A few people are allergic to it and others may not be affected at all. But for many people, cider vinegar opens up a wonderful new chapter in life.

BREWER'S YEAST

Various kinds of brewer's yeast are grown for human consumption. Baker's yeast is not at all the same thing and should not be eaten. Baker's yeast is an active, living yeast which, once ingested, will multiply in the intestines and deplete B vitamins.

Brewer's yeast is a unicellular microorganism, a plant without chlorophyll. Originally it was a by-product of brewing. During the process of fermentation, which converts the sugar in the unfermented beer (wort) to alcohol and carbon dioxide, the yeast multiplies four- or fivefold. Now it is specially grown on cereals, molasses or malt extract, which explains varieties in flavour. One popular variety grown on wood pulp is called Torula yeast and is extremely rich in trace elements (except chromium).[10] Brewer's yeast can be bought in powder, tablet or flake form. Each form has its advantage. Powder is more concentrated than flakes or tablets and mixes well with liquids such as soups, milk and juices. Flakes are better-tasting and are normally sprinkled on food. Some people find tablets more convenient, especially if they do not like the taste of powder or flakes. All forms are normally debittered with sodium carbonate or ammonium carbonate in the final stages of production.

Brewer's yeast is a well-balanced food, containing an excellent concentration of B-complex vitamins. It contains, for example, twenty times more vitamin B1 and B2 than liver,[11] and is up to 45 per cent complete protein, containing 17 amino acids, including all the essential ones. It also contains a very great abundance of minerals and trace elements. All in all, it is a marvellous bargain when you consider its high protein content, which is double that of meat, or compare its great stores of vitamins and minerals to expensive encapsulated supplements. Researcher James Rorty writes: 'Brewer's yeast is not only our cheapest source of B vitamins, it is also our cheapest complete protein. It takes months to grow our best vegetable proteins such as soybeans, peanuts and sunflower seeds. It takes years to grow cattle, but it only takes hours to grow yeast.'[12] In fact, 8 tons of molasses can yield 7 tons of yeast in just 10 hours.[13] A single microscopic yeast cell can produce 50 tons in a fortnight.

Many beneficial values have been attributed to brewer's yeast. One laboratory study showed that yeast powder in daily doses of 60 grams (which constitute a therapeutic dose), dramatically improved the condition of 1,000 people suffering from infectious hepatitis and cirrhosis of the liver.[14] Yeast has also been found to accelerate growth and development in laboratory rats,[15] and to protect mice from bacterial infections. Gayelord Hauser recommends it to prevent constipation,[16] and another study showed that yeast supplements given to men doing hard physical labour relieved fatigue, depression, inefficiency, poor appetite, constipation and irritability within 48 hours.[17]

PROTEIN CONTENT

Brewer's yeast is a concentrated source of complete protein, which means that it contains all the essential amino acids which cannot be synthesized in the body. Protein's biologic role is of the utmost importance, as we saw in Chapter 2. The complete protein of brewer's yeast, a rarity in plant foods, is nutritionally superior to animal protein. It is also a much better source of B vitamins and minerals than any type of meat. And brewer's yeast is not highly contaminated, as meat is, by hormones and antibiotics, nor is its freshness or cleanliness questionable. Vegetarians and people who do not tolerate meat, as well as hypoglycaemics who need a high protein diet, can benefit from regular use of brewer's yeast. It is desirable for dieters, too, because of its low content of carbohydrate calories.

Being a high protein and high nucleic acid food, brewer's yeast is a purine-forming food (purines are the precursors of uric acid). People who are prone to purine-caused gout or arthritis may notice a worsening of these conditions when taking massive doses of yeast. If so, only small amounts should be taken at a time, while eating a high alkaline diet, rich in fruits and vegetables.

B-COMPLEX CONTENT

Since B-complex deficiency impairs metabolic processes in the digestive tract as well as in the nervous system, brewer's yeast is important in maintaining normal appetite, improving digestion, absorption and elimination, and preventing insomnia, depression, nervousness and fatigue.

MINERAL CONTENT

Because of its high iron and copper content, brewer's yeast has long been known to relieve anaemia and its symptoms. Some advocate its use even in baby formulae and for people who live largely on milk,[18] since milk is relatively poor in iron. Brewer's yeast has also been known to benefit diabetics when taken in large doses. The reason for this was revealed only recently by Dr Walter Mertz, who discovered that brewer's yeast is the richest known source of glucose tolerance factor (GTF). This factor improves the impaired glucose and insulin functions of diabetics and hypoglycaemics (see 'Chromium', Chapter 4).

Brewer's yeast has ignited the imagination of health food producers. They 'feed' yeast on minerals, further increasing its mineral content. High-selenium yeast, for example, is yeast fed on selenium salts. This provides naturally bound selenium, which is at least 20 times easier to absorb than regular sodium selenite.[19] The selenium content of processed and refined foods is constantly diminishing, so brewer's yeast is an important and dependable source of this essential element (see 'Selenium', Chapter 4).

CAUTION: when taking large amounts of brewer's yeast or wheat germ, additional calcium should be taken as well, because both have a high phosphorus content and calcium combines with phosphorus and is excreted from the body.

USAGE

There are many kinds of brewer's yeast to suit various tastes and tolerances. Beginners should always start with small amounts, increasing their intake gradually. This is to give the body a chance to adjust. If digestion is weak and there are insufficient bacteria in the gut to deal with yeast effectively, the results of taking large doses of brewer's yeast will be severe indigestion and bloating. Nevertheless people with a weak digestion and depleted gut flora are precisely the ones who derive the most benefit from brewer's yeast. In fact, the poorer the digestion, the greater the need. Indigestion will subside gradually as the yeast begins to take effect.

WHEAT GERM OIL

Wheat germ has been known as a highly nourishing food since antiquity. Psalm 81, verse 16, says: 'He should have fed them also with the finest of the wheat.' It is the best source of vitamin E available, and a fine source of protein – half a cup of raw wheat germ provides the protein equivalent of four eggs. It is also a concentrated source of vitamin B complex, iron, phosphorus, trace elements, oils and essential fatty acids, and natural oestrogen.

Wheat germ occurs as a 'speck' on the wheat kernel, from which it starts to germinate. As the life source of a new plant, it is hardly surprising that wheat germ is such a concentrated source of vital nutrients. Wheat germ oil is pressed from these embryos, and for the best results should be cold pressed (extracted without heat), packed in opaque glass containers, and stored in a cool dark place.

'MIRACULOUS' EFFECTS

The many outstanding effects of wheat germ oil on the human body range from alleviating neurological disorders[20] to lowering liver cholesterol.[21] Wheat germ oil contains octacosanol, a type of waxy alcohol, whose effects on the body are many and varied and include increasing energy, endurance and strength, improving resistance to the effects of stress, reducing muscle spasms, toning up reflexes, alleviating the pain of arthritis, improving heartbeat (affecting the T waves of electrocardiograms), and so on.[22] These and other effects were observed by Dr Thomas K. Cureton, Director of the Physical Fitness Institute at the University of Illinois, after years of controlled experiments using wheat germ oil on youngsters, elderly people and athletes. In one case, a single teaspoon of wheat germ oil a day, taken by a group of sedentary elderly people over a period of two months, resulted in a sharp increase (as much as 51.5 per cent) in their physical fitness and endurance. Dr Cureton believes that middle-aged people can reverse loss of stamina and fitness considerably by combining mild exercise with a daily dose of 1 1/2 teaspoons of wheat germ oil.

One of the experiments conducted under Dr Cureton's supervision was done during a training course for the U.S.

Marines' Underwater Demolition Team, to check the effects of wheat germ oil on fear, dizziness, drowsiness and fatigue. The team was divided into three groups, one receiving wheat germ oil (6 capsules daily), the second pure octacosanol, and the third cottonseed oil as a placebo. It was a double blind experiment with no one knowing what he was receiving or administering. After the course, when all the scores were computed, it was found that those taking the cottonseed oil increased their fitness scores by an average of 7.97 points, those taking wheat germ oil increased theirs by 13.12 points (62 per cent more fitness), and those taking octacosanol pushed their scores up by an average 16.36 points (double fitness!) Ironically, among those who flunked the course those who used cottonseed oil to improve fitness outnumbered wheat germ oil or octacosanol users by three to one.[23]

The effects of wheat germ oil are much greater than those of wheat germ flakes. The oil has a denser concentration of active nutrients such as octacosanol and vitamin E. Moreover, during storage and use, flakes repeatedly come into contact with the air and their oils easily oxidize and turn rancid. Wheat germ oil is normally cold pressed and unrefined, and packed in tightly-capped amber glass bottles to protect it from spoiling

Dr Cureton is not the only researcher to have found significant effects for wheat germ oil and octacosanol, although other research has mostly been done with animals. A very carefully controlled study in 1962 confirmed that giving wheat germ oil to dairy cows considerably increased their pregnancy rates.[24] Minute doses of octacosanol were found to have a powerful effect on the male hormones of roosters.[25] As far back as 1937 wheat germ oil was given to a woman with a history of miscarriages and made it possible for her to give birth to healthy babies. In recent studies, concentrated wheat germ oil has been shown to halve the incidence of toxaemia, miscarriage and prematurity.[26]

Studies conducted by Dr Carlton Fredericks and his medical colleagues have shown that concentrated wheat germ oil, or massive doses of octacosanol prepared from wheat germ oil, have a remarkable therapeutic effect on a particular group of degenerative diseases, the myoneuropathies (nerve-muscle disorders); into this group come multiple sclerosis, epilepsy, cerebral palsy, encephalitis and myasthenia gravis.[27] Durk Pearson, a gerontology researcher, has reported that octacosanol blocks the uncontrolled formation of thromboxanes (blood clotting hormones).[28] Thromboxanes, as well as being produced enzymatically, according to body needs, can be synthesized in large amounts by the oxidative action of free radicals and peroxides, escaping the checks and balances of enzymatic production. The result is abnormal clotting on arterial walls, leading to coronary thrombosis. By using octacosanol, one can literally help to prevent a heart attack.

The energy-releasing function of wheat germ oil is still not fully understood, but one thing is known for sure: any person under physical or mental stress can benefit from it. And you do not have to be on a commando training course to experience stress. Tests conducted by Charlotte Leedy, a professor at the University of Maryland, showed that the heartbeat of a man engaged in a tough game of chess can accelerate as much as an athlete's during a mile run. In fact mental stress can be more damaging than physical stress since it is not accompanied by increased oxygen consumption.

Everyone should use wheat germ oil because modern diets do not usually contain the raw, cold pressed oils which supply so many important nutrients. White flour and white flour products do not contain the germ, the vital life source, of the kernel.

CAUTION: Cold pressed wheat germ oil contains significant amounts of natural oestrogen (female sex hormone). Taking massive doses of more than a few teaspoons daily over a prolonged period of time can cause testicular degeneration and loss of sex drive in some men.[29] For higher levels of supplementation, octacosanol tablets are much safer and more beneficial.

SUNFLOWER OIL

Sunflower seeds are one of those rare foods that have remained unchanged since biblical times. Not only were they used in their natural state as a sustaining food, but also as a source of flour and oil. The stalks of the plant were used to make fire, and the ashes were used as a fertilizer.

In pre-revolutionary Russia, every soldier in the field received a 1 kg (2.2 pounds) bag of sunflower seeds as an emergency ration. Because of their exceptional nutritional value, it was believed that one could subsist on them exclusively for long periods without ill effects.

EFFECTS

Since the sunflower is a strong plant, highly resistant to insects, it is seldom necessary to use toxic insecticide sprays on it. Its seeds are therefore unlikely to be contaminated, except by air-borne pollutants in the growing area. Sunflower seeds have been described as beneficial to eyesight, skin and fingernails, and as useful adjuncts in the treatment of high blood pressure and irritated nerves.[30] The U.S. Department of Agriculture rates their protein content nearly as high as steak and higher than that of all other seeds. Sunflower seeds also contain concentrated amounts of vitamins A, D, E, and B complex. Their vitamin E content is particularly impressive: 100 grams of kernels contain 30 IU. They are also rich in minerals, including iron, potassium, phosphorus, magnesium, manganese, copper and calcium.

Sunflower seed oil contains a high concentration of unsaturated (essential) fatty acids. As we have seen, these help the body to use fats properly, reduce cholesterol levels, and stimulate the burning of stored body fat.[31]

It is because of these essential fatty acids (EFAs) that sunflower oil is such a beneficial food. Only safflower oil has a higher EFA content. In terms of linoleic acid (a principal EFA), sunflower seeds are nearly top of the list, containing 135 grams per pound of hulled seeds. Most edible oils which contain EFAs in their crude state undergo heating, refining or hydrogenation; this destroys EFAs, impairing the body's synthesis of prostaglandins. Hydrogenated oils, as in many types of margarine, have a negative effect on cholesterol levels, as do animal fats. Replacing some saturated fats with cold pressed oils is highly beneficial. If cold pressed oils are unavailable, solvent-extracted oils may be substituted, though they are not as desirable. Traces of solvents may still be present, but no serious heating is involved.

USAGE
Sunflower seed oil can be used as an all-purpose kitchen oil. To take advantage of its full value, it is best used in its raw state as a salad dressing. It can also be incorporated in Dr Donsbach's 'super butter' (see p.43). NOTE: Sunflower oil must be packed in glass bottles, and caps must be tightly secured after use to prevent it oxidizing and turning rancid. It should also be stored in a cool, dark place. Plastic bottles are not advisable as they tend to release vinyl chloride, a gas

which has adverse effects on health.

Excessive use of vegetable oils can cause vitamin E deficiency. To quote Dr Carlton Fredericks 'Moderate intake of vegetable oil means what it says: about 20 per cent of total fat intake derived from such oils, no more'[32]

Sunflower seeds can also be used. A unique way of using them is in sunflower yogurt, used extensively in naturopathic centres. Place a half-cup of sunflower seeds in a sprouter (or soak for 24 hours) until they start to germinate (little shoots will be visible). Put them in a blender, add one half-cup of water, and blend for 20 seconds; then gradually add another half-cup of water while continuing to blend for another 2 minutes, or until the consistency is like heavy cream. Store this cream for 8 to 24 hours at 70-80°F (21-26°C) in a yogurt maker if you have one or by putting the mixture in a container next to an electric light bulb. The container should be closed but not airtight. When the yogurt is ready, it tastes slightly tart. It may even have a 'black cap', which some people eat. If overfermented, it will taste sour. Sunflower yogurt will keep for up to a week in a refrigerator. It makes a delicious and nutritious salad dressing or vegetable dip, particularly when combined with tomatoes and sprinkled with kelp powder (see below). It can be seasoned to taste.

As a supplement, 2 tablespoons a day of sunflower seeds are recommended, even for people on reducing diets.

KELP

Kelp is a particular kind of seaweed harvested by boats which pull the plants out of the sea with huge hooks. Special cutters mow off the tops of the kelp, which is then taken to a processing plant to be finely chopped, cleaned, shredded and dried into powder or pressed into tablets. No boiling is involved, so most of the original nutrients remain in the final product. Kelp contains abundant minerals and trace elements, especially iodine, which is deficient in many agricultural soils.

Fresh kelp contains about 100,000 mcg iodine per pound while dried kelp contains nearly ten times as much.[33] As a seasoning agent, kelp provides ten times as much iodine as iodized salt. Iodine normalizes thyroid secretion. If it is lacking in the diet, thyroid function slows down. This can lead to many and varied disorders. As Dr Carlton Fredericks writes: 'If your thyroid is underactive, your troubles will range from constipation to dry skin, from too many colds to dry, brittle hair, from fatigue to slow-growing nails.'[34] By supplying iodine to the thyroid, kelp can step up basal metabolic rate, improving the burning of food to release energy. This increases body heat and contributes to weight loss. People who always feel cold or who are very sensitive to cold weather might feel warmer with supplemental kelp.

Kelp can replace or supplement iodized salt in treating and preventing goitre, a disorder in which the thyroid gland becomes enlarged due to lack of iodine in the diet. In fact, regular use of iodized salt only has been found inadequate to prevent goitre in many areas,[35] unless kelp is used.

However, kelp is only one of many different types of seaweed, all of which contain iodine. Agar is a seaweed used to thicken jellies and fruit juices in place of animal-derived gelatine. Several other seaweeds imported from Japan, like, nori, hijiki, wakame, kombu, arame and sushi nori are sold extensively in health food shops. Nori is rich in protein and can be used as a condiment, while kombu and arame are extremely rich in iodine and can be added to soups. Wakame and Hijiki contain high amounts of calcium. Another seaweed which is becoming increasingly popular is dulse, which comes from the coast of Maine, and can be added to soups, or used as a chewy snack with a distinctive sea flavour.

COMPOSITION

Kelp, like any other plant, contains carbohydrates (sugar and starches). Its sugar is called mannitol, which is not very sweet, has a mild laxative effect and does not raise blood sugar. It is excellent for diabetics. Proteins and fats are also present in low amounts, as are vitamins A, B and C. It is interesting to note that fresh kelp was at one time the only source of vitamin C for certain Eskimo tribes, but one which contained all the ocean minerals and trace elements as well.

CANCER

A recent study confirmed that there is a connection between breast and ovarian cancer and a low-iodine diet.[36] A comparison was made between a group of Japanese women who had emigrated to the United States and a group of Japanese women living in Japan. The emigrants showed the same high incidence of breast and ovarian cancer as American women, but the non-emigrant group, who ate the traditional Japanese diet, abundant in sea food, fish and seaweed, showed very few instances of either kind of cancer. Their iodine-rich diet protected them. The study showed that a low iodine intake raises the level of estradiol, the type of estrogen which increases the risk of breast and uterine cancer, but reduces the level of estriol, the protective type of estrogen. Since it is difficult to ascertain specific iodine levels in regular laboratory tests, the study recommended supplements of kelp to insure an adequate supply.

RADIOACTIVE FALLOUT

In a recent study at the Gastrointestinal Research Laboratories of McGill University in Montreal, a group of scientists found that kelp contains a substance which is capable of reducing intestinal absorption of radioactive strontium-90 by 50 to 80 per cent.[37] It is no secret that our planet is becoming progressively contaminated by radioactive fallout from experimental nuclear explosions and from nuclear reactor wastes. This radioactivity reaches us through the air, the water supply and our food. Breathing polluted air cannot be helped and some radioactive particles will be absorbed. However, the greatest absorption of radioactive elements comes through our water and our food. Strontium-90 tends to accumulate in calcium-rich foods such as green leafy vegetables, milk and dairy products, and also in human bones, where it destroys the function of the marrow and impairs the formation of red blood cells. A substance in kelp, sodium alginate, binds with strontium-90 in the intestines, preventing its absorption and promoting its natural excretion through the faeces. Some of the danger of radioactivity is thus eliminated. Sodium alginate, by the way, is a product widely used in the food industry as a jellying and thickening agent.

USAGE
In order to receive 100 mcg of iodine (two-thirds of the necessary daily intake) one would have to eat 10 pounds of fresh fruit and vegetables or 8 pounds of grains and nuts! Without a diet rich in seafood, the problem of consuming enough iodine can be solved by eating kelp, which contains about 200,000 mcg iodine per kilogram (2.2 pounds), or dried kelp powder, which contains nearly ten times as much or 0.1 to 0.2 per cent iodine.

Kelp is a convenient and safe food supplement which ensures a proper intake of iodine and trace minerals. It is sold in powder or tablet form, and is often contained in natural multi-mineral capsules. Other seaweeds are also sold in various dried forms for use in cooking.

CAUTION: people with an overactive thyroid condition, pregnant or lactating women, should consult their physician before starting iodine or kelp supplementation.

SPROUTS

Sprouts, mainly soybean sprouts, have been used in diets for thousands of years, especially by the Chinese. They have also been used medicinally in East Asia and Europe. Many ethnic groups, including the Navajo Indians of Arizona and New Mexico, sprouted corn to prepare alcoholic beverages. Over the centuries the benefits of eating sprouts assumed legendary proportions – alertness was improved, the heart was strengthened, immunity was doubled, life was lengthened. . .

The first well-documented trial of sprouted seeds was carried out by a British army doctor, Major H.W. Wiltshire, during World War I. He used sprouts in his attempt to fight scurvy among soldiers. He treated two groups of scorbutic soldiers, giving 4 ounces of kidney bean sprouts boiled for 10 minutes to one group, and 4 ounces of fresh lemon juice to the other group. After four weeks, he found that while only 53.4 per cent of the fresh lemon juice group had recovered, 70.4 per cent of the sprout group were cured![38] He calculated that the vitamins supplied by the sprouts cost only 60 per cent of what they cost if supplied exclusively by lemons. Sprouts surpassed fresh lemons both nutritionally and in value for money.

Bean sprouts made their first appearance in America in the 1940s, in the days of meat shortages, and were widely publicized as a meat alternative. Dr Clive McCay of the

School of Nutrition at Cornell University gave this oft-repeated definition of them: 'A vegetable that will grow in any climate, rivals meat in nutritive value, matures in three to five days, may be planted any day of the year, requires neither soil nor sunshine, rivals tomatoes in vitamin C, has no waste and can be cooked with as little fuel and as quickly as pork chops'.[39]

COMPOSITION

Sprouts are rich in vitamins A, C, D, E, K and B complex, in calcium, phosphorus, potassium, magnesium and iron, and also contain high quality protein and enzymes.[40] Moreover, sprouts are rich in unknown vitality factors because, unlike most vegetables, they can be eaten at their peak of freshness, while they are still growing in fact. Unlike fresh vegetables, whose vitamins begin to break down (enzymatically) the moment they are picked, sprouts keep on forming nutrients until they are eaten or cooked. The noted nutritionist Catharyn Elwood has described them as 'the most living food in the world".

Miraculous things happen when a grain or legume seed starts to germinate. The starches and oils inside it are converted to vitamins, minerals, enzymes, simple sugars and proteins.[41] Given the right amount of moisture, air and heat, the germinal part of the seed starts to feed on the core of the seed, which acts as a depot of vital nutrients. These can increase to many times their amount in the pre-germinated seed, at the expense of less vital substances. Vitamin C, for example, increases by 600 per cent during sprouting,[42] at the expense of sugars. A single average serving (100 grams) of mung bean sprouts, for example, contains 120 mg of vitamin C, which is almost double the RDA for adults.[43] The same weight of chick peas yields 75 mg.[44] The B complex vitamins and many enzymes also increase spectacularly during germination, making sprouts easily digestible, even for people with weak digestion. The protein content of sprouts increases in quantity and quality at the expense of carbohydrates and fats. In fact protein is broken down to amino acids, ready for use by the young plant. This is why sprouted legumes are less gas-producing than dried.[45]

Another reason for eating sprouts daily is the fantastic quantity of enzymes which they contain. As we age, our bodies become less efficient at producing enzymes from food, a condition which often manifests itself as indigestion or flatulence. By offering us lots of enzymes, sprouts also offer more efficient digestion and improved metabolism of food into energy. To dieters, sprouts are a double blessing, being low in calories as well as highly nutritious.

HOW TO GROW SPROUTS

Sprouting requires only water and a sprouting container – a glass jar will do. Sprouting takes between three and six days, depending on the kind of seed, the ambient temperature, and amount of light and water available. Direct sunlight is not needed. The seeds have to be rinsed three or four times a day, or else they rot. However, even this chore is not necessary today. Patent plastic sprouters are available, which maintain all the required conditions. Sprouting then becomes a joy, a private, all-weather garden in the kitchen.

The most popular sprouts today are mung beans, alfalfa, dried peas, chick peas, wheat, sesame seeds and corn kernels. Alfalfa sprouts are considered to be the richest in minerals. Sprouts are best eaten raw in salads or sandwiches. They can also be steamed lightly and eaten as a side dish.

GARLIC

Garlic is a classic combination of food and folk medicine. Like sprouts, garlic has been used as a cure-all for millennia. The Chinese were taught about garlic in the calendar of Hsai, in 2000 B.C. A thousand years earlier the Babylonians were using it. Inscriptions on the Great Pyramid at Gizeh in Egypt mention garlic as one of the foods eaten by its builders. Garlic has a considerable reputation – it stimulates gastric secretions, respiration and digestion, fights colds, lowers blood pressure, stops hair loss. . .

An idea that has gained credence in recent years, especially among naturopathic physicians, is that most common infectious diseases, such as flu and bronchitis, are caused by an over-accumulation of toxins in the body. These toxins gradually undermine the functions of internal organs. Garlic has been found to be an excellent antiseptic, and was used with amazing success in treating soldiers with infected wounds during both World Wars. In World War II, the British treated many of their wounded soldiers with extracts of garlic. Some of their wounds were already gangrenous, but garlic effectively checked the spread of gangrene and resulted in the shedding of gangrenous tissue.[46] Indeed, the Food and Drug Research Laboratories in New York City found that some garlic compounds are very effective bactericides.[47] Russians, as a rule, have a high regard for the healing powers of garlic. As recently as 1965, the Russians are reported to have flown 500 tons of garlic to Moscow to combat a flu epidemic. No wonder some people still call garlic 'Russian penicillin'.

The active ingredient in garlic was traditionally thought to be allicin. Allicin has been researched since 1944, when it was identified as being responsible for garlic's anti-bacterial action. It has since been shown to be particularly effective against the bacteria which cause throat inflammation, typhoid and dysentery.[48] However, recent studies have found that another constituent of garlic, ajoene, isolated by Dr Eric Block in New York, is superior to allicin in antifungal and anti-thrombotic activity.[49] Since the initial studies, garlic extracts have been successfully used to boost immunity,[50] inhibit cancerous tumours,[51] and treat a host of common conditions such as hypertension, high cholesterol levels, diabetes, yeast infections,[52] stress[53] and allergies.[54]

Various studies have confirmed that garlic lowers blood pressure and cholesterol levels. In one group of heart patients, who supplemented their daily diets with the oil of about 1 ounce of garlic for a period of eight months, cholesterol levels decreased by 18 per cent and triglyceride levels also fell 'significantly'.[55] The active factor is believed to be in the oil, which contains various sulphur compounds. Onion, by the way, contains a similar oil, but in much lower concentrations.

In another study, in which healthy people were given garlic along with large amounts of butter, not only did average cholesterol levels fall but blood samples also took longer to clot. We now know that quick blood clotting time is an indicator of high platelet adhesion or 'stickiness'', a factor which favours hypertension, cholesterol deposits and coronary thrombosis. Extending blood coagulation time therefore helps to prevent these severe circulatory disorders. Recent studies have shown that purified extracts of garlic can inhibit the formation of blood clots and provide protection against atherosclerosis by lowering cholesterol and triglyceride levels by about 50 per cent.[56]

Hypertension or high blood pressure is one of the major risks of atherosclerosis. Most drugs for controlling blood pressure have serious side effects, one of which is male impotence. Garlic has been used to treat hypertension in China and Japan for centuries and is officially recognized as an anti-hypertensive by the Japanese Food and Drug Administration. The first scientific studies of garlic's blood pressure lowering effect were done as early as 1921.[57] Numerous studies since have confirmed its anti-hypertensive effect. In a recent study, 61.7 per cent of hypertensive patients given 50 grams of garlic a day reduced their blood pressure.[58] Other studies have shown that people predisposed to cardiovascular diseases through diabetes, hypertension or a family history of heart disease and strokes, can benefit from long-term use of garlic, dispensing with drugs and their side effects.[59] Garlic is abundant in selenium and germanium, two antioxidant trace elements that combat degenerative diseases such as cancer and heart attack. This may explain why garlic not only prevents blood clots, but also suppresses malignant tumours in mice. In one experiment at Howard's School of Human Ecology in Washington, a group of rats with liver cancer were given garlic extract. Tumour growth dropped by 50 per cent.[60] This effect was explained by the fact that garlic prevents the formation of cyclic guanosine monophosphate (cGMP), a substance needed by cancer cells to grow and proliferate.

Garlic has also been reported to act much like an anti-diabetic drug.[61] A chemist and nutritionist with the FDA Bureau of Foods, Dr Glen Shue, says that in view of recent investigations garlic 'could reduce the need for insulin'.[62]

Garlic was also a folk remedy for children with pin-worms, tapeworms and other intestinal parasites, and is still used for the purpose by modern biological practitioners such as Dr Paavo Airola.[63] Dr Michael Tansey of the Department of Plant Sciences at the University of Indiana reports that zoopathogenic fungi, such as those which cause athlete's foot and vaginitis, are inhibited by aqueous solutions of garlic.[64]

Garlic is not a cure-all, but there is a firm scientific basis for the old belief that a few raw garlic cloves a day (or a few garlic oil capsules) are beneficial to health and increase resistance to the above-mentioned diseases.

People who like to eat raw garlic in salads may be pleased to know that fresh parsley eaten simultaneously will inhibit garlic's pungent odour. Weight-watchers can enjoy garlic without worrying about calories – there are only 1 or 2 calories in each clove.

Garlic oil capsules are the easiest way to take garlic if you don't like the taste or smell or are concerned about socializing after eating fresh garlic. The capsules have a gelatine coating that does not dissolve until they reach the intestines, preventing the bad breath typical of garlic eating. The normal dosage is one capsule per meal.

LECITHIN

Lecithin was discovered in 1850 by the French researcher Maurice Gobley. While studying egg yolk, he succeeded in isolating a fatty substance capable of emulsifying water and oil. The new substance was called lecithin, from *lekithos*, Greek for egg yolk. Today lecithin is no longer derived from egg yolks, although egg yolk contains 8 to 10 per cent lecithin. Most of it is produced from soybeans, which contain 0.3 to 0.6 per cent and are much cheaper than eggs. Lecithin is widely used as an emulsifier in food products such as margarine and chocolate, and also in other products such as paint and cosmetics.

COMPOSITION

Lecithin is a waxy substance and belongs to a class of body fats called phospholipids or phosphatides. It is a complete mixture of phospholipids, phosphoric acid, two B vitamins (phosphatidyl choline and phosphatidyl inositol) and the amino acid methionine.

Lecithin is found in all body cells, including those of the brain and nerves, and takes part in various vital processes. It aids the transportation of fats throughout the body and helps to mobilize and disperse unhealthy deposits of fat and cholesterol. With cholesterol, it is essential to the production of bile. In fact it is such an important substance that the liver produces it continuously, as it does cholesterol. Seventy-three per cent of total liver fat is lecithin, and 30 per cent of the dry weight of the brain is lecithin.[65]

EFFECTS

Because of its remarkable emulsifying capacity, lecithin has the effect of reducing the size of lipid particles in circulation, keeping the blood clear and inhibiting atherosclerosis.[66] Lecithin contains essential fatty acids and has been shown by Dr Lester Morrison, Director of Research at Los Angeles County General Hospital, to substantially lower cholesterol levels even at a daily supplemented dosage of just 3 ounces.[67] Dr Morrison's study was particularly impressive, since it was done with a group of high cholesterol patients, none of whom had responded to the usual drugs or to low fat diets.

Although commonly stigmatized as a major cause of atherosclerosis and heart attacks, cholesterol is highly important to the body (see pp.43-7). It is constituent of steroid hormones and a conductor of nerve impulses, it is needed for the formation of bile, and it is converted to vitamin D whenever the body is exposed to sunlight. It is so essential that if you eat less of it, the liver will only produce more. In fact, 80 per cent of the cholesterol in the blood is synthesized by the liver and other organs from carbohydrates, proteins and fats. Only

20 per cent comes directly from cholesterol contained in food.[68] Cholesterol is not all bad. The bile it forms is crucial for fat metabolism and if bile is in short supply, the absorption of fats and fat-soluble vitamins (A, D, E, K), will be impaired, creating devastating deficiencies. When fat digestion is impaired, other foods are also poorly digested – excess fats cover the food particles and prevent digestive enzymes from getting to work on them.[69] Besides, cholesterol behaves according to the various types of lipoproteins present in the blood. High-density lipoproteins (HDL) are the 'good guys'. Low density lipoproteins (LDL) are the 'bad guys' who promote cholesterol deposits. When there is a deficiency of nutrients such as choline, inositol or methionine in the diet, then cholesterol assumes its negative roles.[70] In such conditions, lecithin can emulsify cholesterol and put it back into circulation, and also lower LDL levels, enabling cholesterol to play its many constructive roles.[71] At the same time as it lowers LDLs, lecithin increases HDL levels, thought to protect the cardiovascular system from atherosclerosis and heart attacks.[72]

Lecithin can also help to prevent gallstones. Gallstones are formed when various factors, an infection for example, cause the excess cholesterol in bile to precipitate as crystals. These crystals can then enlarge to form stones.[73] The solubility of cholesterol in bile depends on lecithin, bile salts and cholesterol being present in certain proportions, so an adequate supply of lecithin may help to dissolve gallstones by restoring the correct proportions. Several studies have confirmed lecithin's ability to do this.[74]

To dieters, daily lecithin consumption means two things: first, that body fats are converted into energy more quickly, and second, that existing fat deposits will slowly disperse. Sportsmen and body builders also value lecithin for its ability, in combination with exercise, to shift fat from unwanted places. In addition, lecithin has been found beneficial in treating skin disorders such as eczema, acne and psoriasis.[75]

BRAIN FUNCTION

Lecithin has also been reputed to be a 'brain food". Students who use lecithin before exams, to improve their memory and enhance their ability to study effectively, have been fully vindicated by recent research.[76] In the mid–1970s brain researchers found that lecithin was more intimately involved in mental and nervous functions than previously thought. Choline, a major ingredient of lecithin, was found to be synthesized in the body to acetylcholine, a substance which conveys impulses from one nerve cell to another and therefore plays a vital role in physical and emotional behaviour. Deficiencies of acetylcholine were shown to impair brain function, and recent evidence has indicated that such deficiencies increase with age.[77] This may explain why lecithin is particularly beneficial to elderly people. Supplemental lecithin, which supplies additional choline and therefore boosts acetylcholine levels, has been reported to improve the condition of patients with neurological disorders such as tardive dyskinesia (characterized by jerky movements and sometimes a side effect of certain psychotic drugs), Parkinson's disease (the rhythmic muscle tremors of old age) and Alzheimer's disease or pre-senile dementia (characterized by loss of recent memories, poor concentration and a short attention span).[78]

SOURCES

The best natural sources of lecithin are unrefined, cold pressed vegetable oils, egg yolks, nuts, seeds, and of course soybeans. Food processing largely depletes lecithin. Lecithin is available from health food shops in granule, capsule and liquid form. Granules are mild-flavoured and agreeable, and can be eaten from a spoon or sprinkled over various foods. Capsules, though convenient for travel, are less potent than granules – ten 1,200 mg capsules are equivalent to 1 tablespoon of granules. Liquid lecithin is two-thirds lecithin and one third soybean oil – the oil adds calories of course. However, liquid lecithin can be used as a substitute for cooking or baking oils; it can also be used to grease baking tins.

Lecithin granule containers should be kept tightly closed and stored in a cool, dry place – although granules have a long shelf life, they can become rather rubbery. Liquid lecithin containers should be kept in the refrigerator after opening. Average lecithin granule dosage is 3 teaspoons to 3 tablespoons a day.

BRAN

No health food has received such sustained and widespread publicity as bran. Its virtues as a bowel regulator and disease preventer have been trumpeted in newspaper and magazine ads, and in radio and TV commercials. Is all this publicity justified?

COMPOSITION

Bran is made up of the fibrous husks which cover grain seeds. These contain 9 to 12 per cent complex carbohydrates (polysaccharides), such as cellulose, pectin and lignin, and also protein, fat, vitamins and minerals.

The common, but mistaken, belief that wheat bran is rough and therefore irritating to the bowels, is easily refuted. Whole wheat bran contains 2.5 per cent cellulose (the indigestible part), which compares favourably with apples (3.6 per cent), grapes (7 per cent) and raspberries (6.7 per cent).[79]

EFFECTS

The unique characteristic of bran is not its nutritional value but its ability to absorb water and give bulk to the faeces. It expands in the colon, stimulating the involuntary contractions of evacuation. Many of the degenerative diseases which plague the West are unheard of in rural Africa. This is because the diet of the average Westerner is much lower in fibre. It is a fact that a high-fiber diet speeds up waste transit time through the colon, preventing constipation,[80] appendicitis,[81] diverticulosis (pockets in the colon),[82] haemorrhoids and varicose veins,[83] obesity and high blood pressure,[84] cancer of the colon[85] and coronary heart disease.[86] With slow-moving stools, unfriendly bacteria in the colon have time to convert bile acids to carcinogens,[87] whereas fast-moving stools facilitate bile excretion and therefore the excretion of cholesterol, reducing hypertension and the risk of heart attacks.

In low fibre diets, evacuation is generally incomplete and the stools are relatively dry and hard, and form hard pellets which press on weak parts of the colon, causing it to pouch and bulge. The result is diverticulosis, diverticulitis and appendicitis. Moreover, the strain of evacuating hard stools greatly increases pressure on the surrounding veins, causing haemorrhoids. Veins are simply not designed to withstand pressures two to four times above normal, so they swell and form extremely painful outpouchings filled with blood.

Bran mania is fully justified. It should be noted, however, that when taking bran one should drink plenty of water to enable it to expand. Without adequate water bran can have the opposite effect, hardening stools and contributing to constipation. Bran may produce flatulence in some people but its advantages far outweigh the slight discomfort caused.

A diet rich in high fibre foods is one which contains plenty of raw fibrous vegetables such as celery, cabbage and carrots, fresh fruits and whole grain cereals, and bran supplements. Thorough chewing is essential to ensure optimal fibre function in the intestines and colon. Relying on bran alone to promote swift transit through the colon is not a good idea, since it absorbs zinc and potassium, which are then excreted in the stools.

POLLEN

Pollen is the yellowish dust produced by the anthers of male flowers. It is then transferred to the ovaries of female flowers by bees and other insects. Thus fertilized, the ovaries develop into seeds and fruits. Specific types of pollen are also collected by bees and taken to the hive to be stored for future use. Some of it serves as food for the bees themselves.

COMPOSITION

The composition of pollen varies according to the type of flower it comes from and the region where it grows. But whatever its source, pollen has a unique concentration of nutrients. It contains, on average, 30 per cent amino acids (protein), 50 per cent carbohydrates, 14 per cent polyunsaturated fats, a huge concentration of minerals and trace elements, and vitamins A, C, D, E, B complex and bioflavonoids. Its protein is complete, and weight for weight rates higher in essential amino acids than steak, eggs or cheese.[88] And pollen is the one plant food that contains vitamin B12 in meaningful amounts. All these ingredients, and other unidentified factors, make pollen an ideal food for strict vegetarians, for people always on the go, in fact for anybody who wants to improve his or her nutrition with a natural multi-vitamin and mineral supplement. According to a 1963 report of the Lee Foundation for Nutritional Research in Milwaukee: 'The composition and nutritional value of the collected pollen is so perfectly balanced that it represents a complete survival food by itself, provided it is extended by roughage and water.'

'MIRACULOUS' EFFECTS

In recent decades, pollen has become a source of interest to scientists as well as lay people. The findings are often fascinating. Dr Nicolai Tsitsin, a biologist and botanist with the Longevity Institute in the Soviet Union, discovered more than two decades ago that a large number of centenarian villagers in the state of Georgia ate daily amounts of 'dirty' honey from beehives, which was almost pure pollen. He was able to correlate pollen with longevity.[89] For a long time, pollen has been given to Russian athletes to improve their energy and endurance. Word spread to the West, where pollen repeated its great success. Fighter Mohammed Ali and sprinter Steve Riddick, a gold-medallist in the 1976 Olympics, took pollen. Tom McNab, senior coach with the British Olympic track team, is on record as saying, 'Bee pollen can spell the difference between mediocrity and greatness.'[90] He also found pollen to be a wonderful preventive against colds and flu. In fact, pollen has been found to fortify the body against virus infections,[91] relieve fatigue and increase appetite,[92] improve powers of concentration, increase sexual potency and fertility,[93] alleviate painful menstrual cramps and reduce the hot flashes of the menopause, and relieve headaches and palpitations.[94]

Pollen also has well-known effects on the prostate. A

group of German urologists, who treated 172 prostate sufferers for three months with pollen only, found that 44 per cent
of the group improved.[95]

Pollen has been reported to be an excellent cure for
burns and gangrene when applied externally in poultices or
dressings, or as a cream, or in combination with honey.[96]
Pollen also plays an important role in cosmetics. A prominent
New York physician associated with Bellevue Hospital, Dr
Louis Mucelli, says: '... Bee pollen has virtually all the vitamins, minerals, enzymes, amino acids and trace elements ...
needed for proper growth. So applying bee pollen cream to
your skin is essentially applying all the nutrients that the skin
requires. And this has a dramatic effect, as it will stimulate the
life of the cells and the result is that there is visible improvement in the texture and the youthful look of the skin.'[97]

ALLERGY

Pollen is believed to cause some of the allergic reactions of
hay fever, asthma and eczema. The truth is that wind-borne
pollens cause hay fever, but pollen gathered by bees seldom
provokes adverse reactions. In fact, bee pollen can reduce the
severity of hay fever attacks.[98] So when buying pollen, sensitive people should make sure the label says 'bee pollen'.

USAGE

In order to enjoy pollen's seemingly 'miraculous' effects, it
should be taken regularly for at least one month. Up to 20
grams a day is a normal food supplement, while 40 grams
constitute a therapeutic dose. Pollen is available as granulated
powder or tablets. Its taste varies depending on the flowers it
is derived from.

SPIRULINA

Spirulina is a blue-green, single-celled alga, microscopic in size and spiral in shape, hence its name. It thrives in warm alkaline lakes such as Lake Texcoco in Mexico and Lake Chad in Africa. To the Aztecs it was *tecuitlatl* and so highly valued as a sustaining food that it was used as a currency. Some writers have even attributed the vitality of the Aztecs to its high protein content, since animal foods were scarce.

Credit for the rediscovery of spirulina belongs to a Belgian botanist, Jean Léonard. When his survey team arrived at Lake Chad in 1964, Léonard noticed that the local tribesmen were collecting green scum from the lake, drying it into cakes and using it for food and trade. He found this dried scum to be highly nutritious and rich in protein. In 1967 a Japanese scientist who read Léonard's report about the African survey became so intrigued by the potential of spirulina as cheap source of high quality protein that he started researching its commercial possibilities. Today spirulina is widely used in Japan both as a food and a medicine. In the United States and Europe it is commonly sold as a dietary supplement.

COMPOSITION

Spirulina is 65 to 71 per cent complete protein, providing all the essential amino acids, a rarity among plant foods. This protein is so well-balanced that it is five times easier to digest than meat or soy protein.[99] Grown in alkaline waters, spirulina absorbs and retains an abundance of chelated minerals, chiefly potassium, calcium, zinc, magnesium, manganese, selenium, iron and phosphorus.[100]

Like pollen, spirulina is one of the rare plant foods which supplies usable amounts of vitamin B12. In addition, it contains vitamins A and E, essential fatty acids, and an array of enzymes that aid digestion. Another major constituent of spirulina is chlorophyll, known to detoxify the liver, soothe inflammations and prevent tooth decay. It is regarded by many as the most concentrated plant food in existence.

EFFECTS

Most studies of spirulina's effects on health have been done in Japan. They show that it has great rejuvenating effects and also that it produces substantial increases in energy in athletes. It also has a blood sugar stabilizing effect and can therefore help to control diabetes.[101] Anaemia responds to the B12, folic acid and chlorophyll content of spirulina, and so do liver disorders such as chronic hepatitis. One test showed that just 2 grams of spirulina a day helped to cure ulcers by coating the irritated stomach lining with chlorophyll.[102] Spirulina is praised by many nutritionists as a fasting aid. People who wish to fast, but are worried about nutritional deficiencies, can use spirulina tablets. To strict vegetarians, spirulina is pure 'manna', providing vitamin B12 and complete protein.[103] NOTE: Unlike ocean kelp, spirulina can be used in low sodium diets.

WEIGHT CONTROL

Dieters can also make use of spirulina. Its concentrated low calorie nourishment (2 calories per tablet) enters the blood quickly and raises the blood sugar level, preventing the hypothalamus in the brain from sending out hunger signals.[104] This is because the protein of spirulina contains a high proportion of the amino acid phenylalanine which is transformed into brain neurotransmitter substances which control appetite, alertness, energy level and mood. Not only is the appetite curbed but a state of well-being is maintained. By taking spirulina before a meal, dieters will find themselves eating less but adequately meeting their nutritional requirements. There is no need for starvation diets, extreme self-discipline or fasting. The common dosage is 3 tablets taken half an hour before each meal.

SAFETY
When spirulina started to be distributed on large scale, there were rumours about its safety. Anyone who still harbours doubts should remember that spirulina has been used as a sustaining food for centuries, long before the FDA approved it. Moreover, since spirulina is grown and harvested in unpolluted places, it is free of environmental contaminants, pesticides and other agricultural poisons. Spirulina can be used with a higher degree of safety than many common foods.

EVENING PRIMROSE OIL

Evening primrose is well-known for its beautiful white or yellow flowers, which bloom for one night only, withering the next day. Its healing effects have been known and used for many centuries. Certain American Indian tribes used extract of evening primrose to treat wounds and infections externally, and coughs and colds internally. Chief Two-Trees of the Cherokees reported that evening primrose was used as a sedative and diuretic.

Today, the evening primrose is known principally for the fantastic effects of its oil. This is made from the seeds and has been shown to have the following effects: inducing weight loss without dieting; lowering cholesterol levels and blood pressure; alleviating arthritis; healing or improving eczema; ameliorating acne (with zinc); calming hyperactive children;

strengthening fingernails; and dispelling hangovers.[105] In animals, evening primrose oil has been found to slow down the growth of cancerous tumours and prevent arthritis.

COMPOSITION

Recent research into the chemistry of essential fatty acids has led to an understanding of how evening primrose oil functions in the body and why it achieves impressive results in seemingly unrelated conditions. The 'secret' lies in one of its ingredients, the essential fatty acid gamma linolenic acid (GLA), of which evening primrose oil one of the richest known sources (9 per cent). GLA is the starting point for the synthesis of hormone-like compounds called prostaglandins (PGs). These compounds stimulate and control various functions in all body organs and deficiencies have been reported to cause conditions such as heart attacks and hypertension, arthritis, menstrual cramps, allergies, asthma, migraines, infertility, glaucoma and perhaps cancer.[106] Different types of PGs not only have diverse effects, but sometimes contrasting ones. PGE_1 and PGE_2, for example have opposing actions. PGE_1 inhibits blood clotting and increases urination, while PGE_2 accelerates blood clotting and increases water retention. Proper ratios of opposing PGs are therefore essential to maintaining optimal functioning of various body processes. Lack of specific PGs will cause imbalances and lead to many and varied disorders.

Babies are protected naturally. Human breast milk is one of the richest natural sources of GLA and provides babies with the equivalent of three capsules of evening primrose oil a day.

Until a few years ago, scientists believed that humans could synthesize GLA from linoleic acid in food. Then it was discovered that GLA can only be synthesized from a specific form of linoleic acid, cis-linoleic acid (cLA), provided it is not blocked by another fatty acid, translinoleic acid (tLA). Margarine and refined oils inhibit the formation of adequate GLA because they are high in tLA and low in cLA. Other obstacles to GLA production are vitamin B6, zinc, manganese and insulin deficiencies, alcohol consumption, diabetes, infections, and radiation, even from a colour TV set. Age is also a negative factor – the older we get, the less GLA we synthesize.

Modern lifestyles and eating habits are not conducive to the synthesis of GLA and prostaglandins, so it makes sense to take evening primrose oil. It is the best guarantee of an adequate supply of GLA, and is the only oil which contains 9 per cent GLA, in addition to 73 per cent cLA and only 18 per cent of the blocking fatty acid tLA. Other popular kitchen oils lag way behind in this respect. Soybean oil for example, generally contains 43 per cent tLA, 51 per cent cLA and no GLA at all.[107]

WEIGHT LOSS

Dr David Horrobin of the Institute for Innovative Medicine in Montreal has conducted many studies with evening primrose oil, GLA and prostaglandins.[108] He has found that evening primrose oil can help obese individuals with metabolic problems to lose weight. Usually such people find it hard to lose weight even when dieting properly. Almost 50 per cent of a group of volunteers who were more than 10 per cent overweight lost weight *without any dieting* when taking supplements of evening primrose oil.[109]

Two reasons were put forward. First, special prostaglandins derived from evening primrose oil activate a dormant type of body fat (brown fat) and signal it to burn calories more quickly. Second, other evening primrose oil-derived prostaglandins improve the expulsion of sodium from body cells. This internal activity normally consumes about 20 per cent of the body's energy, so any improvement in efficiency will burn more calories without any physical effort. In one study, in which sodium expulsion was improved by 60 per cent, weight losses of 18 to 22 pounds were observed in six weeks.

OVERCOMING IRRITABLE BOWEL SYNDROME

For many years, sufferers with digestive pains, intestinal gas and bouts of diarrhoea (irritable bowel syndrome or IBS), were assured that their problems stemmed from stress. The possibility of food allergy was usually dismissed by doctors when blood tests failed to show the reactions typical of allergy. Nevertherless, many patients have found that they can reduce the severity and frequency of their symptoms, or even eliminate them altogether, just by avoiding certain foods, and recent studies have shown why. Such people tend to over-produce PGE_2 after eating, and high levels of PGE_2 are closely linked with inflammation of the digestive tract (and mouth), periodontal disease and premenstrual syndrome, among other mischiefs. In fact, the anti-inflammatory effects of aspirin are believed to be due to its ability to suppress the activity of PGE_2. However, many practitioners are reluctant to prescribe aspirin for irritable bowel syndrome, understandably, because aspirin can be a gastric irritant. A better course of action would be to raise the level of PGE_1, which has an opposite effect to PGE_2. Evening primrose oil is one of the richest sources of GLA, from which PGE_1 is synthesized in the body. It is therefore increasingly used by nutritionists to treat irritable bowel syndrome. Those who find evening primrose oil allergy-causing or too expensive, could try linseed oil instead. Linseed oil is rich in linoleic acid, the starting point for both GLA and PGE$_1$ synthesis.

ADDITIONAL EFFECTS

Evening primrose oil has also been found to promote the production of PGI$_2$, a prostaglandin which inhibits clot formation in healthy arteries (vitamin E also protects PGI$_2$ synthesis[110]). Another prostaglandin derived from evening primrose oil GLA, PGI$_1$, has been reported to prevent excessive release of arachidonic acid, a precursor of a group of substances known as leukotrienes. These are the substances which cause the red, swollen, aching joints of rheumatoid arthritis and also painful breast lumps. In trials, PGI$_1$ effectively controlled rheumatoid arthritis in a number of patients.[111]

Certain prostaglandins stimulated by evening primrose oil increase the formation of antibodies against cancer.[112] Antibodies are the body's last line of defence against cancer, after the liver, which detoxifies carcinogens, and the membranes of cells themselves, which prevent the entry of carcinogens. Everyone forms cancer cells many times during their lifetime, but when the immune system is functioning properly, T-suppressor cells from the thymus gland, which supervise immune response, identify cancerous cells as they form and instruct antibodies to kill them. PGI$_1$ is particularly potent in inducing the production of antibodies which kill cancer cells.[113]

Other prostaglandins have been reported as beneficial in schizophrenia,[114] multiple sclerosis,[115] hyperactivity in children,[116] alcoholism,[117] and in diabetes, where PGE$_1$ increases insulin production by improving zinc absorption.[118]

Evening primrose oil was found helpful in relieving women from the discomforting symptoms of premenstrual syndrome (PMS). Feelings of exhaustion, nervousness, irritability, mood swings, tender breasts, abdominal bloating, cramping and weight fluctuations, are only some of the symptoms that plague 73 per cent of women of childbearing age before menstruation. Women who suffered from painful menstruation, depression and headaches, reported that evening primrose oil reduced or stopped these symptoms altogether, especially when taken with vitamins B6 and E.[119] In 1981, in a study done in St. Thomas Hospital in London, 65 women suffering from severe symptoms of PMS were treated with evening primrose oil (Efamol) only. These women were chosen because they had previously tried all types of drugs, hormones, tranquillizers etc. and none had worked. After treatment with evening primrose oil, the results were as follows: 61 per cent had complete relief; 23 per cent partial relief; 15 per cent no change. Breast discomfort responded particularly well, 72 per cent improvement.[120]

USAGE

The average dosage of evening primrose oil is up to a maximum of 1000 mg a day. This amount is mostly taken in two 500 mg capsules, one in the morning and one in the evening. Some feel its benefits with 500 mg a day, and each person has to find the best individual dosage by trial, starting with lower dosages and working up. The results are usually felt within six weeks. NOTE: Evening primrose oil is a safe nutrient, but some people may have an intolerance to it and react with diarrhoea. If this happens, or if you are the sort of person who tends to get headaches from alcohol, take instead blackcurrant oil capsules ('glanolin'), or starflower (borage) oil capsules. These oils, particularly the starflower oil, are higher in GLA content than evening primrose oil. Therefore, a smaller capsule will contain more GLA.

CHLORELLA

Chlorella is a green, freshwater alga which has only recently appeared on the health food market in the West. It is the richest known natural source of chlorophyll, containing 50 times more chlorophyll than alfalfa, hence its name.

Chlorella has been on this earth for at least 2.5 billion years. That it has survived for such an amazing length of time is thought to be due to its strong cell wall and its unusually effective DNA repair mechanism.[121] Although discovered and named by science in 1890, it was not until 1977, when a method was found of breaking down the hard cell wall and making it digestible, that its potential as a health food began to be exploited. Chlorella is now the largest-selling health food in Japan, where it is used both as a nutrient and as a medicine. In 1981 the *Taiwan Medical Science Journal* reported: 'Chlorella has been found to be not only eligible for food, but also effective in treatment and prevention of disease.'

COMPOSITION

About 60 per cent of chlorella is protein (soybeans are only 30 per cent protein). About 20 per cent consists of carbohydrates and 10 per cent of fats. The protein of chlorella contains 19 amino acids, including all the essential ones. It is therefore on a par with animal protein, except that it contains less methionine. However, this can be an advantage in some forms of cancer which depend on methionine for growth. Chlorella is especially rich in lysine, the amino acid lacking in high wheat diets. Because of the quality of its protein, chlorella is now being used as a high protein supplement in weight control diets.[122]

Chlorella also contains more than 20 different vitamins and minerals. It provides, for example, an abundance of beta

-carotene (provitamin A), which combats ultraviolet radiation damage to the skin and prevents lung cancer, and also appreciable amounts of iron, iodine, zinc and cobalt. In fact it contains more B12 than even beef liver and is an excellent, lean source of this vitamin, so often lacking in strict vegetarian diets. Finally, as well as being the richest natural source of chlorophyll, it is also the richest natural source of DNA.

Only some of chlorella's great properties in promoting health and treating disease are cited in the pages which follow. The conditions and symptoms mentioned are by no means the only ones that can benefit from regular use of chlorella. As research continues, new effects will come to light.

EFFECTS

A review of the scientific literature shows that four of the constituents of chlorella have specific health-giving effects: chlorophyll, beta-carotene, chlorella growth factor (CGF), and the cell walls themselves.

There are considerable differences between the effects of chlorella and spirulina, which is also a green alga. Chlorella contains four times more chlorophyll and ten times more iron than spirulina, but that is not all. Chlorella contains many additional factors, such as CGF and cell wall. In fact, spirulina is a much more primitive organism than chlorella and lacks a true nucleus. The result is a higher quality of DNA and RNA in chlorella.

THE BENEFITS OF CHLOROPHYLL

Chlorophyll is an interesting substance with various commercial and therapeutic applications. It is widely used in colouring foods and cosmetics, for example. Its chemical structure is similar to that of haemoglobin (the red blood pigment which carries oxygen), which is why it is used in the treatment of certain anaemias. If neither iron nor copper is lacking, then chlorophyll or its derivatives can promote the formation of red blood cells.[123]

A number of studies have demonstrated that chlorophyll can influence growth, metabolism and respiration. Its ability to stimulate tissue growth was demonstrated as far back as 1930.[124] By 1938, in experiments with artificially inflicted wounds on rabbits and guinea pigs, chlorophyll had been found to stimulate wound healing.[125] In 1943, physicians in New York successfully used chlorophyll ointment to treat skin ulcers.[126] Injected chlorophyll has been found to promote the excretion of free cholesterol from the body, [127] which explains why chlorella has a cholesterol lowering effect. Finally, chlorophyll has a long history as a detoxifier and deodorizer – a common brand of chewing gum for bad breath contains chlorophyll.

CHLORELLA AND CANCER

The immune system defends the body against foreign invaders such as bacteria, viruses and pollutants. Inactivating or detoxifying these substances is done by special white blood cells, by B-cells from the bone-marrow, which form antibodies and fight bacteria, by T-cells from the thymus gland, which fight viruses, and by macrophages, which 'phagocytize' (engulf and kill) harmful substances and cancer cells. One way to fight cancer is therefore to stimulate macrophage production. Interferon, a substance produced by immune cells, stimulates macrophage production and therefore has potent anti-viral and anti-cancer activity, and chlorella is a known stimulator of interferon production. Chlorella injections have been found to stimulate the immune system and detoxify the blood within 72 hours.[128]

A glycoprotein extracted from chlorella was found to have an anti-tumour effect against sarcoma 180 (a type of cancer which occurs in muscles or bones) and also against mouse leukaemia in culture.[129] Hot water extracts of chlorella also inhibited the growth of certain induced types of cancer (fibrosarcomas) in mice when injected into the tumour or surrounding tissue.[130] Other studies with chlorella have shown its activity against breast cancer and liver cancer in mice when given orally or injected into the abdomen.[131]

OTHER EFFECTS

Removing toxins from the body is of the utmost importance in preventing disease, and chlorella has been shown to have remarkable detoxifying capabilities due to its unique cell wall.[132] A very efficient method of cleansing and rejuvenating the body is fasting with chlorella. With its poison–absorbing properties, chlorella can enhance the purifying effects of fasting. Being such a comprehensive food, it can also be used safely in crash diets or fasting to lose weight.

Chlorella is also effective against hypertension and fatigue.[133] In many cases, blood pressure problems disappeared after taking chlorella for periods ranging from three to twelve months.[134]

Diabetic ulcers are often difficult to heal, especially when they are infected. This is why anyone with diabetic ulcers should be under strict medical supervision. However, the empirical use of chlorella and honey has been reported to have definite healing power in such cases, no doubt partly due to CGF). Research is currently being undertaken to substantiate this claim.

The chlorophyll in chlorella has also been found to provide relief from chronic constipation and intestinal gas in about 85 per cent of people tested.[135] Chlorella is now being studied for its effects on the liver, and on allergies, acne, warts and arthritis. Good results are anticipated.

USAGE
Chlorella can be taken alone or with medication. Sometimes intestinal gas is produced and released due to brisker intestinal action, but this usually stops once the intestines have been cleansed. Stools may become greenish in colour, a sign that excess chlorophyll is being excreted. This is quite normal.

Chlorella is non-toxic. However, excessive intake (300 tablets a day or 60 grams for a period of many months, which is most improbable) may cause vitamin A toxicity. In a study performed by the Huntington Research Centre in England, no toxicity was found even with extremely high doses of chlorella.[136]

MELATONIN
The natural sleeping pill
of the nineties

Melatonin has swept the early 1990s with great intensity. First found to enhance sleep, it cheered the 20 million insomniacs in America, especially as they learned that melatonin is not a heavy-handed drug, but a natural, safe substance. Soon afterwards, it was revealed that melatonin can dramatically reduce the symptoms of travelling through different time zones.

Several newspapers and magazines covered the story, including the April 1994 issue of *The Condé Nast Traveler*, the bible of the jet set. The news about melatonin's ability to enhance sleep and relieve jet lag has earned it millions of fans. Twenty-four companies in the U.S. alone are selling the hormone with more coming along constantly.

Most people however, have no idea that melatonin was found to have many other beneficial roles, simply because many of these findings are so new that the ink has barely dried on the scientific reports.

WHAT IS MELATONIN?

Melatonin is a natural hormone produced mainly by the pineal gland, a tiny organ which is the size and shape of a kernel of corn, situated exactly at the centre of the brain. The pineal gland is the first gland to be formed in the body, but was the last to reveal its secrets. In fact, until a couple of decades ago, doctors believed that the pineal gland served no useful purpose in human beings.

Melatonin is also synthesized in other tissues, apart from the pineal gland.[137] It occurs widely in most life forms including one-celled algae and plants such as bananas, beets, cucumbers and tomatoes.[138]

Today, science is beginning to discover that the melatonin molecule has a lot of influence on our health and well-being. Not only does it improve the quality of sleep and relieve the symptoms of jet lag, but also counteracts stress, fights off viruses and bacteria, reduces the risk of heart disease. It may even protect against cancer and help determine how long we live.

Melatonin is made in the pineal gland by enzymes that are activated and depressed, respectively, by darkness and light. Release of the hormone follows a circadian (24-hour) rhythm. It rises and falls in a 24-hour pattern that is controlled by light. During the night (or in darkness) the activity of the pineal gland increases to produce and secrete more melatonin,[139] and during daytime (or in light) this activity is depressed.[140]

However, melatonin, it now appears is a powerful antioxidant. [141] That is, it is able to scavenge free radicals, those unstable molecules with unpaired electrons, which attack and destroy healthy cells, disable enzymes and corrupt the DNA's genetic code, causing disease and aging.

New studies showed that working as an antioxidant, melatonin can effectively prevent cancer by protecting DNA,[142] protect the body against X-ray radiation[143] and prevent cataracts.[144]

Our brain is the organ most susceptible to free radical damage because of its high concentration of fatty acids which are easily oxidized. And free radical damage is now considered to be at the root of brain disorders like Alzheimer's disease, multiple sclerosis and Parkinson's disease.[145] A good preventative method is to take oil-soluble antioxidants like vitamin E. In that respect, melatonin was found to be at least twice as effective as vitamin E.[146]

Boosting the immune system is the best way to prevent disease. A strong immune system can identify and destroy disease-causing organisms, before they develop into a disease. Melatonin was found to enhance the immune response, by increasing the number of natural killer (NK) cells which attack and destroy cancer cells and virus-infected cells,[147] and also, by producing more antibodies. [148]

Immunity is known to decrease with age. Older people have weaker immunity than younger people. Recent studies suggest that melatonin can better protect the immune system of older animals than younger animals.[149] These findings may give new hope for a reduced vulnerability to disease in old age.

In the scientific attempt to help women with breast cancer, studies suggest that when melatonin is combined with other therapies, patients live better and longer.[150]

Research offers hope for heart disease. In one study it was

found, that healthy people were producing five times as much melatonin as people with a diseased heart.[151] Melatonin was also found to lower high blood pressure,[152] and to reduce the tendency of platelets to form life-threatening blood clots that can occlude arteries by 85 per cent.[153]

Low levels of melatonin in the body were associated with depression.[154] There is also evidence that melatonin can help relieve the stressful symptoms of premenstrual syndrome (PMS).[155] This is no surprise, since melatonin is derived in the body from tryptophan, the calming amino acid. The pineal gland synthesizes melatonin by converting tryptophan to serotonin (a calming neurotransmitter) and then to melatonin. Therefore, eating more tryptophan-rich foods, increases production of melatonin.[156] Niacin (vitamin B3) and pyridoxine (vitamin B6) can also help increase melatonin production since they are both involved in the melatonin synthesis.

New studies are providing evidence that melatonin may help you live longer. In one experiment, a study group of animals treated with melatonin, lived 20 per cent longer than a control group.[157] Women were found to produce 25 per cent more melatonin than men.[158] No wonder that according to statistics, women outlive men.

Today's excitement at the scientific research is fully justified. It seems in the best interest of each one of us to retain our full share of melatonin. Apart from taking melatonin tablets and eating more melatonin-rich fruits and vegetables, L–Tryptophan rich foods, vitamins B3 and B6, a great importance is now attributed to our exposure to light during daytime.[159] Spending more time outdoors, walking, exercising or having lunch, is an ideal way to increase light exposure, provided the eyes are protected from ultra violet light by UV sunglasses.

Just as important, is to minimize light exposure at night,

particularly an hour before bedtime. Getting more sleep rewards you with a longer cycle of melatonin production, stimulating your immune system and contributing to a healthier and longer life. [160]

CAUTION: Melatonin should be best taken at bedtime, or prior to retiring. It must not be taken before active periods. A starting daily dose is considered to be 1 mg.

GLUCOSAMINE SULPHATE

This is a new and promising addition to the line of food supplements which is becoming increasingly popular. Studies performed with glucosamine sulphate, have shown its effectiveness in the treatment of osteoarthritis.[161]

Also known as degenerative joint disease, osteoarthritis is the most common form of arthritis, affecting millions of elderly people. The joints of knees and hands which are weight-bearing joints are most affected. Over the years, these joints sustain much cartilage destruction, followed by a hardening of joint margins, causing pain and a limitation of motion.

Glucosamine sulphate is a naturally occurring substance in joints. Its molecule is composed of glucose, an amine (nitrogen plus two molecules of hydrogen) and sulphur. Its main function in the body is to stimulate the growth of cartilage. It does this by serving as a building block for producing cartilage glycosaminoglycans (GAGs). Glucosamine sulphate also promotes the incorporation of sulphur into the cartilage.[162] That means that Glucosamine sulphate is not only necessary for joint function, but also for stimulating its repair.

It appears that glucosamine sulphate synthesis in the body declines with age in many people, as their cartilage loses its flexibility as a shock absorber. And glucosamine sulphate deficiency , it has been suggested, is the major factor in the onset of osteoarthritis.[163] This fact led scientists to experiment with glucosamine sulphate as a food supplement. The results were better than expected.[164]

Glucosamine sulphate was found to produce much better results than non-steroidal anti-inflammatory drugs like aspirin, ibuprofen and indomethacin.[165] These drugs only offer symptomatic relief but in fact inhibit cartilage repair.[166]

Studies have shown that glucosamine sulphate taken orally is very efficiently absorbed, and is preferentially taken up by cartilage where it stimulates production of chondroitin sulphate and other mucopolysaccharides.[167] This is why some researchers prefer glucosamine sulphate over other treatments: chondroitin sulphate, green-lipped mussel or even shark cartilage. In one large study in Portugal, with 1,758 people, a total of 95 per cent of the participants achieved benefits from glucosamine sulphate, which were rated as better than those obtained with other treatments including drugs, vitamins and cartilage extracts.[168]

Glucosamine sulphate is very well tolerated and there are no known contra-indications or adverse interaction with drugs.[169] In rare instances it may cause symptoms such as nausea or heartburn. In such cases, it is advised to take glucosamine sulphate with meals. The standard dose is 500 mg three times a day. Overweight people may need more, based on their body weight (20 mg per kg of body weight per day).

THE SOYA REVOLUTION

Soya bean, an ancient food staple in Asia, and one of the richest sources of vegetable protein, are quickly revolutionising eating habits in the West. Soya beans have developed into one of the world's major sources of vegetable oil and texturised vegetable protein (TVP), improving the healthfulness of foods. Soy sauces and ice cream, tofu and miso (soya bean curds), are used by more and more people who delve into the benefits of the macrobiotic diet. But the biggest craze of the 90s is that of the soya milk. The question arises, why are people moving away from dairy milk to soya milk?

One may think of the mad cow panic as a reason, and that the abusive way cows were treated with antibiotics, hormones, tranquillizers and sprays, could eventually have resulted in polluted milk. But dairy milk was gradually losing its status as the perfect food long before that. Dairy milk has been linked to iron deficiency anaemia in infants; identified as the cause for cramps, bloated stomach, intestinal gas, diarrhoea, allergies and possibly, as a contributing factor in causing atherosclerosis and heart attacks.[170] A recent study concluded that milk from cows injected with recombinant bovine growth hormone (rBGH) may increase the risk of breast and colon cancer in human beings.[171]

In fact, so great was the concern of doctors about the potential hazards of dairy milk, that the Committee on Nutrition of the prestigious American Academy of Pediatrics, released a report entitled, 'Should Milk Drinking by Children be Discouraged?'[172]

Another pitfall is the digestion of milk sugar, lactose. To break down lactose into simpler sugars which the body can use, we all need an enzyme called lactase. Without enough lactase enzyme, lactose ferments in the colon producing gas

(C02) and water, causing a sense of bloating, belching and diarrhoea.[173] In a survey of a population of healthy adults, a high incidence of lactase deficiency in various nations was detected, ranging from 7 per cent in the Swiss, up to 90 per cent in the Philippinos. [174]

Soya milk has none of these problems. Not only is it highly nutritious, rich in vitamins and minerals, but scientific studies have shown soya's great protective effects against cancer, heart attacks and other degenerative diseases of civilization.

The benefits of soya beans are related to their high content of phytochemicals. These compounds, found in vegetables and fruit, are not nutrients, but do affect health. Many such phytochemicals have been researched and found to show anticancer activity.[175] Soya contains several compounds found to reduce cancer risk.

A protein in soya called protease inhibitor, was shown in several studies to inhibit breast cancer by 50 per cent,[176] as well as colon cancer,[177] lung cancer [178] and others. Soya beans are also high in phytates, the form of phosphorus which is stored in the body. These phytates were found to play a role not only in preventing cancer, but also in providing protection from heart disease.[179]

Soya beans contain several antioxidants, which protect us from the damage of free radicals, like, phytosterols, saponins and phenolic acids. And they all have anticancer effects. One type of phytosterol reduced the development of colon cancer by 50 per cent.[180] Another report indicated that when saponins were mixed together with HIV virus, the virus stopped growing.[181] But the best anticarcinogens in soya beans are its bitter-tasting pigments, the isoflavones. These are types of phytoestrogens (plant oestrogens) which act like weak oestrogens. The isoflavones effectively inhibit the action of oestrogen in the body by hooking into the normal estrogen receptors, blocking them, and hence, prevent oestrogen from doing its job. [182] Although oestrogen is needed for various physiological functions, high levels of it are known to increase the risk of breast cancer.

Soya isoflavones were found to be effective against a wider range of cancer. In 1986, the main isoflavone in soya beans, genistein, was shown to have strong anti-cancer effect. When genistein was added to cells growing in a test tube, it inhibited the growth of cancer cells but not of normal cells.[183]

Soya beans have also been shown to have beneficial effects in reducing cholesterol levels and preventing heart disease, which is still the number one killer in the West. High cholesterol levels, atherosclerosis (hardening of the arteries) and heart attacks are now considered to develop mainly due to high protein, meat centred diets. [184] In contrast, the consumption of soya protein was found to significantly reduce total cholesterol levels and triglycerides.[185]

A LITTLE SOYA IS ALL YOU NEED!

In most studies with soya, all animal protein was replaced by soya protein. But what if we only keep our dietary habits and only add some soya product to our diet. Will it work? The answer is yes. In one Japanese study, merely adding a small daily serving of just 20 grams of soya protein to the diet, without any other changes, caused cholesterol levels to drop.[186]

It therefore stands to reason, that regular use of soya milk, soya ice cream, miso, tofu or TVP (texturized vegetable Protein), even in small amounts, can be very beneficial.

OLIVE TREE LEAVES
(Olea Europaea L)

For thousands of years the olive tree was highly regarded traditionally. The bible referred to it as the 'tree of Life'. And indeed, nowadays, it is rediscovered as a health-restoring, anti-viral and anti-bacterial boon to mankind.

As far back as 1855, information started to spread that drinking bitter tea brewed from olive tree leaves, was a potential cure for malaria. Olive leaves were boiled in water and the solution given to malaria patients. Doctors reported of their patients' improvement.

Later on, the active anti-bacterial ingredient in the olive leaves was isolated. It was a phenolic compound, oleuropein. This is a bitter glucoside which imparts bitterness to olives.[187] According to botanists, oleuropein is distributed throughout the olive tree, and protects it against insects and bacteria.[188]

Elenolate, a derivative of oleuropein, was tested for its anti-viral activity on several viruses, and was found to inhibit the growth of every virus it was tested against.[189]

Of its anti-bacterial properties, olive leaf extract was found effective against bacillus cereus, a tough, heat-resisting germ which can cause food poisoning, as from eating re-heated food.[190] The phenolic components of the leaf extract were associated with the inhibition of two types of fermentative bacteria.[191] This, by the way, is the reason olives are cracked before pickling (with lactic acid) to remove oleuropein, since oleuropein has a strong antimicrobial effect which inhibits fermentation.[192]

Dr Donald Gay from Ontario, Canada, uses olive leaf extract successfully for chronic fatigue and immune depression syndrome (the downhill syndrome). Says Dr Gay, 'My observation is that chronic fatigue patients have an impaired immune function leading to assorted infections with viruses and bacteria...' 'What's needed is something that rids the involved person of bacterial and viral infections, and now I have found the appropriate compound. I see that olive extract does very well for patients suffering from these incidental infections.' Dr Gay also recommends the extract against sore throats, coughs and chronic sinus problems. Dr Gay uses the powdered extract supplied by Dr Stephen Levine.

Oleuropein was found effective as an antioxidant, protecting cholesterol from oxidation[193] and lowering the risk of coronary heart disease.[194] Since oxidized cholesterol is more likely to be deposited on the inner walls of blood vessels, it clogs them, gradually blocking the blood flow, eventually causing high blood pressure and an increased risk of heart attack.

From San Mateo, California, Dr Bernard Friedlander, chiropractor, reports about olive leaf extract as a potential treatment against herpes virus II (herpes genitalis) and other conditions ranging from psoriasis to the common cold.

Presently, the only source of olive leaf extract known to the author are powder capsules developed by the research biochemist Dr Stephen Levine, through a special process that ensures the effectivity of the extract. These capsules are available through his Allergy Research Group in San Leandro, California.

GREEN TEA:
More than just a soothing brew a rediscovered health drink

Black tea is a widely consumed traditional beverage. However, the early 90s have seen a huge surge of scientific research on Green Tea. Consequently, exciting claims started to spread. Claims that green tea can reduce the risk of cancer and protect the body against heart attacks, to name only two, served to boost the popularity of green tea in the U.S. and other Western countries.

Since ancient times, tea drinking has been held in high esteem in Asian countries. It was traditionally thought to help keep the body and soul in good health with its soothing effects. The Japanese tea ritual in proposing marriage is well known.

At some point, scientists observed both the Japanese preference for green tea drinking and the reduced cancer rate in Japan. They decided to investigate a possible correlation between the two.

And indeed, as scientific research on tea progressed, many studies linked the various traditional effects of green tea to its specific components. Green tea has been found to contain catechins, which are types of polyphenols, or 'tea tannins', a group of substances with antioxidant and anticarcinogenic (anti cancer-causing) properties. It is these tea tannins that give green tea its astringent taste.

Green tea is made from the same plant as the black tea, Camellia Sinensis, commonly consumed in Western countries. However, green tea is not processed. It is not allowed to ferment after harvest before drying, as black tea. Therefore, it retains high amounts of catechins, 30 to 42 per cent, compared to 3-10 per cent in black tea.

Light processing converts it to Chinese Oolong tea, and more extensive processing produces common black tea. It is during this fermentation that the catechins are oxidized and destroyed in black tea.

In the 90s however, most of the research focused on green tea – the richest in catechin polyphenols. A study with 902 patients, published in the *Journal of the National Cancer Institute* in 1994, reported that green tea provided a protection against oesophageal cancer, and also, that 'green tea has been reported to block the formation of tumours arising in the skin, lung, forestomach, small intestine, colon, liver, pancreas and mammary gland'. [195]

Other studies confirmed the ability of green tea in reducing cholesterol levels,[196] and in preventing oxidative damage to liver and kidney.[197] Research carried out in a Japanese hospital, with a group of volunteers, found that green tea catechins 'significantly' lowered the blood pressure.[198] David Steinman, author of *Diet For a Poisoned Planet* (Ballantine 1992), reports in *Natural Health*, about Japanese studies claiming, that green tea also fights viral colds and flu, and prevents gum disease, cavities and bad breath.[199] Green tea bags are now readily available in health food shops. To reap their benefits it is recommended to drink between 3 and 5 cups a day.

DHEA
The key to health

Although DHEA was known for 50 years, it is only in the last decade that most studies revealed its diverse physiological and biochemical action. Research showed that it is the single most important compound in the body which can determine health or disease. No wonder that it is now being manufactured and sold as a supplement in health food stores.

DHEA (dehydroepiandrosterone) is a most abundant hormone in humans and mammals and is manufactured in the body from cholesterol. However, as cholesterol levels tend to increase with age, DHEA levels tend to decline. Its decline signals age-related diseases. Indeed, DHEA was found deficient in people with major diseases, like diabetes,[200] high blood pressure,[201] coronary heart disease,[202] various cancers[203] and even obesity.[204] DHEA is vitally important in the body for the production of principal hormones, such as oestrogen and testosterone.

Stress is the underlying cause in all diseases. DHEA levels were found to decrease particularly during stress periods, whether physical or emotional. That means, that the body uses up DHEA to combat stress. One of the main factors determining the intensity and duration of stress is cortisol. This is a hormone secreted by the adrenal gland during stress, which elevates blood sugar levels, causing the release of insulin to burn extra glucose. Irregular glucose–insulin response is a stress reaction. DHEA appears to be a major modulator of stress reaction by regulating increased cortisol levels,[205] and at least in animals, it was also found to reduce anxiety.[206] In patients with major depression, DHEA was reported to act as a powerful antidepressant and cognition enhancer, having a beneficial effect with low doses of 30-90 mg a day. [207]

DHEA was found helpful in various diseases. In the early stages of adult onset diabetes, DHEA increased sensitivity to insulin and reduced blood sugar levels to normal.[208] Dr Barrett-Connor of the San Diego School of Medicine found that DHEA lowers the production of fatty acids and cholesterol by inhibiting an enzyme that triggers their production. This of course can benefit cases of obesity and atherosclerosis. In a study done with 242 men aged 50-79 for twelve years, increased levels of DHEA were connected to a 48 per cent reduction in cardiovascular disease and 36 per cent reduction in mortality from any cause.[209] In a study with 5,000 women, the highest risk of breast cancer was linked with low levels of DHEA.[210]

DHEA blood levels are easily measured with a simple blood test. For anyone who is considering DHEA supplementation during an illness, the optimal level of DHEA in the body is considered to be 750ng/dL or above for men, 550 ng/dL or above in women.

Apart from supplementation, DHEA levels were reported to increase naturally in the body with physical exercise,[211] calorie restriction[212] and transcendental meditation.[213] This reconfirms the known truths, that regular exercise, moderate eating and relaxation contribute to our health and well-being.

THE HEALING CARTILAGE

Cartilage capsules became popular, especially after the publication of Dr William Lane's book *Sharks Don't Get Cancer*. Sharks have long been known for their high resistance to disease and remarkable wound-healing abilities. These unique qualities have been attributed to a complex protein-carbohydrate substance found in the shark's skeleton, called glycosaminoglycans. Unlike other vertebrates, the shark's skeleton is composed entirely from cartilage protein, which makes up 6 to 8 per cent of the shark's total weight. Complex carbohydrate molecules, known as mucopolysaccharides, are attached to the cartilage, giving the shark great strength, flexibility and resistance.

Studies have shown that both mucopolysaccharides and glycosaminoglycans in shark cartilage have a strong anti-inflammatory effect.[214] Also, that shark cartilage can contribute additional strength and flexibility to joints.[215] As far as cancer is concerned, shark cartilage was shown to inhibit the growth of malignant tumours. It was found to promote antiangiogenesis, that is, to inhibit formation of new blood vessels. And with impaired blood flow, tumour growth is inhibited.[216]

Recently, however, attention has focused on bovine cartilage. It now appears that most studies were done with bovine cartilage. It all started back in 1954, when Dr John F. Prudden, associate professor of Clinical Surgery at Columbia Presbyterian Medical Center, discovered that cartilage taken from bovine tracheal rings can promote wound healing.[217] During this study Dr Prudden was amazed to observe a dramatic shrinkage in the tumour of a breast cancer patient. This discovery let to further studies with other cancer patients. Since these initial discoveries, more than $7 million have been invested in clinical research under the direction of Dr Prudden. Bovine cartilage preparations were studied for their effect in the treatment of arthritis, rheumatism, skin allergies and acceleration of wound healing.[218]

The effectiveness of bovine cartilage in the treatment of cancer was established in extensive human studies.[219] Dr Prudden showed that bovine cartilage stimulated the immune system by activating macrophages (which devour cancer cells). It also increased the number of T cells and B cells, 'soldiers' of the immune system, creating more immunoglobulins which inhibited tumour growth.[220] Another cancer study by Dr Brian Durie demonstrated the ability of bovine cartilage to inhibit cell division, i.e., to repress the growth of tumours, in several kinds of cancer, like, ovarian, pancreatic and colon cancers.[221]

It was repeatedly shown that while it takes 9 grams of bovine cartilage to produce therapeutic effects, it requires 70 grams of shark cartilage to reach threapeutic levels.[222] Another disadvantage of shark cartilage is its high content of calcium: 22 per cent. A therapeutic daily dose of 70 grams shark cartilage means taking 14 grams of calcium. This is an excessive dose of 14 times the daily allowance, whereas bovine cartilage has less than 1 per cent calcium. Bovine cartilage is also high in chondroitin sulphate, a mucopolyssacharide which removes excess calcium from the body. Chondroitin sulphate is also anti-thrombogenic: it was shown to reduce the risk of heart attacks by inhibiting arteriosclerosis.[223]

More information on the applications of bovine cartilage can be obtained from:

The Foundation for Cartilage and Immunology Research
104 Post Office Road
Waccabuc
New York 10597
U.S.A.

CREATINE

A new dietary supplement, creatine recently caused great excitement among athletes when studies showed its ability to improve athletic performance. It was first used by British and American field and track atheletes around 1992 and its use has since spread to the rest of the sporting world.

Creatine is not a steroid or drug. it is a natural chemical

that is made in the body from three amino acids: arginine, methionine and glycine. It is mainly stored in the muscles as phosphocreatine, the precursor of ATP, the body's primary energy chemical. Creatine is part of a system that supplies energy, and creatine supplements, especially when taken with some carbohydrate, can increase energy and exercise performance. "Creatine loading" of muscles boosts muscle mass building voluminous muscles, which is a great boon to body builders. It also increases energy, endurance and power, and can reduce muscle soreness, enabling an increase in the frequency of exercise.

The richest sources of creatine are meat and fish, especially beef and salmon, which each contain 2 grams per pound. Typically, about 2 grams a day are synthesized by the body and an additional 2 grams can come from food metabolism. To increase sport performance, creatine supplements are usually taken in 5 gram doses, one to four times a day, depending on whether the athlete is starting to load the muscles with creatine or just maintaining its level. Creatine absorption is greatly improved when taken with high insulin-releasing, sugary carbohydrates, such as grape juice. Vegetarians usually have a low intake of creatine.

CHAPTER 6

SUPPLEMENTATION:
GOOD, BAD, OR IRRELEVANT?

Nutritional supplementation is becoming increasingly popular. More and more people are sweeping health food stores and pharmacies, looking for vitamins.

According to a new report in the *OTC foresight* series (from IMS' Self Medication International unit), the worldwide market for supplements in 1995 was estimated to be $5 billion (in ex-manufacturer' prices). This market is set to grow annually by an average compound rate of 8.1 per cent to reach a value of $6.4 billion by 1999.

What is this supplement rush all about? Food supplements include all the vital nutrients, such as vitamins, minerals, trace elements and amino acids, as well as health foods like brewer's yeast, wheat germ oil, spirulina, and so on.

WHAT IS NUTRITIONAL SUPPLEMENTATION?

The purpose of nutritional supplementation is to provide the body with all those nutrients not obtained in adequate amounts from daily food intake and which are important for health. Today it is accepted that people who eat optimally supplemented diets are less susceptible to disease and less affected by pollutants than people whose diet philosophy is 'anything goes'.[1]

Why do people with seemingly sensible eating habits need to supplement their diet at all? First, not all vitamin and mineral needs can be satisfied by food alone.[2] Many people have such high requirements for certain nutrients that no diet could supply them all. This may be due to inborn quirks or errors of metabolism – hereditary conditions present at conception and caused by a faulty or missing gene – or due to congenital defects acquired during development in the uterus of a stressed or malnourished mother. These handicaps are reflected in defective enzyme systems which inhibit absorption and assimilation. Food does not yield all the nutrients it contains if, for example, certain gastric juices are in short supply. Alternatively, if the body uses certain nutrients at an extremely accelerated rate in order to overcome a stressful condition, this also will create a high requirement for those nutrients which cannot be satisfied by food alone. Some schizophrenics, for example, excrete up to ten times more vitamin C in their urine than normal people do,[3] which explains why massive vitamin C supplementation can have a therapeutic effect in some cases.

Many people suffer from chronic fatigue, poor memory and depression for years, not realizing that congenitally low secretion of intrinsic factor by the stomach is inhibiting the absorption of vitamin B12 from their food. A lack of B12 causes precisely these deficiency symptoms. Such individuals will not be able to satisfy their need for B12 from food alone, even by eating to bursting point. Massive supplementation of vitamin B12 will be necessary if they want to feel well.

Metabolic defects, stress conditions and faulty eating habits all contribute to higher nutrient requirements. So do contaminated air and water, smoking (which depletes vitamin C), alcohol (which depletes zinc and magnesium) and oral contraceptives (which deplete vitamin B6, vitamin C and zinc).

Every person is different not only in lifestyle and eating habits, but also in body chemistry. So each individual must determine what nutrients are deficient in his or her diet by carefully noting specific symptoms. This is normally done by consulting a nutritional therapist and by experimenting with different nutrients and their effects.

DEFICIENT AND DANGEROUS FOODS

Of course, everything would be easier if we could satisfy all our requirements just by sensible eating and a little common sense in choosing foods. However, very few people are capable of this. Most of us eat to satisfy our taste buds rather than our nutritional needs.

A hundred years ago it was much simpler. All produce was grown on compost-fertilized soils, with no chemical sprays. Chemical additives had yet to be invented. Vegetables and fruits were eaten ripe, fresh and in season, at the peak of their nutritional value. Refrigerated transport and storage, which lead to vitamin loss, were still in the future. All flours were stone ground, and white sugar was so expensive that few people could afford it.

There is no doubt that our food today is very inferior in nutritional value. This is mainly due to intensive farming which depletes the soil. In 1940, for example, Kansas wheat contained as much as 17 per cent protein. By 1951, only 11 years later, the best Kansas wheat had no more than 14 per cent protein, while most other wheats contained only 11 to 12 per cent.[4]

The dramatic increase in life expectancy since the turn of century, which is sometimes put forward as 'proof' that the modern diet is highly nutritious, has little to do with nutrition. Life expectancy is longer because more children are surviving into adulthood due to antibiotics, immunization and better sanitation.

Today, fields are sprayed with toxic herbicides, pesticides and fungicides – convenience foods contain the residues of many toxins. Cereals and sugars are stripped of their nutrients. The practice of eating fruits and vegetables out of season has led to fruits being picked before they ripen; this ensures that they do not spoil before they reach the supermarket and that they last a long time on the shelf, but they have only a fraction of their peak nutritional value. Animals are injected with antibiotics and hormones, and meats are kept fresh with nitrates and nitrites, which are converted in the body to cancer-causing substances called nitrosamines. Freezing, preserving and processing destroy many nutrients. To quote the distinguished nutritionist Robert Rodale: 'To believe that food sold in supermarkets can build health is a dangerous illusion.'[5]

WE DON'T EAT ENOUGH VEGGIES
The US Government takes action

Due to our reliance on convenience foods, most of the Western population, mainly in the U.S. and U.K, eat too much fat and too little fruit, vegetables and whole grains. We are overfed but undernourished. As a result, we are plagued by many degenerative diseases of aging not found in those countries where consumption of fruit and vegetables are much higher.

In 1992, new Dietary Guidelines were issued by the U.S. Department of Agriculture (USDA), recommending increased consumption of fruits, vegetables and grains. In addition, the USDA revised their former dietary guidelines by replacing the Basic Four Food Groups (which promoted a diet rich in fatty milk and beef products) with the new Food Pyramid, reflecting a need for increased consumption of vegetables, fruit and fibre (below).

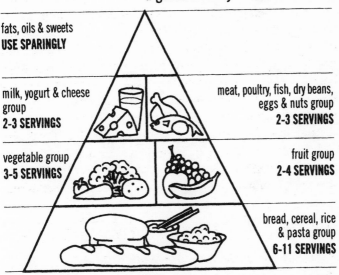

FOOD GUIDE PYRAMID
a guide to daily food choices

fats, oils & sweets
USE SPARINGLY

milk, yogurt & cheese group
2-3 SERVINGS

meat, poultry, fish, dry beans, eggs & nuts group
2-3 SERVINGS

vegetable group
3-5 SERVINGS

fruit group
2-4 SERVINGS

bread, cereal, rice & pasta group
6-11 SERVINGS

Do you eat five servings of vegetables and three servings of fruit every single day?

In order to meet the new USDA guidelines, you would have to eat, as an example, 1 apple, 1 banana, 1 orange, 4 ounces of broccoli, 4 ounces of brussel sprouts, 4 ounces of cauliflower and 4 ounces of spinach each day.

Few of us eat according to these average guidelines. Therefore, even our *average* nutritional needs are not being met, let alone our specific needs. This creates a deficiency in dietary nutrients that are very important to good health. Food supplements can be a very practical solution. No wonder that demand for multivitamins is growing by leaps and bounds.

SYNTHETIC VERSUS NATURAL SUPPLEMENTS

Chemically speaking, a vitamin is a vitamin whether synthetic or natural, because its chemical structure is identical in both cases. The vitamins which occur naturally in fresh food and in health foods, however, are in many cases accompanied by co-factors which help their function – vitamin C, for example, is often accompanied by bioflavonoids. Not all complex factors are known.

In a laboratory experiment, a fish placed in artificial seawater quickly began to die in spite of the fact that the water was chemically identical to seawater. Once put back in natural seawater it quickly recovered.[6] In other words, nature contains special factors vital to life, which cannot necessarily be reproduced in a laboratory.

A group of patients suffering from digestive disorders were given brewer's yeast extract, a natural concentrated source of B complex vitamins. Their distressing symptoms were greatly alleviated or completely cured. But when brewer's yeast was replaced with synthetic B vitamins, all of the distressing symptoms returned.[7]

When the effects of natural vitamin E (d–Alpha tocopherol) were compared with those of its synthetic ester (dl–

Alpha tocopherol acetate) over a two-year period, the synthetic ester was found to have only 20.6 per cent of the activity of the natural vitamin. In other words, the natural vitamin was five times more efficient than its synthetic twin.[8] In fact, Israeli nutritionist Eli Kari has suggested that the synthetic vitamins sold in drug stores may actually contribute to deficiencies.[9] This can occur when synthetic vitamins convert to antagonistic isomers (chemical twins) and actually prevent natural vitamins from performing their beneficial functions.

An exception to this, however, is when higher doses of nutrients are required for specific dietary supplementation or megavitamin therapy. As we have seen, plants and even health foods can be relatively poor as vitamin sources for supplemental purposes, which of course makes their use highly expensive and impractical. Dried rosehips or acerola cherries for example, the richest natural sources of vitamin C, contain so little vitamin C, industrially speaking, that the vitamin extracted from them would cost over $1,000 per kilogram to the manufacturer. That is why the higher potencies of vitamin C sold in health food shops are made up mostly of ascorbic acid acid with only a little acerola or rosehip powder added. However, it is always best to buy a vitamin C preparation that contains a large proportion of bioflavonoids.

In the case of vitamin E, although the pure d-Alpha tocopherol is better than its esters, it is very unstable and readily oxidizes, which makes it impractical for domestic use. An esterified form of vitamin E, such as tocopherol acetate, phosphate or succinate, is preferable. The dry tablet form is safer and much more stable than oil-filled capsules.

By all means let us make the most use of natural health foods and vitamins which are perfectly balanced, but let us not hestitate to use high doses of less natural nutrients when required for specific supplementation. Supplementation can benefit us in three ways: it can prevent and replenish deficiencies; it can have therapeutic effects against a range of established or incipient conditions; and it can protect the body from the effects of environmental pollution.

A BASIC PROGRAMME FOR BEGINNERS

All supplementation programmes should be tailored to the individual. However, if you have never supplemented before, here are some of the supplements you should consider.

◆ VITAMIN C, as found in rosehip or acerola tablets (or powder), between 300 and 1000 mg per day; this should be stepped up to several grams a day during colds or infections.

◆ VITAMIN B COMPLEX, as found in brewer's yeast or desiccated liver tablets or powder, between 3 and 15 tablets a day or 3 teaspoons.

◆ VITAMIN E, as found in natural mixed tocopherol capsules or esterified tablets, starting with 100 IU a day, and going up to 400 IU.
CAUTION: Vitamin E in daily doses of a few hundred IUs can modify blood pressure and affect people with heart conditions. Susceptible people should consult their doctors before taking it.
◆ CALCIUM AND PHOSPHORUS, as found in bonemeal tablets, 1 to 3 tablets a day.

◆ CALCIUM AND MAGNESIUM, as found in dolomite tablets, 1 to 3 tablets a day. Dolomite is best taken with a protein meal. For higher calcium dosages, use calcium lactate or oyster shell calcium with supplemental magnesium tablets to keep calcium soluble and reduce the risk of kidney stones.

◆ IODINE AND TRACE ELEMENTS, as found in kelp tablets, 1 to 3 tablets a day.

◆ LECITHIN, preferably pure granules, 1 to 3 teaspoons a day.

◆ PROTEIN, mainly for vegetarians, convalescents, growing children and body builders.
   Preferably natural protein powder, 2 to 6 tablespoons a day in a protein drink or sprinkled on food.

◆ NATURAL OILS. Fish oils (preferably cod liver oil) supply vitamins A and D. Vegetable oils such as cold pressed sunflower or safflower oil supply essential fatty acids.

NUTRITIONAL FORMULAS
Preventing and treating conditions the easy way
To make supplementation easier for the general public, vitamin manufacturers have been developing nutritional formulas for a wide variety of specific conditions, from thinning hair to low sex drive.

In the case of hair loss, for example, one does not have to scan the scientific literature for nutritional solutions. The manufacturers take care of that. They use all the latest available information to compose a capsule which contains the specific nutrients known to encourage hair growth. These can include, for example, amino acids (like cysteine), vitamins (like biotin) and minerals (like zinc). All these ingredients come in average potencies to stimulate hair growth by correcting deficiencies and improving nourishment to the hair roots.

Similarly, stress tablets contain the necessary vitamins, mainly B and C, which the body uses up rapidly during stressful conditions. Taking additional amounts of these vitamins, supplements the increased nutritional needs of the nervous system, caused by the stress. The nerves become 'stronger', better able to cope with stressful conditions.

Obviously, formulas are not the perfect solution in every case and for everyone. If, for example, hair loss is caused by stress, it is much more beneficial to use a B Stress supplement, before attempting to use the more expensive hair formula. These issues are best discussed with a nutritionist or with a nutrition-oriented doctor.

MEGAVITAMIN THERAPY

When vitamins are given in megadoses, they have a range of therapeutic effects. They are given orally or injected. However, **these treatments should be undertaken only under medical supervision.** Here are three typical examples.

VITAMIN E

The normal daily requirement is between 100 and 150 IU, although the RDA is much less. However, after 40 years of clinical tests, we know that in doses of more than 400 IU daily vitamin E acts as a powerful drug rather than as a vitamin.[10] Here are some of its therapeutic effects:

•It helps to heal wounds and burns, without scars; burns do not blister; much safer and more efficient in this respect than steroids.

•It helps to dissolve blood clots, and therefore helps to prevent heart attacks.

•It cures thrombophlebitis (varicose veins with blood clots in them), since it is an anticoagulant; a clot which breaks loose can be life-threatening.
•It helps to heal diabetic gangrene, sometimes making amputations unnecessary.
•It is beneficial (with vitamin C) in certain forms of cancer.
•It helps to prevent retrolental fibroplasia, a cause of blindness in low birth weight premature babies.
•It assists treatment of jaundice, liver and gallbladder problems.
•It assists treatment of haemolytic anaemia in children.

VITAMIN C
A normal minimal intake of vitamin C is between 60 and 100 mg a day, but according to Dr Linus Pauling, in doses of 5,000 mg a day and over, vitamin C becomes a medicine.[11] These are some of its beneficial effects:
•It stimulates the immune system, and therefore combats infections such as tonsillitis and hepatitis.
•It heals wounds by increasing the body's production of collagen; this can reduce the length of time one needs to stay in hospital after an operation.
•It is believed to assist in fighting cancer and to increase survival time of terminal cancer patients.
•It assists treatment of allergies by acting as a potent anti-histamine.

NIACIN (vitamin B3)
Taken in megadoses, and in combination with vitamin C, niacin has the following therapeutic effects:[12]
•It assists in the treatment of schizophrenia.
•It assists in the treatment of alcoholism.
•It reduces cholesterol levels.
•It helps smokers to cut back.

COMBATING ENVIRONMENTAL POLLUTION

Environmental poisons can cause various disorders, from headaches and nervousness to cancer and brain damage. Yet plastics factories continue to dump mercury effluents into rivers and poison edible fish, battery plants continue to dump cadmium and nickel, cars continue to pollute the air with lead, and people continue smoking, and in the process poison themselves with cadmium, a major cause of hypertension and heart disease.[13] In fact, the more pollution-caused diseases develop, the more products the chemical and pharmaceutical industries develop to help combat the effects of pollution.

However, there are foods and supplements which can help to neutralize the effects of pollution.

•CULTURED MILKS (yogurt, acidophilus milk, buttermilk). The beneficial bacteria in these products fortify the intestinal flora and help to eliminate DDT and other toxins,[14] residues of which persist despite their banning many years ago.

•KELP. As already explained, kelp contains sodium alginate which combines with radioactive strontium-90 and assists its excretion in the faeces.

•ZINC. Foods rich in zinc, such as brewer's yeast, liver, pollen and chelated zinc tablets, will prevent the accumulation of cadmium,[15] and may help to prevent heart disease.

•SELENIUM. Foods rich in selenium, such as brewer's yeast, assist the excretion of cadmium and mercury.[16]

•VITAMIN E. This helps to protect the body against infection.

•VITAMIN A. This protects the mucous membranes of the eyes, nose, throat and ears.

•CALCIUM. This helps the body to rid itself of lead and

mercury. Bonemeal is a very good source of calcium. Calcium lactate (as in milk) also binds with strontium-90 from radioactive fallout and eliminates it from the body.[17]

•LECITHIN. This also helps to minimize the toxicity of many poisons in the body.[18]

GENERAL NOTES ON SUPPLEMENT TAKING

• As a general rule, supplements are best taken during or after meals. It also is best to divide the total daily dosage into three equal parts, to be taken with each meal. This enables the body to use them with maximum efficiency.

•For maximum benefit, supplements should be taken regularly, not at odd or infrequent intervals. When water-soluble vitamins are taken in normal doses, there is no danger of adverse effects, since excesses are excreted by urine. However, vitamins A, D, E and K are fat-soluble and caution is advised since they tend to accumulate in the body with prolonged overdosing.

• Megadoses of vitamins should only be taken after consultation with a doctor.

•Each person's body chemistry has individual requirements. So never follow someone else's supplementation habits. His or her needs are likely to be quite different from yours.

•If you have a specific health problem, such as high blood pressure, heart disease, diabetes, etc., you should consult a doctor or a nutritionist before starting high-dose supplementation. For example, if you have rheumatic heart disease, you may be vulnerable to high vitamin E intake; large amounts of vitamin E doses might unbalance heart function and aggravate the condition. If you are diabetic you should not take GTF chromium without consulting your doctor, as your medication may need to be changed.

•High doses (1 gram or more a day) of acidic vitamins such as niacin or vitamin C can cause indigestion in people susceptible to stomach over-aciditiy. This extra acidity should therefore be neutralized with dolomite or bicarbonate tablets or powder. It is best to chew the tablets rather than swallow them.

•Always use supplements of natural origin; read labels carefully.

•Last, but not least, never forget that eating whole foods, natural foods and health foods comes first. Supplements are, as their name implies, only supplements, not staples.

CHAPTER 7

DIGESTION, ABSORPTION, AND ASSIMILATION

Once people put food in their mouths they think they have done their nutritional duty, that the process of digestion is entirely automatic, beyond their control and none of their concern. This is a mistake. To eat properly, one needs to understand something about the digestive processes. The alimentary canal is a fascinating, miraculous mechanism which can deal simultaneously with different foods, subjecting them to various and sometimes opposing processes.

The digestive system consists of the mouth, oesophagus, stomach, duodenum, small intestine and colon. These are helped by the salivary glands, pancreas, liver and gallbladder.

THE MOUTH

The digestive process begins in the mouth. As food is chewed, it is mixed with saliva, which is secreted by the salivary glands. Saliva softens the food and makes it easy to swallow, and also initiates the breakdown of starches into dextrin. This is because saliva contains a starch-digesting enzyme called ptyalin. When starchy foods such as bread, potatoes and rice are swallowed hurriedly, however, this enzyme does not have enough time to convert starch to dextrin, and so it descends to the stomach unchanged. This interferes with the efficiency of the stomach, which does not contain starch-splitting enzymes, and may cause fermentation and flatulence. Starch is not acted upon again until it reaches the small intestine.

Cellulose, as found in vegetables, must be broken down by thorough chewing. There is no enzyme that acts upon it. If cellulose is not broken down in the mouth, instead of benefiting elimination, it will produce gas, putrefaction and bloating.[1] For efficient digestion to take place, food must be masticated thoroughly.

OESOPHAGUS AND STOMACH

From the mouth, food goes down the oesophagus to the stomach. The oesophagus is a thin tube which pushes food down by rhythmic, wavelike motions called peristalsis. These peristaltic motions continue throughout the digestive tract, and are controlled by the autonomic nervous system.[2] This is an involuntary system and not under our conscious control, although it is affected indirectly by the condition of our central nervous system and by stress, or the lack of it. Peace of mind is important to proper digestion, since enzymatic secretions of the intestines are influenced by mood.[3] In fact, an effective way to prevent indigestion and flatulence is to eat in a relaxed and pleasant atmosphere, chewing everything thoroughly. A group of expert dieticians has correlated tension, worry and apprehension with indigestion, heartburn and stomach pains. 'Better a dry morsel and quietness therewith, than a house full of sacrifices with strife,'(Proverbs 17:1).

The stomach is a muscular J-shaped bag which secretes gastric juice. Gastric juice consists mainly of pepsin, the enzyme which hydrolyzes proteins to proteoses, hydrochloric acid (HCL), which both sterilizes food and supplies the acid medium in which pepsin works, and mucin for lubrication. Children have an additional enzyme in their stomachs, rennin, which curdles milk and enables its protein to be digested. This same enzyme is used to curdle milk in cheese-making. In adults, pepsin plays the milk-curdling role.[4] Incidentally, milk intolerance in adults is due to a lack of lactase, an intestinal enzyme which breaks down milk sugar (lactose).

Through muscular and enzymatic action, the food in the stomach is reduced to an acidic soup called chyme. This encourages the stomach exit to open, and the contents of the stomach pass into the duodenum. It takes 3 to 5 hours for an average meal to be digested in the stomach.

THE SMALL INTESTINE

The small intestine is a much-coiled tube whose total length averages about 22.5 feet (6.5 metres). It extends from the stomach exit (pyloric valve) to the entry of the colon (ileo-cecal valve). The first 10 inches (25 cm) of the small intestine are called the duodenum. This receives pancreatic juice from the pancreas and bile from the gallbladder. Bile emulsifies fats and provides the alkaline medium necessary for pancreatic juice to function. In addition, the intestine itself secretes enzymes (sucrase and lactase) which metabolize sugar and milk sugar. All of these juices have the ability to break down various types of foods so that they can be absorbed into the body through the intestinal linings.

Intestinal absorption is aided by friendly bacteria (flora)

and by tiny finger-like projections called villi, which line the walls of the intestine. These increase the absorption surface. As the broken-down food is slowly pushed along by peristaltic motion, its nutrients are absorbed.[5]

It is most important that the flora in the small intestine are kept in a healthy, flourishing state. These 'friendly' bacteria not only help in the absorption of food, but also synthesize certain vitamins, such as vitamin K, which enables blood to clot.[6] Unfortunately, antibiotic drugs kill bacteria without discriminating between friend or foe, so when taking antibiotics, it is advisable to eat live yogurt and take supplements of acidophilus and brewer's yeast. These help to recolonize the intestine with friendly bacteria.

THE PANCREAS

The pancreas is a tubular gland just below the stomach. It consists of an exocrine portion and an endocrine portion. The exocrine portion secretes the pancreatic juice which enters the duodenum through the pancreatic duct. This juice contains several important enzymes: trypsin, chymotrypsin and erepsin, which break down proteins to amino acids; steapsin, which breaks down emulsified fats to fatty acids and glycerol; amylopsin, which breaks down starch to maltose; and maltase, which breaks down maltose to glucose.

Only simple, basic molecules are able to pass through the intestinal wall into the bloodstream and go on to feed the cells. Proteins, fats, and carbohydrates are made up of molecules which are too big to be utilized by the body. Proteins are the biggest and most complex; the only way for them to get into the blood and to the cells which need them is as amino acids, molecules which are small enough to be absorbed through the intestinal wall into the bloodstream.

Once delivered to the body cells, they are reassembled into the various proteins the body needs. In similar fashion, body cells can only use fats as fatty acids and carbohydrates as glucose.

The other part of the pancreas, the endocrine portion, secretes two hormones, insulin and glucagon, directly into the bloodstream. Between them, these two hormones control blood sugar levels.

Diabetes is a condition in which the pancreas fails to secrete enough insulin; without insulin, the body cannot absorb sugar from the blood, and so blood sugar levels rise and diabetes symptoms appear. In such cases sugar consumption must be avoided. Special diets, insulin injections and herbal therapy may be needed. Excess sugar consumption, which overworks the pancreas, is considered to be a factor in the development of diabetes and hypoglycaemia.

LIVER AND GALLBLADDER

The liver is the largest gland in the body, and is located in the upper right portion of the abdomen. It weighs 3.3 pounds (1.5kg) on average, and comprises two lobes.[7] It receives its blood supply from both the hepatic artery and portal vein,[8] which provide it with the large amounts of oxygen it needs for the many tasks it performs. The liver is often likened to a giant industrial plant, in which incredibly complex and diverse reactions take place simultaneously and continuously.

One of the chief functions of the liver is the production of bile, which is either stored in the gallbladder or enters the duodenum directly to help emulsify fats. We cannot digest fatty foods without bile.[9]

Liver cells help to control blood sugar level. On the one hand, they convert excess glucose to glycogen and store it.

On the other hand, when the blood sugar level drops, they convert glycogen to glucose and release it into the bloodstream. In addition, the liver converts excess sugar to fat, and synthesizes and stores fat. It also synthesizes amino acids, forming urea, uric acid, and other waste products, preventing the accumulation of ammonia. It detoxifies the poisonous wastes of metabolism and uses bile to excrete excess toxic elements, which ultimately end up in the faeces.[10] Special cells in the liver called Kupffer cells engulf disease-causing bacteria.[11] The liver also forms vitamin A from carotene, and stores vitamins A, D and B12 and iron and copper. Last but not least, it plays a role in the production of core body heat and also activates certain hormones.[12]

THE COLON

The digestive process is concluded in the colon. The colon, or large intestine, which is larger in diameter than the small intestine, receives the food after digestion and prepares it for elimination.

The colon absorbs water from the fluid mass which arrives from the small intestine and converts it to semi-solid faeces. Eliminated faeces contain the unabsorbed parts of foods such as cellulose, inorganic matter, toxic substances and dead bacteria, and the residues of digestive secretions. Gases and the waste products of protein metabolism are responsible for the typical odour.[13] NOTE: A high fibre diet and healthy intestinal flora can prevent the offensive putrefactive odoor of faeces, and speed up the digestive process.

ASSIMILATION

Assimilation is the final stage of food utilization. Food factors are assimilated (become part of the body) in the cells, where they are used for maintenance, repair, new growth and energy. Check your food before you eat! Is it fit to become a part of you? Is it natural, wholesome and nutritious, or refined, processed and denatured?

We have seen the complexity of metabolic processes and their interdependence. The body needs a balanced supply of all nutrients to function optimally and to produce a feeling of well-being, with all organs and processes working in harmony. When the diet is not balanced, when certain nutrients are undersupplied or oversupplied, as in the case of a low carbohydrate or high protein diet, we are, in fact, destroying the delicate physiologic balance in our bodies. Destroying this balance not only stresses the body, reducing alertness and increasing fatigue, it also increases waste products, disturbs the acid-alkaline balance and leads to dietary deficiencies. All of these things predispose us to the various disorders typical of an overfed but undernourished lifestyle.

CHAPTER 8

FOOD COMBINATIONS
OR HOW TO AVOID FOODS THAT FIGHT

As we noted in the last chapter, proteins require an acid medium (the stomach) for their digestion. Starches require an alkaline medium, which is supplied partly by the mouth and by the intestines. Fats and oils are digested slowly, mostly in the intestines, and do not interfere much with either protein or starch digestion. Sugars are the quickest food to digest; some are even absorbed in the stomach,[1] while most are absorbed through the intestines.

This means that proteins and fats, or starches and fats may be eaten together. Their digestion does not interfere with each other. However, proteins and starches are a poor food combination because proteins need an acid medium and starches an alkaline one. Their digestive processes are chemically opposed, so when they are eaten together, they stress the system by producing fermentation, flatulence and indigestion.

Young and healthy people with a strong digestion and plenty of stomach acid, may not be affected by protein-starch combinations. However, older people or those with a weak digestion can easily develop indigestion, particularly if food is not thoroughly chewed. Most modern meals include protein and starch combinations – hamburgers and French fries, or steak and potatoes. The potatoes ferment in the stomach and stress it, while waiting for the steak to be digested.

Correct food combinations are regarded by many nutritionists as the simplest, most effective way to prevent such common problems as stomach acidity, heartburn, bloating, dyspepsia, headaches, allergies and nervousness. In the author's practice, correct food combinations almost invariably result in weight loss. Most overweight patients report considerable weight loss, ranging from 5 to 20 pounds, during the first month.

Drugs can bring only temporary relief to these symptoms, not permanent cure. People who use over-the-counter antacids to combat over-acidity or heartburn, should know that the symptoms of too much acid in the stomach are similar to those of too little.[2] Taking antacids could be the worst thing to do. In addition, some antacids contain aluminium, which has been found to disturb calcium-phosphorus metabolism.[3] In fact, many cases of heartburn resulting from a low acid stomach can be relieved by betaine HCl tablets. Some health authorities even recommend these tablets, one after each meal, for every person over 40 years of age, when stomach secretions are known to diminish. In other cases of indigestion, digestive enzymes in the form of tablets are preferable; these are prepared from extracts of animal digestive secretions and can be of great help to people with a weak digestion. The author has found a cold glass of milk or a few raw almonds most effective for heartburn.

People with an extremely sensitive digestion may find the common practice of combining high sugar foods with protein distressing. When one eats a sweet dessert after a juicy steak, for example, the sugar is held up in the stomach until the steak has been digested. In the meantime, for 3 to 5 hours the sugars ferment and bloat, causing indigestion and heartburn. Sugary desserts are best avoided.

KIND FOOD COMBINATIONS

The basic principle of proper food combining is to avoid eating protein and starch meals. Starches, fats, green vegetables and sugars can be combined together in one meal, since they all require either an alkaline or a neutral medium for their digestion. Proteins, fats, green vegetables and acid fruits can be combined together, since they need an acid or a neutral medium for digestion. However, as a general rule, proteins and starches, or starches and acid fruits should not be eaten together.

There is one exception however. Eggs and flour (protein and starch), when cooked together to form simple foods such as pancakes and bread, are quite permissible, the reason being that the proteins and starches are chemically blended into an integrated food which can be properly digested. All natural foods, even starchy carbohydrates like potatoes, contain some protein which is easily digested.[4]

The list overleaf shows acceptable food combinations. Naturally, it is quite impossible to detail all the possibilities that exist for every combination. Meals should be planned according to individual taste and tolerance. People who suffer from indigestion, heartburn and other digestive disorders are often the first to benefit from experimenting with food combinations. Correct food combining may be the key to easing long-time distress and embarking on a new chapter of personal well-being.

- PROTEIN/VEGETABLES
  Salad with steak, fish or eggs; chicken salad.
- PROTEIN/ACID FRUITS
  Milk shake with fruits; fruit and cheese salad.
- PROTEIN/FATS
  Fish with butter sauce; meat and marrow bone stew.
- PROTEIN/FATS/ VEGETABLES
  Salad with oil dressing; roast beef and vegetables.
- PROTEIN/FATS/ACID FRUITS
  Roast meat with apple sauce; nuts and apples;
  grilled fish with butter and lemon sauce.
- FATS/ACID FRUITS
  Fresh fruit with heavy cream.
- FATS/SUGARS
  Dried fruit and nuts; dried fruit and cream
- PROTEINS/SUGARS
  Hot milk sweetened with honey; high-protein drink
  blended with fruit.
- STARCHES/FATS
  Bread and butter; banana and cream; baked potatoes
  with butter.
- STARCHES/VEGETABLES
  Salad and baked potato; lettuce sandwich with nutmeg.
- STARCHES, FATS/ VEGETABLES
  Salad with oil dressing, eaten with bread and butter.
- STARCHES/SUGARS
  Bread and honey; cereals and honey.
- STARCHES/DRIED FRUITS
  Granolas; raisin sandwiches; date sandwiches.
- STARCHES/SUGARS/ DRIED FRUIT
  Bread and honey, with raisins, dates or figs.
- STARCHES, FATS/ VEGETABLES
  Salad with oil dressing, eaten with bread and butter.

10 TIPS FOR SENSITIVE STOMACHS

Meals, as a rule, should be as simple as possible. Many people who have a sensitive stomach find small, one-course meals preferable to large meals consisting of many foods.

1. Fruits (not acid fruits) are best eaten alone because they are highly alkaline.

2. Oranges, grapefruits, melons, bananas and potatoes are best eaten separately, as a small meal on their own, because of their special structure.[5] (Eating watermelon and cantaloupe at the same meal can, in the experience of many of the author's patients, cause severe indigestion.)

3. Cooked animal proteins and vegetables, or cooked starches with vegetables, are easy on sensitive stomachs.

4. In general, grains combine very well with dried and fresh vegetables and fruits.

5. When sugar and protein are combined together, they form waste enzymes which rot protein in the stomach and inhibit its metabolism.[6]

6. Cheese and fruit combinations are OK *only* if sour fruits are eaten, i.e. grapefruit, limes, lemons, oranges, etc.

7. Pineapple and papaya (pawpaw) can be combined with lean animal protein (cheese, chicken, fish) because pineapple contains bromelain and papaya contains papain, two powerful protein-digesting enzymes.

8. Fruits and vegetables are not compatible at the same meal.

9. Drinking right after meals, or up to two hours later, dilutes digestive juices and can impair digestion, causing stomach pains and heartburn. During meals, soup and milk are the least troublesome beverages.[7]

10. Hot condiments, such as chili, paprika and mustard, increase gastric juice secretions, irritate the stomach lining and can lead to ulcers.[8]

COFFEE AND TEA

As drinking is an integral part of most meals, something must be said about today's drinking habits. Huge amounts of coffee and tea are consumed in the West and consumption is on the increase. Wherever one goes, in offices, homes and factories, coffee and tea are everywhere, an integral part of the culture. Coffee, tea and soft drinks are stimulating drinks due to their caffeine content, but caffeine is a poison (the lethal dose is around 10 grams), and the 'lift' it gives, lessening fatigue and brightening thoughts, is very temporary and far outweighed by its long-term side effects.

Caffeine has been repeatedly reported to increase stomach acid secretion and promote ulcers.[9] A recent study showed that it also produces anxiety, irritability and depression.[10] It also raises blood pressure, damages blood vessels and causes heart attacks.[11] Birth defects have recently been correlated to coffee consumption during pregnancy.[12] Women who attempt to become pregnant and consume more caffeine than the equivalent of one cup a day decrease their fertility; they are half as likely to become pregnant as low caffeine consumers.[13] And, finally, caffeine has been shown to promote breast cancer,[14] bladder cancer [15] and infertility.[16]

Theophylline, which is contained in tea, is five times more potent than caffeine as an irritant to the nervous system.[17] Tea also contains tannin, which is an astringent drug. Tannin contributes to constipation and impairs the secretion of digestive enzymes. In fact, drinking coffee or tea after a heavy meal is a common cause of heartburn.

The undesirable effects of tea and coffee do not stop here, however. The huge amounts of sugar which are normally taken with them promote tooth decay. And cigarette smoking, which is often part of tea and coffee breaks, promotes high cholesterol levels [18] and aggravates duodenal ulcers. [19]

Caffeine is also a known diuretic, i.e., it increases urination. In his own practice, the author observed that people who urinated frequently, were able to urinate less frequently by cutting down their caffeine consumption. This was especially beneficial for older people who woke up at night several times for nocturnal urination.

It is therefore in the benefit of each of us to reduce our caffeine intake, by drinking less coffee, tea and caffeine-laden soft drinks. Instead, there are numerous types of cereal beverages and herb teas available in many flavours and fragrances to suit practically any taste. Each herb has its own beneficial effects: peppermint is refreshing and digestive, camomile is carminative, lime flower a sedative, and so on. Herbs also contribute to health by supplying trace elements and vitamins. What more could one ask?

CHAPTER 9

FOOD ALLERGIES
GLUTEN, LACTOSE, ET AL.

Many people think of food allergies in terms of strawberry rash, the kind of minor inconvenience which troubles a few sensitive people and usually fades away of its own accord. They are wrong. Over 20 million Americans are being treated for allergies.[1] Food allergies are on the increase and represent more of a problem than ever before due to the many additives now used in food production.

Food allergies cause a variety of disorders for which there seem to be no obvious causes. Inexplicable weight gain, water retention (oedema), headache, fatigue, drowsiness, nasal congestion, constipation, diarrhoea, ulcers and heart palpitations can be common symptoms.[2] More serious symptoms of food allergies are believed to include high blood pressure, heart disease, schizophrenia[3] and suicidal depression.[4] Common disorders in children include poor learning ability, clumsiness, mood swings, short attention span and hyperactivity, now collectively known as 'cerebral allergy syndrome'.[5]

WHAT CAUSES FOOD ALLERGIES?

Although allergies have afflicted the human race for millennia, their causes and disguises are still not fully understood. In the absence of correct diagnosis, many sufferers are labeled hypochondriacs, and because they are misdiagnosed they are not successfully treated. Dr Claude Frazier, who has studied allergies for years, warns his fellow doctors; 'Do not be quick to decide that your patient is a neurotic or a hypochondriac. He may simply be allergic to his daily bread.'[6] Some allergic people may be fortunate enough to learn the underlying reasons for their symptoms by chance. Others may improve their tolerance to allergens (allergy–causing factors) by changing their eating habits. But many sufferers have no recourse.

Food allergies are commonly described as being a result of an impaired immune system. The white blood cells which mount the body's immune response produce specific antibodies (immunoglobulins) whenever food allergens are ingested. Normally, when antigens (hostile substances) enter the blood, the immune system promptly reacts by producing antibodies to engulf and destroy them, thus protecting the body against invading bacteria and carcinogens. In allergic conditions, however, the immune system reacts with the same hostility to certain food substances, producing histamine and causing a variety of distressing symptoms.

Studies[7] have shown that two unsuspected but common causes of food allergies are low levels of stomach acid and a shortage of certain digestive enzymes.[8] The latter can be caused by deficiencies of the B complex vitamins. Stress[9] and hypoglycaemia[10] can also cause allergies. In fact, the role of emotional stress in allergy diseases is more prevalent than many people imagine. In a way, stress and allergies revolve in the same circle, since food allergies can produce neurotic symptoms.

More specifically, pancreatic insufficiency has been suggested as a cause of allergy, or food hypersensitivity. Protein-splitting enzymes, secreted by the pancreas, break down complex protein into their components, the amino acids. Insufficient secretion of enzymes by the pancreas, results in by-products of partly digested dietary protein. These protein fragments can induce a food allergy in the intestines, which is manifested in symptoms like skin problems, headaches, recurrent infections or even psychiatric disturbances.[11] Another study showed that incompletely digested protein absorbed by the blood after a meal, weakens the immune system, leading to long-term allergic reactions.[12] Such allergies can also be passed on to breast-fed babies, by mothers with pancreatic insufficiency. Newborn infants are particularly vulnerable because they can absorb food antigens more than older infants or children.[13] Apart from B complex supplementation, this problem can be taken care of by enzyme replacement therapy. Pancretain tablets taken orally after each meal, can solve the problem.

Although people have always suffered from allergies, logic suggests that they were a relatively minor disorder in the past. Dr Carlton Fredericks[14] and others[15] claim that allergies began to increase when mothers substituted the bottle for the breast, and fed their babies on formulae based on cow's milk and cereals. It was not known until recently that children do not have the necessary starch-splitting enzymes to cope with cereals until they are two or three years of age,[16] and that cow's milk is a common allergen. Many modern babies have not had a chance to develop a tolerance for these foods and so become allergic, occasionally suffering from diarrhoea, ear infections and swollen tonsils.[17] Paediatricians today advise nursing mothers to introduce solid, cooked foods gradually to give babies a chance to adjust. Many people, already allergic as babies, grow up exposed to a vast array of food additives, which further complicate the picture. Allergists have already documented adverse reactions to BHA and BHT (powerful synthetic antioxidants), sodium nitrite (used in meats), bleaching chemicals, chlorine (in water) and many other commonly used additives.

In many cases foods which are the subject of craving, such as chocolate, milk, alcohol or candies, are likely to be allergenic. That is why the first thing an allergist studies in a patient is his or her reaction to foods which are craved. As well as triggering off a bout of allergy, these may also be addictive. Why? Because after the enjoyment of eating craved foods, allergic reactions such as headaches, irritability and nasal congestion appear. Then to stave off these distressing symptoms, the body develops a craving for the very foods which caused them.[18] This explains why some people can spend all evening drinking, only to wake up the next morning reaching for the bottle. The same is true of cigarettes, coffee and chocolate.

Reactions to allergenic foods are by no means limited to the body. Cerebral allergies, due to high levels of histamine in the blood, are known to lead to mental disorders ranging from irritability to schizophrenia. Some specialists claim that 92 per cent of schizophrenics are allergic, and that they can be suffering from as many as ten allergies![19] In children, the most common symptoms of allergy are learning disabilities, clumsiness, hyperactivity, irritability, aggressiveness, antisocial behaviour, short attention span and mood swings.[20]

A more recent study done in England with children demonstrated that keeping to a simple diet and omitting common food additives from the diet can often cure severe chronic conditions for which medication is normally prescribed. Eighty-eight children suffering from frequent, severe migraine headaches were put on a diet consisting of four basic foods, plus water and a vitamin supplement. Four weeks later, 89 per cent of them had no migraine symptoms and 5 per cent reported great improvement. Other symptoms such as abdominal pain, diarrhoea, flatulence, hyperactivity, aching limbs, epileptic fits, runny noses, mouth ulcers, vaginal discharges, asthma and eczema also decreased dramatically. [21] But when excluded foods were reintroduced into the diet at the rate of one a week, many of the children manifested a recurrence of their former symptoms. Benzoic acid (a food preservative) and tartrazine (a food colour) were among the culprit additives. Tartrazine, also known as Yellow No.5, is widely used in the food industry and in drugs. Sensitive individuals would do well to read food labels carefully and avoid products which contain it.

Interestingly, blood tests of the children involved in this study did not show the findings typical of allergy, such as elevated levels of IgE antibodies. Nevertheless, given the wide range of foods tested, researchers believe that the children's symptoms were provoked by allergy rather than by individual metabolic intolerances. Although this seems to contradict the orthodox concept of allergies, the fact remains that those children who continued to avoid suspect foods and additives remained symptom-free and had no need of migraine medication.

The most common allergenic foods in this study were found to be cow's milk, eggs, chocolate, oranges, wheat, benzoic acid, cheese, tomatoes, tartrazine, rye, fish, pork, beef and maize. Goat's milk was found to be much less allergenic than cow's. In some cases the processing of a food affected its ability to cause symptoms; for example, some children reacted to white wheat flour but not to brown. Rice, peas and avocados are among the foods considered to be least allergy-causing.

IDENTIFYING ALLERGY-CAUSING FOODS

Allergists try to prevent allergies by identifying the foods responsible and advising their patients to avoid them, in an elimination diet. To confirm an allergy, they use the scratch and patch test. This involves applying a small amount of the suspect substance to the skin and watching for reddening or swelling. However, as many sufferers know, skin tests have only limited accuracy.[22]

Other tests for food allergies include a 4-6 day fast to cleanse the system, after which extracts of the suspect food are placed under the tongue,[23] and the pulse test. The latter is an efficient and simple test based on the principle that allergic foods cause an increase in the pulse rate.[24] When a meal is found to speed up the pulse, its ingredients should be eaten separately as one-food meals. Then, by checking the pulse before and after these meals, the offending foods can be identified. When using this method, it is most important to keep an accurate and complete record of all foods eaten and to follow a rotation diet. More information about this method can be obtained from Dr Arthur Coca's book, *The Pulse Test*.

Sometimes an elimination diet of specific allergenic foods may fail to help. For example, if you were found to be allergic to pistachio nuts and eliminated them from your diet, you might still develop a reaction to cashew nuts and mangoes. This is because these three foods belong to the same botanical family, the cashew family. Similarly, an allergic reaction to peanuts may mean an allergy to all the legume family, which includes beans, peas, chickpeas, lentils and licorice. Once a plant is found to cause a reaction, all of its botanical relatives should be suspected.[25]

Cytotoxic tests have also been introduced in recent years to identify allergens. Live white blood cells, taken from a small sample of blood, are mixed with various suspect food extracts; if the food extract is an allergen, the white blood cells will be destroyed or damaged as they come into contact with it.[26] Cytotoxic tests are done on an empty stomach, after a night's fast. The results, however, are often inaccurate, and many doctors refuse to make a diagnosis on the basis of a cytotoxic test alone.

HOW TO INCREASE YOUR TOLERANCE TO PROBLEM FOODS

The best way to avoid allergic reactions is to identify the offending foods and abstain from them. Allergies come in varying degrees of severity. Foods which cause acute allergies should be completely avoided; less irritating foods can be eaten safely once a week, or just occasionally, without any particular reaction. However, food tolerances can be increased by improving the diet and using nutritional supplementation. A high protein diet of the kind described in Chapter 10, for example, can cure those allergies which are triggered by hypoglycaemia.[27]

Recently, greater use has been made of nutrients which are known to reduce toxicity and histamine levels in the blood. One study showed that although histamine is quickly absorbed from the alimentary tract into the blood, a healthy liver can deactivate much of it, thus protecting the body from its harmful effects.[28] Massive doses of vitamin C have been hailed by many nutritionists as an effective means of fighting allergies.[29] Vitamin C has potent antihistamine properties. Vitamin B6, zinc, calcium and vitamin E are also known to neutralize histamines, thus reducing the increased permeability of cell membranes which histamine causes. It is this increase in permeability that is responsible for the various symptoms of allergy, from skin eruptions to irritability.

Pantothenic acid, the famous anti-stress vitamin, is very effective in high doses and highly recommended in treating allergies,[30] particularly those which arise during periods of emotional stress. Vitamins A, D and B12, along with B complex, have also been found to be helpful.[31]

A lack of stomach acid (HCl) is known to cause allergies.[32] As people age, their production of HCl and of digestive enzymes decreases. Dr Alan Nittler, author of *A New Breed of Doctor*, states that everyone over the age of 40 should take HCl supplements. A betaine HCl tablet taken after meals, along with other digestive enzymes such as pancreatin, papain and bromelain,[33] improves food tolerance and digestion. Regular use of cider vinegar has a similar effect.

To conclude, let us remember that allergies can manifest themselves in the most unexpected disguises. Sometimes even the specialists are baffled. But nutrition has much to offer and nutritional supplements can often produce surprising benefits. Says Dr Carlton Fredericks: 'I have seen a child's asthma disappear with injections of B12. I have seen hay fever, which did not respond to vitamin C, markedly mitigated by supplements of vitamin E. I have seen eczema of allergic origin disappear with feedings of unsaturated fat, vitamin B6 and vitamin E.' [34]

CHAPTER 10

HYPOGLYCAEMIA:
THE ENERGY GAP

Hypoglycaemia, low sugar levels in the blood, was first discovered by Dr Seale Harris in 1924. The condition was then called hyperinsulinism because it was considered to be caused by excessive insulin secretion due to an overactive pancreas. The excess insulin causes rapid uptake of glucose by the cells and tissues of the body, leaving the blood very depleted of glucose. This is just the opposite of diabetes, in which the pancreas secretes less insulin than required, resulting in high blood glucose levels.

Sugar is the body's source of energy and heat (calories) and the carrier of energy to every cell, especially the cells of the brain, nerves and heart,[1] which need a constant, second by second supply of glucose for proper functioning. When glucose is in short supply, cell function is impaired, leading to both physical and mental disorders.

Recently, public interest has focused on hypoglycaemia, particuarlly functional hypoglycaemia which is caused by an overactive pancreas. In the United States, approximately one person in ten is thought to be hypoglycaemic.[2] Hypoglycaemia has a variety of symptoms, and this has led to difficulties in diagnosis. According to Dr Carlton Fredericks, symptoms can not only mimic emotional disorders such as neurosis or psychosis, but also epilepsy, migraine headaches, peptic ulcers, arthritis, insomnia, asthma and allergies.[3] In one study it was even reported that angina pectoris and coronary thrombosis were triggered by hypoglycaemic fits.[4] Hypoglocaemia may even be a factor in juvenile delinquency.

THE SYMPTOMS OF HYPOGLYCAEMIA

Fatigue, which is so prevalent in our times, is considered to be one of hypoglycaemia's major afflictions. Dr Sam Roberts, in his book *Exhaustion*, estimates that at least 50 per cent of the work done in the United States is done by people who suffer from fatigue but do not think it sufficiently out of the ordinary to complain. Low blood sugar may impair mental health even more than physical health, since it deprives the delicate brain and nervous system of much-needed oxygen.

Hypoglycaemia has been called 'the great imitator' because it imitates so many mental and emotional disorders. As a result, many hypoglycaemics are mistakenly diagnosed as neurotic. Conversely, it has been shown that a large proportion of patients receiving psychotherapy, more than half in fact, are hypoglycaemic.[5] The table below, based on one doctor's records of 1,100 hypoglycaemic patients, shows the bewildering variety of symptoms associated with hypoglycaemia and their frequency.[6]

Symptom	Per cent
Nervousness	94
Irritability	89
Exhaustion	87
Faintness, dizziness, trembling, cold sweats, weakness spells	86
Depression	77
Vertigo, dizziness	73
Drowsiness	72
Headaches	71
Digestive disturbances	69
Forgetfulness	67
Insomnia (waking and not being able to sleep again)	62
Constant worrying, unprovoked anxiety	62
Mental confusion	57
Internal trembling ('butterflies in stomach')	57
Palpitation of the heart, rapid pulse	54
Muscle pains	53
Numbness	51
Unsocial, asocial or antisocial behaviour	47
Indecisiveness	50
Crying spells	46
Lack of sex drive (females)	44
Allergies	43
Lack of coordination	43
Lack of concentration	42

Leg cramps	43
Blurred vision	40
Twitching and jerking of muscles	40
Itching and crawling sensations on skin	39
Gasping for breath	37
Sudden feelings of breathlessness or asphyxiation	34
Staggering	34
Sighing and yawning	30
Impotence (males)	29
Unconsciousness	27
Night terrors, nightmares	27
Rheumatoid arthritis	24
Phobias, fears	23
Neurodermatitis	21
Suicidal intent	20
Nervous breakdown	17
Convulsions	2

WHAT CAUSES HYPOGLYCAEMIA?

During digestion, all ingested carbohydrates (sugars and starches) are converted to glucose, which is the only carbohydrate the body can utilize. After a meal, particularly one with a high sugar content, surges of glucose enter the blood, causing the pancreas to secrete insulin. Insulin causes rapid uptake of glucose by almost all the tissues of the body and also promotes the conversion of excess glucose to glycogen, a more compact form of glucose which can be stored in the liver for future use. But the pancreas is only part of the mechanism which controls blood sugar. The whole process originates in glucoreceptor (glucose-sensitive) nerve cells in the brain from which impulses travel to the pituitary gland, adrenal glands, liver and finally the pancreas.[7] In this sophisticated sugar-control chain, in which too little glucose can be as harmful as too much (although not as lethal), there are also hormones that convert glycogen back to glucose to raise the blood glucose level. The hormones that do this are glucagon, also secreted by the pancreas, and adrenalin, secreted by the adrenal glands. In this manner, opposing forces are constantly at work, balancing each other, so that blood sugar levels are kept within fairly narrow limits. They do not always succeed. If the blood sugar level gets too low, hypoglycaemia occurs.

Apart from cases in which there is overproduction of insulin due to a tumour in the pancreas, there are few functional reasons for hypoglycaemia. Some people inherit or develop an overactive pancreas, which secretes excessive amounts of insulin even when only small amounts of sugar enter the blood. Sometimes, the pancreas may react slowly and insulin does not enter the blood until the sugar level has already fallen – this is known as retarded hypoglycaemia. On the other hand, secretion of glucagon and adrenalin, the hormones which balance the action of insulin, may be too low. Hypoglycaemia can also be caused by allergies [8] or by an imbalance in the autonomic nervous system.[9] Other causative factors are excessive consumption of alcohol, tobacco, coffee and soft drinks containing caffeine, overeating, and emotional stress.[10] Whatever the reason, hypoglycaemia develops when the delicate balance of the systems and substances which control blood sugar is upset.

Theoretically, sugar would appear to be the ideal food to raise blood sugar levels. However, sugar is the one food which hypoglycaemics should *avoid*. In fact, sugar will eventually contribute to *lower* blood sugar levels. Why?

SUGAR CONSUMPTION

When we eat sugar, it is readily absorbed into the blood, where it raises blood sugar levels, triggering the pancreas to secrete insulin, which will cause glucose to be absorbed into the tissues. So, in normal circumstances, excess sugar is quickly used up, but insulin, because it breaks down much more slowly than sugar, remains circulating in the blood for several hours, lowering blood sugar level to below even the original level.[11] Thus, it triggers the hypoglycemic symptoms again, creating a craving for more sugar. So the hypogly-caemic eats *more* sugar, which deepens the vicious circle. In fact, it is the gluttonous consumption of refined sugar, which has now reached an incredible 125 pounds per year per person in the United States, that is believed to be the main cause for higher rates of hypoglycaemia.[12]

Sugar, as already explained, is the fuel which provides the body with heat and energy. Proteins, fats, and complex carbohydrates such as corn, beans, potatoes and bread also provide fuel, but they are broken down slowly in the body because they are very complex molecules. Slow breakdown means that glucose is released gradually into the blood stream, not in great surges which cause the pancreas to go into overdrive to produce insulin.

This is where the real trouble begins, when we start consuming large amounts of white sugar and highly stressing our pancreas. But not only the pancreas. White sugar is a known stressing food. Its consumption has been linked with anxiety and panic disorders in some individuals.[13] The occasional binge can be handled more or less effectively, but when large intakes of refined carbohydrates are the norm, the strain on the sugar-regulating mechanism becomes intolerable and it breaks down. The pancreas may develop an oversensitivity to sugar and produce more insulin than is really required to keep a normal sugar level. The result is a consistently low blood sugar level, depriving the brain and nervous system of vital oxygen and producing the numerous symptoms of hypoglycaemia.

But there are other factors in the development of hypoglycaemia apart from sugar. Coffee (particularly the coffee-sugar combination) and soft drinks (high in caffeine) contribute to hypoglycaemia by acting on the adrenal glands, brain and liver while sugar is flooding the blood stream.[14] Other contributing factors include cigarette smoking (absorption of tars and acids),[15] too much salt in the diet (salt depletes potassium), alcohol,[16] and stress and allergies which overtax the adrenal glands.[17] Deficiencies of zinc, chromium (GTF), certain B vitamins (particularly pantothenic acid),[18] magnesium, potassium, vitamin E and vitamin B6[19] can also contribute to hypoglycaemia. All of which goes to show that hypoglycaemia is mainly a nutritional disorder.

The influence of sugar in the body goes far beyond carbohydrate metabolism. It is becoming apparent that fatty acid synthesis and oxidation, cholesterol synthesis and the accumulation of ketone bodies, are all in part controlled by the rate at which glucose is broken down within cells.[20]

Evidence indicates that refined sugar causes more build-up of fat than any other carbohydrate except alcohol.[21] In other words, more sugar means more cholesterol and a greater susceptibility to heart attacks and high blood pressure. Changes in Western eating habits during the last 70 years have been in the direction of fewer complex carbohydrates (cereals, potatoes, etc.) and more simple sugars. Studies have repeatedly shown that it is the increased consumption of sugar, and not fat, which is implicated in the increased incidence of coronary heart disease.[22]

Life stresses can also be an important factor. In stressful

conditions, more adrenalin is secreted, releasing more sugar from the liver. Repeated stress can impair the function of the adrenal glands, reducing the body's ability to cope with stress. When this occurs we get depressed easily, and develop hypoglycaemic symptoms into the bargain. Many people suffer from depression without realizing that persistent stress is the cause. It is estimated that one adult in seven has symptoms of depression.[23]

DIAGNOSIS AND TREATMENT

Like diabetes, hypoglycaemia is diagnosed by means of the glucose tolerance test (GTT). Dr Robert Atkins describes GTT as the most important test anyone can take in his or her life. The test is done in the morning on an empty stomach. A blood sample is taken, after which a solution containing 100 grams of glucose is drunk. Two blood samples are then taken, the second 30 minutes after the first, and then five more samples at hourly intervals. A shortened version of the test, taking just two hours, is an adequate check for diabetes, but hypoglycaemia is rarely detectable in such a short time, with the result that not a few hypoglocaemics are labeled hypochondriacs because their doctors fail to consider hypoglycaemia. Many physicians still insist that hypoglycaemia is a rare condition, yet when large numbers of patients have been studied, it has been found to be anything but rare.[24] To give a correct result as far as hypoglycaemia is concerned, the glucose tolerance test should last not less than six hours. If the test takes only one or two hours the main hypoglocaemic conclusions will be missed. The results of the GTT should be evaluated by a nutrition-oriented doctor or by a qualified nutritionist, who can also recommend the proper individual diet and supplements.

DIETARY TREATMENT OF HYPOGLYCAEMIA

The anti-hypoglycaemia diet recommended by leading nutritionists Carlton Fredericks and Robert Atkins is a high protein, moderate fat, low carbohydrate régime, supplemented by vitamins and minerals according to individual requirements. Sugar, alcohol and smoking are strictly forbidden. Vegetables can be eaten freely, but fruits should be eaten in moderation, with small quantities preferable to large and sour fruits preferable to sweet. Consumption of complex carbohydrates such as beans, corn, potatoes and rice is controversial and depends on individual reactions to them.

The over-consumption of meat in hypoglycaemia diets has aroused a great deal of opposition recently. Although it helps to control the symptoms of hypoglycaemia, excessive protein consumption, especially meat, has been claimed to cause deficiencies of vitamin B3, calcium and magnesium, and also excessive production of wastes such as ammonia, which is considered to be a carcinogen, and uric acid.[25] High meat consumption has been found to contribute to heart disease[26] and cancer of the colon,[27] to name but two common diseases. It has also been argued that, in the long run, a high protein diet may actually aggravate hypoglycaemia and make it incurable.[28] For vegetarians and people who are allergic to meat or cannot tolerate it, a high meat diet is out of the question, but all is not lost. Dr Paavo Airola has devised a new dietary approach to hypoglycaemia after many years of study and experimentation[29] and it is a vegetarian diet, based on grains, seeds and nuts, vegetables and fruit. He recommends cooked flax seeds, buckwheat and millet, which, he claims, digest slowly and therefore release sugar gradually. He also recommends milk and milk products. A bowl of buckwheat or millet with a dab of butter and a glass of milk or a cup of yogurt, for example, is the kind of meal which takes hours to digest, is completely satisfying, and keeps a proper sugar level. It also avoids the hazards associated with excessive meat.

A comprehensive supplement of multivitamins and multiminerals is also recommended, as are certain herbs, such as licorice root, golden seal, lobelia, dandelion, horsetail, chicory and garlic. Raw pancreas and raw thyroid tablets are also prescribed by some practitioners. These are tablets made from desiccated and powdered glands, freeze-dried or manufactured under vacuum. The producers claim that they retain all the goodness of the raw glands.

The good news is that hypoglycaemics can avoid all symptoms and lead a perfectly normal life provided they take the trouble to find a suitable diet and stick to it and take a comprehensive multivitamin and multimineral supplement. They can even feel better than most healthy people who subsist on junk food. The main thing is perseverance, for unless a special diet is persevered with the symptoms will return. In short, hypoglycaemics must give up junk food for good.

CHAPTER 11

INTESTINAL FITNESS

Ilya Ilich Metchnikoff (1845-1916) was a famous non-conformist Russian biologist, a Linus Pauling of his time, who worked in the Pasteur Institute in Paris doing immunity research. He won the 1908 Nobel Prize for establishing the theory of phagocytosis (phagocytosis is the process by which white blood cells engulf and destroy hostile bacteria, forming the body's first line of defence against infectious diseases). Later, however, his interest focused on the bacteria which infest the human intestine and particularly on the bacteria which cause fermentation and putrefaction in the colon.

Like Pauling, Metchnikoff wrote a small booklet which became a minor sensation. It was entitled *The Prolongation of Life* and became very controversial in medical circles. In it Metchnikoff expressed his conviction that excess wastes and poisons in the intestines are damaging to health. He believed that the residues of food not digested properly accumulate in the colon, forming an alkaline environment in which colonies of putrefactive bacteria thrive. Toxins liberated during fermentation and putrefaction pass through the intestinal walls and into the bloodstream, causing self-toxification of the body and increased susceptibility to disease. This is particularly true when stool transit time is overly prolonged, as in the case of chronic constipation. Claiming that lack of acidity in the colon adversely affects health, Metchnikoff enthusiastically recommended the daily consumption of yogurt and other fermented milks, which contain acidic bacteria. 'Yogurt', he claimed, 'also stimulates bowel movement, promoting regular elimination.'

To prove his point, he referred to the famous longevity of rural Bulgarians, who eat large amounts of yogurt daily, maintaining their health and vitality to an exceptionally old age. In fact Metchnikoff initiated the wide use of yogurt as a health food. More importantly, he was the first scientist to bring the intimate subject of colonic cleanliness and the danger of self-poisoning to the attention of the public. He made colonic health a 'decent' subject of conversation.

A common side effect of intestinal putrefaction is halitosis or bad breath. The manufacturers of mouthwashes and mouth fresheners would have us believe that all bad breath is due to dental decay, but apart from the occasional mouth infection most cases of bad breath can be traced to intestinal putrefaction, which can be rectified by yogurt or acidopilus milk.[1]

YOGURT TO THE RESCUE

Yogurt is simply milk which has been fermented by a species of bacteria called *Lactobacillus bulgaricus*. These bacteria curdle milk, converting milk sugar (lactose) to lactic acid. Yogurt is made by adding the bacillus, or a spoonful of pre-made yogurt, to heated milk and letting it incubate at a temperature of about 140°F (60°C). Excessively high temperatures kill the bacilli. Those who dislike commercial yogurt can buy a domestic yogurt-maker and make their own. A point to remember is that the acidity of yogurt increases with incubation or storage.

Acidophilus milk, which is soured by *Acidophilus* bacteria, is similar to yogurt, but has a less pleasant taste. That is why acidophilus milk does not match the popularity of yogurt. Whey, which has become popular recently, is another promoter of healthy intestinal flora due to its lactic acid and lactose content. Whey is the liquid left over from cheese-making, just as buttermilk is the residue of butter-making. Soured milks are a traditional food in many countries. Siberians have *kumiss*, Russians have *kefir*, Finns have *piima* and Israelis have *leben*. In fact, several biblical scholars have interpreted the 'butter' which Abraham served to his heavenly guests in Genesis 18:8 as soured milk.[2]

Today there is no doubt that Metchnikoff was correct in relating health to acidity in the colon. He was ahead of his time in preaching the benefits of yogurt, which does indeed contain many health-promoting properties. Modern studies have shown that cultured milks, and especially acidophilus milk, are extremely valuable in the treatment of gastroenteritis, colitis, constipation, biliary disorders, flatulence, migraine and nervous fatigue.[3] Yogurt is also highly digestible. While only 32 per cent of regular milk is digested after an hour in the digestive tract, 91 per cent of yogurt is digested after the same time.[4] In addition, yogurt and acidophilus milk can often be taken by people who cannot have ordinary milk due to lactose intolerance.

Dr Boris Sokoloff, in his book *Middle Age is What You Make It*, writes that yogurt's friendly bacteria protect the colon from hostile microbes, destroying them with lactic acid. The friendly yogurt bacteria join the beneficial bacteria already in the colon and fortify them. So yogurt promotes digestion as well as preventing constipation. Its laxative effect is enhanced when prunes are added, but for most people plain yogurt is usually sufficient.

Yogurt has also been found to possess potent anti-tumour activity.[5] Researchers at the Bulgarian Academy of Sciences in Sofia found that they could cure several types of experimentally induced cancer in animals with *Lactobacillus bulgaricus*, injections of which have also been found effective against human skin cancers.[6] It has also been suggested that meat eaters should take acidophilus capsules (or yogurt), in addition to bran, if they want to eliminate the enzymes that predispose the colon to cancer. Other studies have shown that yogurt can lower cholesterol levels, in spite of the fact that it contains cholesterol.[7] In one study, yogurt reduced cholesterol levels by 5-10 per cent after just one week's consumption.[8]

Yogurt also helps the intestines to synthesize vitamins K and B6.[9] Calcium is also better absorbed from yogurt than from milk, because of its acidity.[10]

Yogurt or supplemental lactobacillus acidophilus capsules should be taken when taking antibiotics in order to replace the intestinal flora killed off by the antibiotics.

Today the benefits of yogurt, as outlined by Metchnikoff, are widely known in connection with intestinal health. However, there are other foods which are also essential to healthy elimination.

FRUCTO-OLIGOSACCHARIDES (FOS)

These are a new class of carbohydrates, which are becoming increasingly popular. FOS are a totally natural substance, and are present in small amounts in many fruits, vegetables and grains we eat every day, like bananas, tomatoes, artichokes, onions, garlic, wheat and oats.

However, recent studies have shown that FOS are a kind of nondigestible sugar: they are not digested and absorbed in the body, like normal sugars. It is as if they are 'immune' to digestive enzymes, much like fibre.[11]

Instead, FOS have a great beneficial effect on intestinal flora. They were found to feed selectively only friendly intestinal bacteria, like bifidobacteria, bacteroides Fragilis group, peptostreptococcus, and lactobacillus acidophilus, but not unfriendly bacteria such as Clostridium perfringens, salmonella or E. coli.[12] In this study, a daily addition of 8 grams FOS to the diet, resulted in a tenfold increase of the friendly bifidobacteria.

These findings have far-reaching implications. They mean that by improving intestinal flora, and keeping it slightly acidic, FOS can help relieve constipation, prevent intestinal putrefaction, neutralize body odours or bad breath, and improve nutrient absorption from food.

These qualities are even more beneficial when taking antibiotics, since antibiotics kill both bad bacteria and friendly intestinal bacteria. As a result, some people experience diarrhoea, yeast infections and low energy levels. These symptoms can be helped by using FOS.

But this is not all. In a study done with diabetic patients, FOS were also found to reduce both sugar levels and cholesterol levels by using 5 or 8 grams of FOS a day.[13] The researchers also remarked that 'FOS can be useful as a low energy sweetener in the replacement of sucrose for those subjects with either diabetes mellitus or obesity.'

FOS are sold as a mildly sweet, white crystalline powder, which dissolves very easily in various drinks and foods, like cereals. It is a stable powder which requires no refrigeration if it is stored in a cool dry place. It is a low calorie food, contributing only about 1.5 calories per gram, whereas digestible carbohydrates like sugar contain 4 calories per gram.

FOS are processed from sugar by using a special enzyme (fructosyltransferase). However, in contrast to sucrose which is composed from one molecule of glucose and one of fructose, FOS are composed of one molecule glucose and one to three molecules of fructose.

One gram of FOS equals only about a half teaspoon, and by adding it to the diet for eight weeks, one may increase beneficial bacteria up to fivefold. Between a half teaspoon to one teaspoon is considered optimal intake. Regular supplementation can ensure that a healthful intestinal flora is maintained. Some FOS manfacturers claim that a higher daily intake of 1–3 teaspoons is needed to relieve constipation.

FABULOUS FIBRE

People who emphasize processed foods in their diet – people who shy away from fresh fruit and vegetables and consume large quantities of refined sugar and starch – create a deficiency of dietary fibre in their bodies. Refined carbohydrates are low in bulk; most are absorbed by the small intestine, leaving hardly any bulk left to fill the colon and stimulate bowel movement and elimination. Dietary fibre provides bulk.

Chemically speaking, dietary fibres are polysaccharides such as cellulose, hemicellulose, and pectin, and other plant substances such as lignin, gums and waxes, all of which differ in their metabolic properties. Some, like hemicellulose, have the well-known capacity to absorb seven or eight times their weight in water,[14] promoting large, soft stools and shortening stool transit time. Adding just 1 oz of dry wheat bran to the daily diet will increase stool weight by 60 per cent and bind with harmful bacteria and other substances so that they are eliminated as quickly as possible.[15] Dietary fibres maintain a clean colon, free from unfriendly bacteria, and prevent a host of diseases, from piles to cancer. Pectin, a polysaccharide contained in citrus fruits and apples, can reduce blood cholesterol levels if it forms 2.5–5 per cent of the diet.[16] Lignin, an insoluble non-carbohydrate fibre, seems to act as a structural binding agent.

Fresh vegetables and fruit, whole cereals and legumes provide us with all of the naturally occurring types of fibre, with their different cleansing effects on the body. Moreover, a diet high in natural fibres leaves scant space for refined sugary foods. Candies and biscuits are less tempting on a high fibre diet.

High fibre vegetables include celery, the leafy greens (broccoli, cabbage, lettuce, spinach, parsley, asparagus) and root vegetables (carrots, kohlrabi). As a rule, fruits are higher in calories for the fibre they supply. Apples and bananas are two of the best fibre fruits because of the varied fibres they contain. All legumes, whole cereals, nuts and seeds provide good fibre but are high in calories. Bran is always recommended as the most concentrated and the most useful fibre supplement. NOTE: Dietary fibre as found in vegetables and other foods should be broken down by thorough chewing, otherwise it can have quite the opposite effect on the colon, producing gas, putrefaction and bloating.[17]

As with other foods, individuals differ in their reactions to the various fibres in the intestines. Some people have so many hostile bacteria that many fibres are decomposed and fail to stimulate bowel movements. These people will not benefit much from fibres. Other people may not be able to tolerate excess roughage. In all these cases, mucilaginous plant substances, also called hydrophilic colloids, can be used. Some well-known plant sources for these are Guar gum, psyllium seeds, flax seeds, comfrey, agar-agar, Irish moss and some seaweeds. Like bran, these substances absorb many times their weight in water, but act more gently, producing a jelly-like mucus which helps to bind intestinal mucosal secretions. One popular commercial laxative makes use of psyllium seed powder, mixing it with dextrose (sugar) in almost equal parts. Pure psyllium powder brands are sugar-free and more beneficial. NOTE: Since dietary fibres absorb many times their weight in water, it is important that an increased consumption of water accompanies their use. If insufficient water is drunk, constipation may be aggravated.

EXERCISES TO IMPROVE ELIMINATION

Daily elimination is most important for health. It can prevent all the dreadful diseases caused by the prolonged storage of toxic wastes in the body. A special effort must be made to have at least one bowel movement a day, without straining. Over-the-counter laxatives should not be used as they irritate the delicate lining of the colon. Elimination should take place naturally, by means of unforced bowel movements, stimulated by a diet high in fibre and soured milk and low in processed foods.

The results of switching to a high fibre diet are not instant, especially if chronic constipation and long-term use of laxatives have weakened colonic muscle tone. Elimination depends a great deal on the condition of the muscles of the colon. However, muscle tone can be improved by exercise. The exercises shown opposite involve the use of the colon muscles and will help to strengthen them. They are very effective and have been recommended by the author to literally hundreds of people over the years, with great success.

Daily practice of these exercises will promote regular elimination without the need for laxatives. NOTE: People with colon diseases (colitis, diverticulosis, etc.) should consult a doctor before attempting these exercises.

Over a three-year period 376 people with varying degrees of constipation performed these exercises daily for periods ranging from one week to two months – they did not take laxatives during this time, nor did they make any drastic dietary changes beyond cutting down on white sugar and white flour products. The results speak for themselves: 207 reported good daily elimination without straining, 136 reported some improvement in elimination, and 33 reported no improvement.

If these exercises seem difficult to start with, do not be discouraged. Do the best you can, however humble your performance, and persevere with daily practice. Results are bound to come.

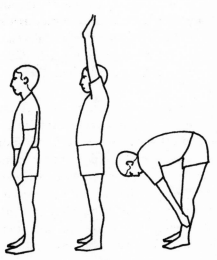

Stand erect, arms hanging loose by your sides. Start inhaling through your nose and at the same time raise your arms above your head. By the time your arms are at full stretch, your lungs should be full. Hold your breath and swiftly bend over as if trying to put your head between your knees. Make a real effort – grab your calves if it helps you to bend lower – but do not bend your knees. Now start to unbend, exhaling slowly, until you are upright again. Repeat three times. This exercise helps to promote elimination and also relieves feelings of fullness or bloating after overeating.

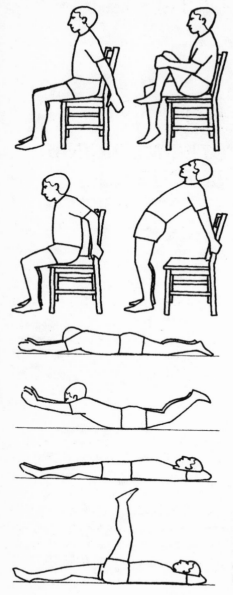

Sit upright in a chair, arms outstretched behind you. With both hands, vigorously pull your left knee up to your chest, grasping the leg below the kneecap, and inhale as you do so. Hold for a second or two, then exhale and lower the leg. Repeat with the right leg.

Sit upright in a chair, with your knees together. Grasp the back of the chair on both sides at seat level. Supporting your weight on your hands, push yourself out of the chair, inhaling as you do so. Arch your body forwards as far as possible – make a peak effort! Hold this position for a second or two, also holding your breath. Now exhale and return to your original sitting position. Repeat as many times as feels comfortable.

Lie on your stomach, arms outstretched in front of you. Inhale and as you do so lift your feet and arms away from the floor, so that your body makes a bow shape. Hold the bow shape for a second or two, then exhale and relax.

Lie flat on your back, with your legs straight and together, and your head resting on the palms of your hands. As you inhale, raise your left leg to 90°, hold for a second or two, then exhale and lower the leg. Repeat with the other leg.

CHAPTER 12

HERBS:
A NEGLECTED MEDICINAL BOUNTY

Nature provides an inexhaustible bounty of healing sources: roots, tubers, bulbs, leaves, berries, fruits, petals, shoots and barks. 'The fruit therefore shall be for meat and the leaf for medicine,' (Ezekiel 47:12).

Plants and herbs have always been humanity's drugstore. Phytotherapy, or healing with herbs, was prevalent in the ancient cultures of the Middle and Far East, Greece and Rome. The ancient doctors were herbalists. Even our grandparents knew a lot about plants and herbs, and how to prepare decoctions, infusions, poultices or ointments to cure common disorders. During the thousands of years of human existence, people have been attracted to the properties of various plants, and tried, and often succeeded, in using them to heal themselves.

The first evidence of a medicinal use of herbs goes back to ancient Assyria, 6,000 years ago. An Assyrian herbal (herb inventory) describes 250 healing plants, including licorice, opium poppy and oil of almond. Hippocrates (377-462 BC), the father of modern medicine, described 400 plants, of which 200 are still in use. But it is the first-century Roman healer Pedanius Dioscorides, author of a *materia medica* which lists 500 herbs, who is considered to be the father of modern pharmacology.

Knowledge of folk medicine and herbs, a knowledge based on practical observation, was passed from generation to generation. American Indians, for example, learned of botanical remedies by experimenting with plants sought out by animals suffering from wounds, fevers or bellyache, by watching how wild turkeys, during a cold spell, fed their chicks with leaves of the spicebush, or how forest bears smeared their wounds with spruce resin. They are believed to have avoided scurvy and vitamin C deficiency by drinking large quantities of black spruce leaf tea. The Rappanhannock tribe of Virginia used an infusion of sassafras roots to lower fever and to bring out the rash which accompanies measles. They also used witch hazel, as a treatment for skin eruptions and open sores, boiling the bark to the consistency of jelly and spreading it over the infected area.

The old herbalists believed that all plants were intended to be used by humans. The shape, colour and habitat of plants were clues to their healing properties. Yellow flowers were tried for jaundice, red flowers for cleansing the blood, and ginseng as a panacea because its roots are shaped like the human body. Habitat was also important. The ancients assumed, for example, that plants growing in wet places, along rivers or in swamps, could cure colds and rheumatism. In one case at least they were perfectly correct: willow bark, used for centuries to cure colds, headaches and rheumatism, was found to contain salicin, a glycoside which is the precursor of salicylic acid, the substance later isolated and used in aspirin.

As various herbal lists make clear, every healing herb was

supposed to treat several disorders, not just one. Each herb was thought to influence several organs and improve general constitution. Garlic, for example, was used to cure no fewer than 22 disorders. Fennel was considered effective as a carminative (expelling gas from the stomach and intestines), as a diuretic (increasing the flow of urine), and as a general tonic. It was also used to stimulate milk production in nursing mothers, to alleviate sore throats, heal ulcers and prevent convulsions.

Throughout history herbs have been used as spices, for preserving foods. Many spices such as cloves, oregano, sage, rosemary and vanilla, are antioxidants.[1] They preserve foods in much the same way as synthetic antioxidants such as BHT or BHA. Herbal spices are so effective that in 1937 and 1938 a patent was granted for a mixture made of small amounts of celery, sage and clove. Extracts of rosemary have been found to be more effective than BHA or BHT in preventing lard from going rancid.[2]

In addition to herbal therapy, ancient folk medicine used faith, autosuggestion and mysticism. Indeed, faith was, and still is, a very effective factor, especially in psychosomatic disorders. Today scientists call it the placebo effect.

FOLK MEDICINE AND PHARMACOLOGY

With the advent of organic chemistry in the nineteenth century, plants began to be studied scientifically. Chemists extracted the active ingredients, isolated them and identified their effects and chemical structure. Thanks to the 'phytochemical revolution' it became possible to treat disorders with small doses of active ingredients, without using the entire plant. Pharmacology, the study of the effects of drugs on living organisms, was to follow.

By isolating active ingredients, specific drugs came to be used for specific ailments. Until the beginning of the nineteenth century, there were very few specific drugs. It was known, for example, that bark of the cinchona tree could cure malaria; it contains quinine, the alkaloid that acts against *Plasmodium*, the parasite that causes malaria. It was also known that the shrub ipecacuanha, which grows in South America, is effective against dysentery; it was found to contain emetine, an alkaloid which destroys the amoebae which cause dysentery.[3]

The father of experimental pharmacology was the French physiologist François Magendie (1783-1855). He isolated strychnine from the seeds of the poison nut tree (*Strychnos nux vomica*) and emetine from the roots of ipecacuanha; emetine, by the way, can also induce vomiting and is used as an emetic to this day. Magendie was followed by many other researchers, all of whom isolated the active ingredients of plants.

The next step in pharmacology was the production of synthetic drugs, drugs manufactured artificially in the laboratory by chemically duplicating the natural substance. Direct use of plants became a thing of the past. Synthetic drugs were cheaper – there was no need to process many tons of plant material in order to extract a few grains of the active substance – and their effects were quicker and more specific. As a result, today's pharmacopoeias or official lists of drugs contain mostly synthetic drugs. Safe, natural cures were neglected in favour of quick-acting, highly specific modern preparations. But after a few years of use, questions of safety were raised. Some of the new drugs had bad side effects which outweighed their beneficial effects.

The second half of the twentieth century, however, has

seen a revival of herbalism. It is now realized that, in many cases, plants can contribute to health more safely than synthetic drugs. In fact many plant remedies cannot be made artificially. Morphine and codeine, for example, which dull pain and alleviate coughing, are still derived from the opium poppy. Reserpine, a common sedative, which reduces high blood pressure, is still derived from *Rauwolfia serpentina*.

What is the reason behind the present trend toward using plants again rather than synthetics? Part of the reason is that some synthetic drugs have severe side effects, but there are also gargantuan costs involved in developing sophisticated drugs, and many years are needed to test the safety of new drugs and approve them. Natural substances are, by contrast, safer and cheaper.

Today's 'new' herbal remedies come from all over the world, many of them from areas inhabited by tribes whose culture is very primitive. Among such peoples the collecting of herbs and the preparation of medicines is the prerogative of the local medicine man, who does not willingly share his secrets. Of the 600,000 or so plant species on earth, only about 5 per cent have ever been studied in the laboratory and, so far, only 677 medicinally useful substances have been isolated.

ACTIVE INGREDIENTS IN PLANTS

Many herbs are now grown by modern agricultural methods, using cross-breeding, hormones and controlled fertilization to increase the levels of their active ingredients. These are at their peak at certain hours of the day and on certain days of the month, according to the biological clock of the plant concerned. For example, at 9:00 a.m. the opium poppy contains four times as much morphine as it contains at 12:00 noon.

The most prevalent active ingredients in plants are the ALKALOIDS, which have varying toxic effects on humans and animals. Alkaloids are complex compounds which contain nitrogen and possess an alkaline reaction. They can be stimulants, hallucinogens, depressants or painkillers (opiates), and are difficult to synthesize artificially. Common examples include theophylline (in tea), caffeine (in coffee), theobromine (in cocoa) and nicotine (in tobacco).

Most hallucinogenic drugs (narcotics) are composed of a few basic alkaloids. Contrary to common belief, NARCOTIC PRINCIPLES are not restricted to plants such as hemp (marihuana), poppy (opium) and ergot fungus (LSD). They occur in many common and 'innocent' foods. Nutmeg, found in most kitchens, contains a powerful drug, myristicin, which can cause hallucinations in doses of over a few grams.[4] Mescaline, an alkaloid which causes hallucinations and convulsions, is found in some species of cactus. Indians chew peyote cactus buttons (mescal buttons) for their hallucinogenic effects.[5]

The GLYCOSIDES are compounds of glucose with other substances. For example, there are the cardiac glycosides digoxin and digitoxin, derived from foxglove (*Digitalis*), for which no synthetic substitutes have been found; these are used to treat congestive heart failure. There is also amygdalin (laetrile), derived from apricot kernels, which has been claimed as a treatment for cancer. Other glycosides which form foam in water are called SAPONINS (*sapo* means soap), and they are highly toxic. Saponins cause red blood cells to disintegrate (haemolysis), but they can also be beneficial as expectorants. The saponin glycyrrhizin, for example, which is found in licorice root, has a function similar to that of the hormone cortisone and is an effective treatment for mild inflammations.

ESSENTIAL OILS, unlike regular oils, are the volatile and aromatic compounds that give plants their fragrance. As such, they have been used as food additives and perfumes since antiquity. A few common plant sources of essential oil are angelica, citrus rinds, hibiscus, gardenia, lemon grass, rose, vanilla and violet. Apart from enhancing the aroma and taste of foods, many essential oils have a stimulating effect.[6] Some, like garlic, onion and thyme, are antiseptics – thyme is often used in mouthwashes and gargles. Aromatic bitters, found in yarrow, chamomile and peppermint, for example, stimulate the appetite. Essential oil of camphor stimulates the heart and raises blood pressure. Anise (aniseed), caraway and peppermint oil are known to stimulate gastric and bile secretions, alleviate digestive disorders and improve appetite.

Another group of active ingredients in plants are the STEROIDS, widely used in medicine and animal husbandry. In humans and animals steroids are secreted by the adrenal glands. Steroids were originally produced, at great expense, from animal glands or from horse's urine, but in the 1940s it was discovered that SAPONIN GLYCOSIDES (*sapogenins*) derived from plants could be converted to steroids. One such sapogenin, diosgenin, was found to be a very convenient industrial precursor of oestrogen and progesterone, the essential ingredients of the birth control pill. In 1952 it was discovered that the wild Mexican yam contains high concentrations of diosgenin in its rhizomes.[7] Today it is the main plant source for estrogens.

CAUTION: Women who have aching breast lumps caused by overproduction of oestrogen would do well to avoid yams (and also wheat germ oil and orange rinds). Any woman finding a breast lump should see a physician at once and not try to self-medicate.

The TANNINS are highly astringent, that is they have

the power to contract soft tissues and blood vessels, checking blood flow and secretions. They are therefore used to treat diarrhoea, intestinal convulsions and ulcers. Applied externally, they stop bleeding. Chinese tea leaves are a rich source of tannin.

Some plants, like psyllium (plantain) and comfrey, contain MUCILAGINOUS SUBSTANCES. These are polysaccharide-like and are destroyed by heat. When they dissolve in water (or in saliva) a sticky gel is formed which soothes and heals mucous membranes, such as those of the respiratory and digestive systems. Mucilages are also mildly laxative and used by some people in preference to bran.

Many herbs are rich in BITTER PRINCIPLES which stimulate the appetite an help to relieve digestive disorders. Hops, for example, contain lupulin, which imparts bitterness to beer. Many plants also contain ORGANIC ACIDS which destroy bacteria and stimulate elimination – citrus fruits contain citric acid, apples malic acid, leafy vegetables oxalic acid and ripe fruit tartaric acid.

HERBS FOR THE HEART AND BLOOD VESSELS

FOXGLOVE (*Digitalis*) contains the glycosides digoxin and digitoxin, which stimulate the heart. Long before digitalis was adopted by modern medicine, illiterate farmers and housewives throughout Europe were treating dropsy (watery sickness) and congestive heart failure with concoctions of foxglove leaves.[8] Digitalis is most effective in cases where heart failure is due to hypertension or atherosclerosis.[9] SQUILL bulbs (sea onion) contain proscillaridine, an alkaloid similar to digoxin and digitoxin which is also an expectorant. STROPHANTUS seeds, from East Africa, contains the alkaloid strophantin K, which is similar to digoxin and digitoxin. All these alkaloids, however, are very poisonous in higher doses.

SWEET CLOVER contains coumarin, a vitamin K antagonist which inhibits blood clotting and may prevent coronary thrombosis. This effect was first observed when cattle eating sweet clover developed haemorrhages.[10]

VALERIAN is an effective sedative which reduces heart palpitations. BISHOP WEED, which grows along the Nile, reduces muscle cramps and relieves angina pectoris by dilating the arteries of the heart. Vitamin K, found in ALFALFA and many leafy green vegetables promotes blood clotting, while dicumarol, found in many plants, is an anticoagulant.

In 1968 it was demonstrated that ONIONS and GARLIC can help to dissolve blood clots, reduce cholesterol and prevent arteriosclerosis.[11] Garlic is particularly effective in reducing high blood pressure. Another effective reducer of high blood pressure is reserpine, an alkaloid occurring in *Rauwolfia serpentina*, a shrub growing mainly in India and the Far East.[12]

CAUTION: An overdose of reserpine can cause low pulse rate and exhaustion.

HERBS FOR THE DIGESTIVE SYSTEM

MOUTH

An infusion of SAGE is a good antiseptic gargle for mouth and throat. Oil of CLOVE alleviates toothache. In Yemenite folk medicine THYME leaves are chewed for the same purpose. EUCALYPTUS oil fights tooth decay and bad breath.

STOMACH OVERACIDITY

Some Native American tribes used HOPS to counteract excess acidity.

CONSTIPATION

There are many plant laxatives – PSYLLIUM seeds or SENNA leaves and pods are common. Fresh ALOE leaves are high in laxative glycosides. GARDENIA fruit has been used for thousands of years in China to overcome constipation. Recently, the laxative effect of its active principle, geniposide, was substantiated by a modern study. [13]

DIARRHOEA

CHINA TEA, POMEGRANATE juice, CACTUS fruit and YARROW tea are all effective.

INTESTINAL WORMS

WORMSEED oil (*Chenopodium* oil) and GARLIC oil have been commonly used to expel worms. In Thailand, PERSIMMON fruit is used for the same purpose. The active ingredient in persimmons is diospyrol; a recent study with diospyrol has validated its effectiveness against parasitic infections.[14]

CAUTION: Anyone who suspects that he or she has intestinal parasites should consult a physician.

ULCERS

LICORICE promotes healing of mucous membranes. In fact, two derivatives of its roots can reduce the size of ulcers by 70-90 per cent after only one month of treatment.[15] Folk medicine also uses licorice to relieve indigestion. CABBAGE and cabbage juice have long been used to cure stomach and duodenal ulcers – the active therapeutic factor in cabbage is a substance called vitamin U.[16] FENNEL or VERVAIN (verbena) tea and LETTUCE or POTATO juice are also very helpful. Crude vegetable oils and also ARROWROOT, COMFREY and IRISH MOSS are good lubricators.

HERBS FOR THE PANCREAS

SALT BUSH *(Artiplex halimus)* is used by the Bedouins of Israel to fight diabetes – it stimulates the pancreas to secrete insulin.[17] Another effective herb in this respect is FENU-GREEK. Drinking a glass of water in which a tablespoon of fenugreek seeds have been soaked overnight is very beneficial in many cases; three glasses a day is the average dose.

HERBS FOR THE LIVER AND GALLBLADDER

Fasting for one to two weeks, taking only GRAPE juice, cleanses the liver and the kidneys. SHEPHERD'S PURSE, YARROW, LEMON BALM tea and PARSLEY all cleanse the liver. MILK THISTLE is effective against hepatitis. Jaundice is alleviated by HYSSOP, particularly in the early stages, and by HOPS. BARBERRY is believed to help the ducts to the gallbladder from becoming blocked, while COMFREY, PARSLEY and NETTLE are often recommended as part of treatment for gallstones.

HERBS FOR THE KIDNEYS

Water-rich fruits (WATERMELONS, GRAPES) help to prevent kidney stones. CELERY stimulates urination, as do ASPARAGUS and KELP. Caffeine found in COFFEE, and theobromine, found in COCOA, are efficient diuretics (induce urination). ONION and GARLIC are effective against infections of the urinary tract, as is CIDER VINE-GAR. BEARBERRY leaf tea helps to stop internal bleed-ings, flush out kidney stones and heal kidney inflammation. BARBERRY bark tea or powder is highly antiseptic and is used to prevent urinary tract infections. The mucilaginous nature of MARSHMALLOW can help to remove stones from the kidneys. SAGE, COMFREY and NETTLE infusions can have the same effect.

HERBS FOR THE RESPIRATORY TRACT

LEMON juice, CIDER VINEGAR and EUCALYPTUS oil are recommended, as are infusions of ROSEHIPS, LEMON-SCENTED VERVAIN (verbena), SAGE, LEMON BALM, LINDEN flowers, MARSHMALLOW, COMFREY, LICORICE and CHAMOMILE.

HERBS FOR ASTHMA

THORN APPLE *(Datura stramonium)* and DEADLY NIGHTSHADE *(Atropa belladonna)* are two herbs containing atropine, an alkaloid which alleviates asthma attacks. Another effective alkaloid against asthma is ephedrine, derived from the *Ephedra vulgaris.*

HERBS FOR THE NERVOUS SYSTEM
SEDATIVES

VALERIAN, ROSEMARY and PASSION FLOWER have a calming effect. CATNIP tea is recommended for hyperactive children. CHAMOMILE and LINDEN can relieve insomnia in a safe way. Passion flower is a well-known sedative, and is commonly used to relieve nervousness, insomnia, hysteria and neuromuscular disorders.

ANALGESICS

The Solanaceae family, to which deadly nightshade, potato, sweet pepper, tomato, eggplant and tobacco belong, provides many effective analgesics. DEADLY NIGHTSHADE contains atropine and scopolamine, highly toxic alkaloids which act on the autonomous nervous system and relax muscle cramps when taken in tiny amounts. MANDRAKE, a plant mentioned in the Bible, was used in the Middle Ages to relieve pain and induce sleep. Last but not least are morphine and codeine, potent analgesics derived from the OPIUM POPPY.

STIMULANTS

Andean Indians chew dry COCA leaves which contain cocaine. Cocaine stimulates the nervous system, suppresses appetite and promotes alertness, but can lead to dependency. Coca-Cola contained cocaine until 1904, when the use of this ingredient was prohibited. CAFFEINE (in coffee, tea and maté) is another stimulating alkaloid, but like most alkaloids it is poisonous in high doses. Even in lesser amounts it can cause anxiety, depression,[18], headaches and ulcers.[19] THEOBROMINE is a similarly stimulating alkaloid found in cocoa (too much cocoa depletes the body of calcium and can cause kidney stones due to its oxalic acid content).

HERBS FOR THE SKIN

Mucilaginous substances such as powdered COMFREY, PSYLLIUM and QUINCE seeds can speed up the healing of wounds. YARROW leaves can stop wounds bleeding and promote healing. Eczema can be helped by CIDER VINEGAR or infusions of CHAMOMILE. Infusions of ROSEMARY, YARROW, SAGE or NETTLE can help prevent the hair from breaking if applied regularly.

HERBS FOR LOSING WEIGHT

Some herbs can reduce the desire for food, among them CHICKWEED, FENNEL and SPIRULINA algae. Other diet-helpers include EVENING PRIMROSE seed oil, KELP (powder or tablets) and SEAWEEDS such as *kombu*, *wakame* or *nori* which are available in health food stores. GUAR GUM is a recent and efficient slimming discovery which helps to reduce hunger; it also binds with dietary fats and helps to excrete them from the body.

There is still a mountain of research to be done on medicinal plants. They are an amazing field of study and have already produced solutions to many human afflictions. Many people still associate herbal medicine with folklore, faith healing and even witchcraft, but over and over again experimental studies have demonstrated that certain herbs can be as effective as laboratory-manufactured drugs. Herbs are increasingly used today in conjunction with other therapeutic modalities such as megavitamin therapy, macrobiotic diets, homeopathy and acupuncture. There is absolutely no doubt that many plant benefits are still waiting to be discovered.

WARNING: Amateur use of plants and their derivatives can be dangerous. Remember, some species used for medicinal purposes are highly poisonous even in small doses. Do not self-treat! A knowledgeable professional should be consulted before attempting a specific treatment.

HERBS FOR HEALTH

The alphabetical list which follows contains over 100 commonly used plants. Most are used as infusions or tisanes, that is, as herb teas; others are boiled and simmered to form more concentrated decoctions; a few can be eaten raw in salads, others as spices or flavourings. The author's own researches into Middle Eastern folk medicine are reflected in a few of the entries.

ACACIA (Acacia senegal)
The gum arabic which exudes from the stem of the gum arabic tree is collected and used to soothe inflammation of the respiratory, digestive and urinary tracts. It helps coughs and sore throats, diarrhoea and dysentery. Gum arabic is usually dissolved in water to make a mucilage. In the Middle East, it is used in cooking and in the making of sweetmeats.

AGAVE (Agave americana)
This is a perennial plant which grows in deserts. Its fibres are mainly used to make threads and ropes. Agave is antiseptic, diuretic and laxative. Its sap is disinfectant and prevents intestinal putrefaction.

AGRIMONY (Agrimonia eupatoria)
A perennial herb with astringent, anti-inflammatory properties. As an infusion (herbal tea), it has a very beneficial effect on the digestive organs – stomach, intestines, gallbladder and liver. It can prevent inflammations of the intestinal tract caused by irritating food or infection (enteritis). An infusion is also used as a gargle for treating mouth infections.

ALDER (Alnus glutinosa)
Infusions of shredded bark relieve constipation and stimulate bile secretion. Decoctions (boiled and simmered teas) are used to make poultices for rheumatic joints.

ALFALFA (Medicago sativa)
Seeds and sprouts are rich in minerals and vitamins

(potassium, iron, phosphorus, magnesium, calcium, carotene, vitamins Bl, B3, B12, D, C, E, K). The seeds are commonly used in sprouted form and to make alfalfa tea. Alfalfa is a tonic, stimulant, appetizer and diuretic, and also relieves urinary disorders and oedema.

ALOE *(Aloe vera)*
Soothes inflammations of the digestive tract and relieves constipation. Normally taken in powder or capsule form due to its repellent taste. Infusions are good for bathing wounds and eyes.

AMARANTH *(Amaranthus hypochondriacus)*
Amaranth, also known as Inca wheat, was the main staple of the Aztec diet due to its high protein content. It is now cultivated in the American Midwest. Infusions have an astringent property, and are therefore effective against diarrhoea and dysentery; they can also be used to reduce excessive menstrual bleeding.

ANGELICA *(Angelica archangelica)*
Angelica tea aids digestion, relieves flatulence and stimulates the appetite. It is useful for all sorts of digestive problems, including ulcers, vomiting and colic. Applied externally, angelica lotion can relieve rheumatic pain. A decoction of the root can be applied to the skin to treat scabies or itching. **CAUTION:** Angelica must not be taken by diabetics as it tends to elevate blood sugar level.

ANISE, ANISEED *(Pimpinella anisum)*
Anise is an aromatic plant, the seeds of which are used mainly in Mediterranean cooking. As an infusion, anise helps the digestion, relieves flatulence, improves appetite and

alleviates cramps, nausea and colic in children. Anise water stimulates milk production in nursing mothers and is also said to bring on delayed menstruation.

ARNICA (Arnica montana)
Also called mountain tobacco. Infusions stimulate perspiration in the case of feverish colds, soothe inflamed mucous membranes and the nasal passages, and act as a diuretic and general stimulant. Infusions can also be used externally as a hair tonic, but should never be used on broken skin or open wounds.

ARTICHOKE (Cynara scolymus)
Stimulates bile evacuation and is a diuretic. The flower heads are commonly eaten as vegetables, but extracts of the leaves and roots were once used to treat arteriosclerosis, jaundice and post-operative anaemia. Some cultures consider artichokes to be an aphrodisiac.

ASPARAGUS (Asparagus officinalis)
The young shoots, mainly used in cooking, are a rich source of minerals and vitamins. Asparagus is a potent diuretic and a mild laxative; it also increases perspiration.

BALM, LEMON BALM (Melissa officinalis)
Infusions of the leaves have a pleasant lemony odour. Dulls pain, eases toothache, and relieves flatulence, cramps, indigestion and colic. Increases perspiration and is useful in treating the symptoms of colds. Traditionally used to treat nervousness, depression and insomnia. Also claimed to stimulate the onset of menstruation and to relieve period pains.

BARBERRY *(Berberis vulgaris)*

The roots, bark and berries are used in infusions. Promotes secretion of bile and is therefore beneficial in liver disorders. Also tends to dilate blood vessels and therefore helps to lower blood pressure. The bark of the roots has a laxative effect. Decoctions make a good mouthwash or gargle for mouth or throat irritations.

CAUTION: Do not self-treat high or low blood pressure with barberry.

BASIL *(Ocimum basilicum)*

The leaves, which have appetite-stimulating properties, are generally used as a culinary herb. Infusions of the leaves can also be used to relieve flatulence, stomach cramps, constipation and enteritis.

BEARBERRY *(Arctostaphylos uva-ursi)*

The leaves contain tannins (astringent) and glycosides such as arbutin, which have excellent antiseptic properties. Even today modern medicine uses bearberry as a urinary antiseptic. Infusions help to alleviate diarrhoea and bleeding, and heal mucous membranes. Bearberry is also a diuretic, reduces uric acid levels, relieves the pain caused by kidney stones and gravel, and alleviates the symptoms of chronic cystitis. North American Indians traditionally used an infusion made from the fruit as an appetite suppressant in weight control.[20]

CAUTION: Excessive use can cause stomach pain.

BELLADONNA, DEADLY NIGHTSHADE
(Atropa belladonna)

This is a poisonous plant, available on prescription in tinctures and extracts. It contains several alkaloids: atropine, which relieves asthma; hyoscyamine, which induces sleep and can cause paralysis; belladonnine, which is a narcotic and painkiller; and scopolamine, another painkiller, which reduces high blood pressure and produces twilight sleep. The narcotic action of belladonna affects the central nervous system and can cause paralysis. It should only be used under medical supervision.

BILBERRY *(Vaccinium myrtillus)*

A small, wild plant whose leaves are rich in flavonoids, particularly in anthocyanidins which are powerful antioxidants and have an anti-inflammatory effect, strengthening capillaries and collagen. Bilberry extracts are now increasingly used to treat eye conditions such as near-sightedness, and to improve night vision and reverse diabetic retinopathy. An infusion of the leaves is antiseptic. Capsules of bilberry extracts and formulas containing them for improving eyesight are available in health food shops.

BIRCH, WHITE BIRCH *(Betula alba)*

Astringent, diuretic which promotes perspiration. Infusions of the leaves are claimed to dissolve kidney stones and eliminate gravel. The decoction is a mild sedative when taken at bedtime.

BIRTHWORT *(Aristolochia longa)*

Birthwort is an ancient Egyptian remedy for snake bite. Infusions of the roots heal ulcers and also arrest tumours in animals. Infusions also stimulate perspiration, raise blood pressure, act as a diuretic, reduce fever, and stimulate delayed menstruation. Birthwort is also claimed to relieve the symptoms of rheumatism and gout.

BISHOP WEED (Ammi visnaga)

A Middle Eastern plant commonly used in Yemenite and other Arab folk medicines. It contains the glycoside khellin, which has been found to reduce the pain of kidney stones by relieving muscle spasms due to stone pressure, and also the pain of angina pectoris by dilating the arteries of the heart.

BLACKBERRY (Rubus villosus)

Blackberry leaf infusions have long been known as a remedy for diarrhoea. They also have tonic and decongestant properties, and can relieve the symptoms of enteritis.

BLACK NIGHTSHADE (Solanum nigrum)

Contains several alkaloids – atropine, solanine and solasodine a derivative of diosgenin from which plant steroids are manufactured. All nightshades (see Belladonna) are highly poisonous and must only be used under strict medical supervision.

BLUE FLAG (Iris versicolor)

Infusions of the root are diuretic, tonic, purify the blood, expel intestinal worms and relieve vaginal infections. Because of its diuretic properties, the American Indians used blue flag to treat oedema. It is recommended for migraines caused by stomach disorders.

BORAGE (Borago officinalis)

Reduces fever by increasing perspiration, stimulates adrenal gland secretions, and acts as a general tonic. Infusions are reputed to alleviate the symptoms of rheumatism and inflammations of the urinary tract. Borage used to be a popular home remedy. The tops were also used in salads with dill.

BUCHU (Borosma betulina)
Makes an excellent herb tea for those who suffer from cystitis, urinary gravel or other urinary troubles. In South Africa, from where it originates, it is drunk as a tonic.

CARAWAY (Carum carvi)
Seeds used for flavouring foods, mainly bread. They stimulate the appetite, relieve flatulence and improve digestion, and are also a mild expectorant (releasing phlegm). They also promote the onset of menstruation and relieve uterine cramps.

CAT'S CLAW (Uncaria Tomentosa)
A herb from the amazon rainforest, which was hailed in recent years as an immune system booster. It was found to be particularly beneficial in the treatment of cancer and AIDS. Dr Keplinger of the Austrian laboratory Immodel, reported that he was able to reverse the progression of both AIDS and cancer in the majority of his patients, using Krallendorn, the pharmaceutical name for cat's claw root extract.[21] Dr Brent Davis, who has been working with Cat's Claw in the U.S., says that *Uncaria tomentosa* is a world–class herb which has the power to arrest and reverse deep-seated pathology, allowing more rapid return to health.[22]

Research into Cat's Claw is currently being conducted in England, Germany and Switzerland, checking evidence of Cat's Claw benefit in the treatment of arthritis, allergies, ulcers, cancer and acne.

There is an increasing demand for Cat's Claw which is sold freely in health food shops as teas and capsules.

CATNIP (Nepeta cataria)
The leaves make an effective and aromatic infusion for upset stomach, colic and flatulence. Can also be used in enemas.

CAYENNE PEPPER (Capsicum frutescens)

One of the oldest herbal remedies. The fruits, commonly known as chilis, can be used to stimulate the appetite and digestion, release phlegm, and increase resistance to colds. Powdered chilis have repeatedly been claimed to heal ulcers in the stomach and intestines, presumably by promoting tissue growth through the release of histamine. In fact, some people rub chili powder into the scalp to promote hair growth. Also effective for high blood pressure, diabetes, hangovers, arthritis, asthma, kidney infections, and sinus and other respiratory problems.

CELERY (Apium graveolens)

The stems are rich in iron, magnesium and carotene. Used mainly in salads or soups, as a condiment and as a salt substitute in low sodium diets. The leaves stimulate the appetite, are diuretic and bring on menstruation. The seeds are sedative and relieve flatulence.

CENTAURY (Centaurium erythraea)

As an infusion before meals, centaury stimulates the appetite and aids digestion by encouraging the liver to secrete bile. Applied externally, centaury is reputed to drive away fleas and lice.

CHAMOMILE (Matricaria chamomilla)

Very popular as a herb tea, effective against indigestion, flatulence, colic, spasms, stomach cramps and insomnia. It is also an antiseptic. Reduces inflammations of the gastrointestinal tract. Used in mouthwashes and gargles, in sitz baths to alleviate haemorrhoids, and also in enema solutions.

CHICKWEED (Stellaria media)
Found abundantly everywhere. Infusions relieve flatulence
and constipation, and can also be used to bathe bruises and
skin irritations, with soothing effects. Can also be used as a
vegetable, like spinach. The potassium in chickweed reduces
food cravings, so regular infusions taken three times a day
may be beneficial to slimmers.

CHICORY (Chicorium intybus)
Widely used in coffee substitutes. Infusions of the roots stimulate the appetite, aid digestion, promote bile secretion and
help to relieve the pain and discomfort caused by gallstones.

CINNAMON (Cinnamonum zeylanicum)
The powdered bark is used as a spice and also to make
aromatic infusions. Cinnamon is a disinfectant, stimulant, and
anti-flatulent. Some people find cinnamon tea helpful for
nausea, if sipped slowly when warm. In Yemenite folk
medicine strong infusions of cinnamon are used to relieve
menstrual cramps.

COMFREY (Symphytum officinalis)
Rich in calcium and mucilaginous substances, comfrey root
acts as a demulcent and lubricant of the intestines as well as a
deterrent against intestinal microorganisms such as *E. coli,*
which it absorbs and excretes.[23] Comfrey root is also rich in
allantoin, a substance which stimulates cell proliferation,
speeding up the healing of burns and wounds[24] when applied
topically in poultices. It can also be used in bath water to
improve skin tone.

 Comfrey is used in infusions, and also in powder or tablet
form. It is an astringent, and as such stops diarrhoea and
bleeding; in particular, it helps gastric and duodenal ulcers to

heal. It is also an expectorant, loosening phlegm so that it can be coughed up. It has been used to treat liver disorders and also to expel kidney stones and gravel. Can also reduce excessive menstrual flow.

CAUTION: Excessive use may cause tumours of the liver and gallbladder due to certain alkaloids present in the leaves.

CORIANDER (Coriandrum sativum)
A Mediterranean herb used mainly as a spice. It relieves flatulence.

COFFEE (Coffea)
In Yemenite folk medicine the shells of coffee berries (gisher) are used to treat kidney stones. The beverage made from them – half a spoonful of shredded shells to one cup of water, brought to the boil and simmered for three minutes – is strained, sweetened with a little honey and sipped while hot. It is a pleasant, low caffeine drink, mildly stimulating and diuretic. Three or four cups a day solve many cases of kidney stones, but it is best to start with one cup a day, increasing the dose gradually.

CORNSILK (Zea mays)
The fine tassel at the top of the corn cob is made into infusions which soothe the urinary passages and act as a diuretic. Very beneficial in cases of kidney stones and cystitis. To be effective, several cups a day should be drunk.

COTTON (Gossypium herbaceum)
The powdered root stimulates labour, inducing uterine contractions. It also helps in cases of delayed menstruation and sexual dysfunction in women.

CUMIN *(Cuminum cyminum)*

The seeds and essential oil are used as a spice to stimulate the gastric juices and relieve flatulence. Also said to increase milk secretion in nursing mothers.

DANDELION *(Taraxacum officinalis)*

Laxative, diuretic and tonic. Infusions stimulate bile formation, relieve oedema, and cleanse the body of poisons. Dandelion is also said to relieve the symptoms of jaundice and gallstones. Can also be consumed as a juice, and the leaves added to salads.

DONG QUAI *(Angelica Sinensis)*

Very popular in Asia. Traditionally regarded as a 'female' remedy. Dong quai was found to have a balancing effect on oestrogen activity and a tonic effect on the uterus. *The Concise Materia Medica* cites the use of dong quai in conditions such as painful menstruation and for menopausal symptoms. It is also used to promote a healthy pregnancy and easy delivery.

ECHINACEA *(Echinacea Angustifolia)*

A recently popular herb in health food stores. Despite its sudden popularity it has a long pedigree. Echinacea was traditionally used by American Indian tribes as a medicine for a variety of conditions, from colds to snake bites. It was considered a blood purifier, analgesic and antiseptic. Another variety, *Echinacea Purpurea,* was used in Europe.

Various studies have shown that Echinacea helps overcome many and varied disorders by enhancing the immune system.[25] The root contains a group of polysaccharides that activate immunity and restrain infection.

The root, flower and leaves all contain a group of glycosides collectively known as Echinacosides. These powerful substances inhibit hyaluronidase, an enzyme which is used by bacteria and viruses to help penetrate cell membranes and cause disease. Collectively, the active factors in Echinacea strengthen the body's defence systems by increasing the number and activity of white blood cells (WBC) which engulf and destroy diseased cells, tumours, fungi and parasites.

The immune stimulation effect of Echinacea was also shown in cancer cases. Echinacea extract given to outpatients with inoperable cancer, clearly showed increased number and activity of WBC, especially natural killer (NK) cells.[26]

While the therapeutic effects of Echinacea are still unknown to many doctors, consumers have learned to recognize it as a powerful remedy. Echinacea is now used to increase resistance to infections and can be used in the prevention of colds and flu.[27] Taken at the onset of symptoms, Echinacea can often stop the infection from developing.[28]

Due to its broad-range effect on the immune system, Echinacea is also recommended in cases of herpes, tonsil and throat infections including strep throat, candidiasis or vaginal yeast infection,[29] staph infections, urinary tract infections, pelvic inflammatory disease and bronchitis.[30] It is contraindicated for autoimmune diseases like AIDS or multiple sclerosis.

ELM, SLIPPERY ELM (Ulmus fulva)

Decoctions of the bark, leaves and powder are an old home remedy for many disorders. Elm is an astringent and abounds in mucilaginous matter which lubricates and soothes mucous membranes. It is mainly used to soothe inflammations of the throat, stomach (ulcers), intestines, urinary tract and lungs. Externally, it can be applied to cold sores, boils and burns. 'Slippery elm food' is very nutritious; mixed with milk, it is easily digestible for those with sensitive stomachs.

ERGOT (Claviceps purpurea)
Ergot is a fungus that parasitizes the growing kernels of wheat and rye. Extract of ergot contains several important alkaloids: ergometrine, which induces uterine contractions during childbirth; ergotanine, which stops bleeding and is effective against migraines if used in the early stages; and bromocriptine, which is used to treat female infertility, stop excessive milk production in lactating mothers, and relieve the symptoms of prostatitis and Parkinson's disease.
CAUTION: Ergot is highly toxic. It contains derivatives of lysergic acid, the active ingredient of LSD, which produces dangerous hallucinations and delusions. Not to be used except under strict medical supervision.

EUCALYPTUS, BLUE GUM TREE (Eucalyptus globulus)
The leaves are used to produce extracts and essential oils, and as disinfectants in many mouthwashes and toothpastes. Eucalyptus is also an expectorant, soothes ulcers and relaxes muscle cramps. An infusion of fresh leaves rubbed into the scalp promotes hair growth.

EVENING PRIMROSE (Oenothera biennis)
An edible mucilaginous plant which has sedative, diuretic and astringent properties. Infusions soothe coughs, relieve asthma, help to lift depression, and also stimulate the liver, spleen and digestive system. Also makes a soothing ointment for rashes and skin inflammations. The North American Indians used the plant for its wound-healing properties. Recently it was found that the oil of the seeds is rich in gamma linolenic acid (GLA), from which prostaglandins are formed (see Chapter 5). Evening primrose oil is now used to treat obesity without the need for dieting, lower cholesterol and blood pressure, cure some types of arthritis and alleviate period pains. It has

also been found to help acne, strengthen fingernails, and calm hyperactive children.

FENNEL (Foeniculum vulgare)

Infusions relieve flatulence, strengthen the digestion, loosen phlegm and help to suppress appetite and therefore aid weight loss. Fennel is also effective in the treatment of colics and ulcers. The seeds and leaves are used to flavour fish dishes and the stems are used as a vegetable.

FENUGREEK(Trigonella foenumgraecum)

One of the oldest medicinal plants known. The seeds are used as a spice, and help convalescents to regain their strength. In Yemenite folk medicine fenugreek is used to treat diabetes. A tablespoon of seeds is soaked overnight in a glass of water and drunk in the morning. In mild to medium cases, fenugreek can make insulin injections unnecessary, or at least reduce the need for them.

FEVERFEW (Chrysanthemum parthenium)

Infusions of the dried flowers are a traditional European remedy for delayed menstruation. The well-known nutritionist and author Barbara Cartland claims that feverfew tablets and crushed leaves are a wonderful cure for certain types of migraine and arthritis. In one study, involving 17 migraine patients, freeze-dried feverfew powder prevented repeated attacks of migraine headache.[31] It should be stressed, though, that migraine sufferers must first be sure that their problems are not due to food allergy. Feverfew leaves have also been reported to alleviate depression and nervous disorders.

FLAX (Linum usitatissimum)

The seeds are mucilaginous and therefore a mild laxative, and also soothing to the respiratory and digestive tracts. Linseed oil is reputed to dissolve gallstones when taken in doses of 1½-2 tablespoons a day.

GINGER (Zingiber officinalis)
Used fresh and powdered as a spice, and also in infusions. It relieves flatulence, discharges mucus, stimulates glandular secretions, and relieves indigestion, seasickness and vomiting. Blended with cinnamon powder in an infusion, it makes a pleasant bedtime beverage.

GINSENG (Panax ginseng)
A very popular plant, available in teas, powders, extracts and capsules. It contains saponin glycosides which improve resilience and resistance to stress. Ginseng is the great cure-all of Chinese medicine. The tea is a stimulant and relieves fatigue. It also normalizes blood pressure and improves blood flow. In Korean medicine, ginseng is recommended for a variety of female complaints, from irregular menstruation to painful contractions during labour. Some men claim that ginseng is an aphrodisiac. In both sexes it promotes physical and mental vigour.

GOTU KOLA (Hydrocotyle Asiatica; Centella Asiatica)
Gotu kola has been receiving a lot of attention as an energy booster and for its ability to accelerate the healing of wounds.

Gotu kola is a native plant of India and Asia. Traditionally, it was used in India for improving memory. Studies done by Dr Daniel Mowrey, a behavioural scientist, showed that gotu kola, in combination with capsicum (cayenne) and ginseng, has a long-term tonic effect. It promoted activity by stimulating strength and energy.[32] The same combination was also found to improve learning ability and memory. A more recent

Indian study done with underdeveloped children, showed the extract of gotu kola (centella) leaves, caused an increase in their mental aptitude after a period of six months.[33]

This is explained by the ability of gotu kola to decrease brain levels of neurotransmitters, such as norepinephrine, dopamine and serotonin, which were found to interfere with learning.[34]

Throughout Europe gotu kola is used to promote self-healing of the skin, in conditions like skin ulcerations or bedsores from a prolonged confinement to bed.[35] Centella extracts have also been reported effective in the treatment of cellulitis, an inflammatory condition of tissues, characterized by swelling, redness and pain (not to be confused with cellulite).[36] In fact, centella can be useful in treating any skin infection or inflammation.

The active factors in centella include triterpenes and saponins. Most studies were done with a preparation containing 25 mg total triterpenes. A normal daily intake for such a dose would be two to three powdered capsules. NOTE:Gotu kola does not contain caffeine (not to be confused with kola nut which does).

GUAR GUM *(Cyamopsis tetragonolobus)*

The valuable substance in this plant, grown for centuries in Eastern countries, is a complex carbohydrate called galactomannan, which is a bulking agent. This means that it delays stomach emptying and also the passage of food through the intestines, contributing to a feeling of satiety and therefore reducing the craving for food.[37] Slow transit time through the stomach and small intestine reduces insulin secretion and therefore the amount of sugar absorbed from the blood into the tissues[38] – a great help if you are trying to keep your weight down. Guar gum also contains a special jelly which has a high affinity for fats (fatty acids, triglycerides and cholesterol), whether they are in the gut or in the blood, and promotes their excretion,[39] another bonus for slimmers.

HAWTHORN (Crataegus monogyna)

A shrub whose flowers and fruits are medicinal. Infusions, or a few drops of tincture, are used in the treatment of heart disorders of nervous origin, insomnia and hypertension. Hawthorn regulates blood pressure by regulating heartbeat. People under stress may find hawthorn tea beneficial.

HOPS (Humulus lupulus)

The flowers secrete lupulin, which gives beer its bitterness and aroma. Infusions of the flowers have a calming effect on the nervous system, improve appetite and strengthen digestion, cleanse the blood, stimulate bile secretion and eliminate intestinal worms.

HYSSOP (Hyssopus officinalis)

Has astringent properties, relieves flatulence and stimulates menstruation. Infusions can be used to improve digestion, suppress coughs and relieve intestinal congestion. Decoctions are said to relieve inflammation.
CAUTION: Do not use for periods of more than a few weeks.

ICELAND MOSS (Centraria islandica)

Relieves nausea, soothes and decongests tissues, and stimulates milk secretion in nursing mothers. Infusions can be used for catarrhal conditions and inflammation of the digestive tract, to regulate gastric juice secretion and to treat anaemia.
CAUTION: Prolonged use can cause liver or intestinal problems.

JASMINE   (Jasminum officinalis)
Jasmine tea, which is highly scented, stimulates perspiration and helps to reduce fever, and calms the nerves.

JUNIPER   (Juniperus communis)
Juniper berries are so rich in natural sugars that they are used in the fermentation of gin, which partly retains the flavour of juniper oil. The berries can be used in cooking, to add flavour and stimulate the appetite, or made into infusions. Apart from sugars, they contain bitter principles and terpenes (essential oils). The former stimulate stomach acid secretion and improve digestion, while the latter are antiseptic and help sufferers from respiratory diseases to clear their lungs of accumulated phlegm. Juniper is also beneficial for digestive tract infections and cramps.
CAUTION: Juniper is not recommended for people with kidney problems.

KAVA-KAVA (Piper methysticum)
A Polynesian and Hawaiian shrub, its roots were traditionally used in ritual ceremonies to prepare a relaxing drink. Nowadays, kava is used to alleviate anxiety, stress and tension. Its rhizomes contain kava lactones, active sedating ingredients which promote relaxation without the loss of mental acuity, which makes it very useful for stress management in daytime.[40] Kava was also reported to alleviate headaches and back pains in combination with ginger and to promote restful sleep. Available in health food stores in tea bags and capsule form, kava is increasingly used as an alternative to anti-anxiety drugs.
CAUTION: Kava-kava is not recommended for pregnant or lactating women. Prolonged use can cause skin yellowing, which indicates that it should be discontinued.

KUDZU *(Radix Puerariae)*
A Chinese herb, known in the southern U.S. as a nuisance
weed. Kudzu has long been used in the traditional Chinese
medicine for the management of alcohol abuse. Recently, a
study performed in Harvard Medical School, proved its ability to suppress alcohol intake in hamsters. When given Kudzu
extract, the animals seemed to prefer water over alcohol.
Two compounds in Kudzu were identified as responsible for
the anti-alcohol effect, daidzein and daidzin, both
isoflavones.[41] It has recently been marketed by some U.S. vitamin manufacturers.

LAVENDER *(Lavendula officinalis)*
The pleasantly aromatic flowers have sedative properties and
can be used in infusions to alleviate cramps and muscle pain.
Flatulence, headaches and dizziness also respond to infusions
of lavender. Due to its antiseptic properties, lavender can also
be used to treat intestinal putrefaction.

LEEK *(Allium porrum)*
Resembles garlic in its properties, but to a lesser degree.
Stimulates the appetite, relieves respiratory congestion, and is
also a diuretic.

LEMON *(Citrus limon)*
Lemon juice is a home remedy for many disorders, particularly colds, sore throats and rheumatism. A course of lemon
juice treatment can often dislodge kidney stones and gravel.
Dilute the juice of 5-10 lemons in water and drink it
throughout the day, for 2-4 weeks. The high vitamin C
content of lemon juice is responsible for its disinfectant and
allergy-fighting properties. Diluted lemon juice can also be
used as a hair rinse.

LEMON GRASS (Cymbopogon citratus),
A fragrant wild herb rich in two volatile oils, citral and cit-
ronellal, and some terpenes. Used mainly for its antiseptic and
bactericidal qualities and also in the treatment of fevers.
Lemon grass has been scientifically studied and found to be
highly effective against influenza and cholera.[42]

LETTUCE (Lactuca sativa)
The leaves contain a bitter secretion which is highly sedative.
Eating a large bowl of fresh lettuce leaves calms nervousness
and induces sleep, particularly when eaten before bedtime.

LICORICE (Glycyrrhiza glabra)
The root contains a glycoside (glycyrrhizin) which acts like
cortisone. Being 50 times sweeter than sugar, it is used to
sweeten medicines and as a flavouring agent. The Arabs use it
to prepare an infusion, served cool, called 'soos'. Licorice is an
expectorant and soothes the mucous membranes of the respiratory and digestive tracts. It also helps to heal ulcers. It
contains oestrogen precursors and is used in Middle Eastern
countries for such problems as menstrual irregularity. It is
available in infusions, syrups and candies.
CAUTION: Excessive consumption of licorice can lead to
cardiac dysfunction and severe hypertension.[43]

LINDEN (Tilia platyphyllos)
Infusions of the leaves and bark are pleasantly aromatic.
Linden is a traditional home remedy for colds, coughs and
sore throats, promotes perspiration, and is a mild sedative.

MANDRAKE (Mandragora officinalis)
Mandrake root contains several alkaloids – mandragorin,
hyoscyamine and scopolamine – which are narcotic and pain-

relieving. All are toxic and should be used under medical supervision only.

MARJORAM *(Origanum vulgare)*
Infusions of the leaves are beneficial for upset stomachs and intestinal colic, headaches, nervousness, coughs, whooping cough and other respiratory disorders. Marjoram also promotes perspiration, relieves flatulence, loosens phlegm and calms the nervous system. It also relieves abdominal cramps in women and regulates the menstrual cycle when taken three or four days before a period is due.
CAUTION: Marjoram should not be taken during pregnancy.

MARSHMALLOW *(Althea officinalis)*
The leaves and roots are high in mucilaginous substances which soothe mucous membranes and are therefore used in syrups or infusions to treat respiratory diseases (coughs, bronchitis). Marshmallow is also a diuretic, and highly recommended to eliminate kidney stones and stop urinary tract bleeding.

MATÉ *(Ilex paraguayiensis)*
Used as a stimulating beverage throughout much of Latin America. Maté has a high caffeine content, though less than tea or coffee. It stimulates alertness, helps iron deficiency anaemia (it contains iron), is effective against arthritis and gout, and stimulates the kidneys. It is a good diuretic.
CAUTION: People who have cardiovascular or nervous complaints, or who are sensitive to caffeine, should avoid maté. Excessive consumption can cause diarrhoea.

MEADOW SAFFRON *(Colchicum autumnale)*

Contains the alkaloid colchicine, which is a dangerous poison, although in very tiny amounts it is effective against gout. In fact, the seeds of meadow saffron have been used as a specific for gout since the time of the ancient Greeks.[44] Colchicine inhibits cell multiplication and may one day be valuable in the treatment of malignant tumours.

MILK THISTLE *(Carduus marianus)*

The leaves are a bitter tonic. The seeds contain the flavones silydanin and silymarin which are used in liver diseases. Silymarin has been found to protect the liver against potent toxins.[45] Both flavones stimulate the evacuation of bile.

MINT, PEPPERMINT, SPEARMINT *(Mentha spp.)*

A popular herb used as a food flavouring and in tisanes. It contains menthol, which is used to reduce pain, and is also a disinfectant, carminative, digestive, appetite stimulant and a sedative. Prevents cramps, insomnia and vomiting, and warms the body in conditions of shock and fainting. It also claims to be an aphrodisiac. Peppermint also has remarkable anti-viral properties – its tannins have been found to suppress the activity of the flu virus and inhibit the *Herpes simplex* virus.[46]

MUSTARD *(Brassica nigra)*

A popular culinary herb, both appetite-stimulating and digestive. The seeds contain glycosides which yield a strong volatile oil. Used externally in poultices for treating rheumatism and inflammation of the respiratory tract – it heats and increases local blood flow.

CAUTION: Large amounts or prolonged use either internally or externally can cause severe irritation or inflammation. In poultices, mustard powder should be mixed in equal proportions with flour. Never let undiluted mustard oil come into contact with the skin.

NETTLE, STINGING NETTLE (Urtica urens)

Rich in vitamins and minerals, the leaves are used to flavour salads and make infusions. Nettle is a disinfectant, stimulates digestion, and promotes milk flow in nursing mothers. It is also an astringent and inhibits urinary tract bleeding, haemorrhoids and excessive menstrual flow. It can also be used to eliminate intestinal worms. Decoctions can be used as a hair tonic.

CAUTION: Handle with care. The fresh leaves have bristly hairs which inject an irritant substance when touched. This disappears after cooking and within a few hours of picking.

OAT (Avena sativa)

Tincture of oats has been reported to reduce the craving for cigarettes.[47]

ONION (Allium cepa)

Antiseptic, diuretic, expectorant and digestive. Onion also tends to reduce blood pressure, act as an anticoagulant and lower cholesterol level.[48]

PAPAYA, PAWPAW (Carica papaya)

A tropical fruit, normally eaten raw, which is rich in carotene (provitamin A) and vitamins B and C. Also contains papain, an enzyme similar to the stomach enzyme pepsin, which helps to digest proteins. In the tropics papaya has long been used as a meat tenderizer. Internally it aids digestion and expels worms, and externally it helps to heal wounds. Increasingly used in commercial digestives and in skin creams. Recently, papain has been acclaimed as a pain-reliever. Injections of papain into the lower spine to alleviate the pain caused by slipped discs were recently approved by the FDA.[49] Continuing research indicates that papaya may be the wonder fruit of the 1990s.

PARSLEY (Carum petroselinum)
The leaves, seeds and roots are used for culinary purposes. Parsley is rich in carotene, vitamin C and minerals. It is diuretic, carminative, promotes appetite, improves digestion and purifies the liver and kidneys. Infusions (two or three cups a day) were once a very popular treatment for dislodging and eliminating kidney stones.

PASSION FLOWER (Passiflora incarnata)
The flowers and fruits are used, mainly to calm nervousness and hysteria, relieve headaches and promote sleep. They are effective against involuntary cramps and also for asthma or high blood pressure caused by nervous conditions.

POMEGRANATE (Punica granatum)
As an astringent, pomegranate prevents diarrhoea and effectively eliminates intestinal worms. The ancient Greeks used the seeds to treat tapeworms.

POPPY (Papaver somniferum)
The seeds and oil are used in cooking. When the unripe seed pods are crushed, they yield a milky juice which quickly hardens – this is opium, which contains 25 different alkaloids, the main one being morphine. Morphine is a narcotic which relieves pain, relaxes muscles, reduces glandular secretions, lowers respiration rate and represses hunger. Injections are used to neutralize local pain. However, an excess can cause dependency. A derivative of morphine, acetylmorphine (heroin), is a much stronger drug, which causes greater

dependency and even death. Another alkaloid in opium is methyl morphine (codeine), to which dependency is very low. Codeine is used to relieve coughing, respiratory infections and asthma. It is interesting to note that morphine was recently found in cow's and human milk, and also in alfalfa, lettuce and other plants.[50] This has made scientists ponder whether morphine plays a more important role in behaviour than previously thought.

POTERIUM *(Sarcopoterium spinosum)*

A perennial plant prevalent in Mediterranean countries. The bark of the roots contains substances which reduce blood sugar level and relieve diabetes. Following successful experiments with animals, the Israeli Polytechnical Institute is now testing poterium on human diabetics.

PSYLLIUM, PLANTAIN *(Plantago ovata or P. major)*

Rich in mucilaginous substances, particularly the seeds. The leaves of *P. major* also contain tannins. Psyllium is an astringent, an intestinal lubricant, and soothes the mucous membranes of digestive and respiratory tracts, relieving coughs, hoarseness, gastritis and enteritis. Decoctions promote blood clotting, hence their use on wounds, scratches, insect bites and haemorrhoids. Mixed with water, the powdered seeds make an excellent laxative; like bran, they absorb water in the intestine and swell, increasing faecal bulk and stimulating evacuation. The effect is usually produced overnight. Many people respond better to psyllium than to bran, and psyllium laxatives are now widely available. Pick brands that contain pure psyllium powder only, not those which have added sugar or dextrose.

RADISH (Raphanus sativus)

Grown for their succulent roots, radishes are mainly used in salads. In Yemenite folk medicine, however, fresh radishes are used to eliminate kidney stones. Half a cup of fresh radish juice each morning on an empty stomach usually dissolves even the most stubborn kidney stones, enabling them to pass out of the body in the urine.

CAUTION: Large kidney stones can scratch the urinary passages and cause bleeding on their way out. Two table-spoons of vegetable oil can supply lubrication. Older Yemenites use radish leaves as well in their salads. These have been found to contain almost ten times as much vitamin C as the roots, and also calcium, iron, sodium, phosphorus, sulphur and potassium.

RASPBERRY (Rubus idaeus)

The leaves are rich in vitamins, minerals and a substance called fragarine, which prevents uterine contractions. Thus, an infusion of the leaves may be useful to prevent premature birth and menstrual pain. Raspberry is also an astringent and used as a gargle. Fresh raspberry juice is an excellent cooling beverage in fevers.

RHUBARB (Rheum palmatum)

An appetite stimulant and astringent, rhubarb is effective for both constipation and diarrhoea, depending on the amount used. Large amounts can promote diarrhoea while tiny amounts will have a constipative effect.

CAUTION: The leaves are high in oxalic acid, which tends to bind with calcium to form insoluble crystals, the precursors of certain types of kidney stones. People with kidney stones or gravel should avoid rhubarb.

ROSEHIP (Rosa spp.)

Rosehips are high in vitamin C and are used to make tisanes and syrups. These are mild laxatives and nerve tonics. They are usually taken for headaches and dizziness, to purify the blood, to treat mouth sores and as a mouthwash.

ROSEMARY (Rosmarinus officinalis)

The leaves are used in cooking and also to make a scented oil and medicinal infusions. The latter are sedative, promote perspiration, relieve headaches, improve circulation, and stimulate menstruation and bile secretion. Also used externally, mainly in shampoos.

RUE (Ruta graveolens)

The aromatic leaves are high in the glycoside rutin, which strengthens capillaries and blood vessels. Infusions increase blood pressure slightly and have abortifacient and diuretic properties. Yemenite folk medicine uses rue for nervous breakdowns and to stimulate the onset of menstruation.
CAUTION: Rue must not be taken during pregnancy.

SAGE (Salvia officinalis)

The leaves are used as a food flavouring and in infusions. Sage is a disinfectant and sedative; it clears the respiratory tract and effectively reduces perspiration, especially at night (night sweats). It reduces milk flow in nursing mothers prior to weaning, prevents the formation of kidney stones by dissolving residues of uric acid, and regularizes menstruation. It can be applied to the scalp to reduce dandruff.

SALT BUSH (Artiplex halimus)

A plant which grows in deserts and around the shores of the Mediterranean. The leaves have a high salt content and are rich in minerals. Two minerals in the leaves, chromium and manganese, have been found beneficial in diabetes and in some cases even cure it.[51]

SARSAPARILLA (Smilax officinalis)

A popular herb beverage used in root beers; also a tonic and blood purifier. In Spanish folk medicine sarsaparilla was claimed to have a regenerative effect on the genital organs, and was used to cure venereal diseases such as syphilis and gonorrhea.[52]

SAW PALMETTO (Serenoa Repens)

Saw palmetto, also known as dwarf palm, was traditionally used as food by the southeastern American Indians. Recently, it was making headlines as a treatment of choice for an enlarged prostate.

Its value lies in its berries, which contain a peculiar mix of fatty acids, phytosterols and alcohols. This particular mix was found to have a beneficial effect on the prostate gland.[53]

The prostate gland can be a potential problem for any man over 50, due to age-related changes. The prostate usually enlarges, and can produce discomforting symptoms like difficult or frequent urination, interrupted sleep patterns because of frequent night-time visits to the toilets, or incomplete emptying of the bladder.

The prostate is a muscular, glandular organ that surrounds the urethra of males at the base of the bladder, and becomes enlarged when its cells reproduce at a greater than normal rate. The swelling of the prostate was tracked down, particularly, to the increased action of dihydrotestosterone (DHT), which is a male hormone derivative. DHT causes the prostate cells to reproduce at an accelerated rate. Saw palmetto berries were found to lower DHT levels by inhibiting the responsible enzyme (5-alpha-reductase) and relieving much of the discomfort.[54]

Extracts of saw palmetto berries are available in capsules through health food shops. The normal daily dose that proved beneficial in studies was 160 mg, once or twice daily.[55] The studies reported that usually, the saw palmetto capsules were well tolerated.

SENNA (Cassia acutifolia)

Senna leaf infusions are an effective and well-known remedy against chronic constipation. Used in many laxative preparations. The active ingredients are two glycosides (sennosides A and B). Senna is often combined with other substances to eliminate intestinal worms. It is also effective against bad breath.

SHEPHERD'S PURSE (Capsella bursa-pastoris)

Middle Eastern Arabs used to eat the fresh plant and also prepared infusions from it. Shepherd's purse is rich in calcium, sodium, and vitamins C and K. An effective blood coagulant, it is used to stop bleeding, both external and internal, including excessive menstrual bleeding. It is also a diuretic.

ST. JOHN'S WORT (Hypericum perforatum)

The flowering tops contain hypericin and related constituents which have antiviral and anti-inflammatory action. However, St. John's Wort extracts and tisanes are now mostly used to alleviate mild depression and anxiety without the side-effects of conventional antidepressant medications. Infusions of the flowers can also be used externally to bathe wounds, burns and haemorrhoids.

TARRAGON (*Artemisia dracunculus*)

Infusions of tarragon stimulate digestive secretions and appetite, relieve digestive disorders, bring on delayed menstruation, and promote urination by stimulating the kidneys. Drinking an infusion at bedtime relieves insomnia. The fresh leaves and oil are also used in tarragon mustard and tarragon vinegar, and when cooking fish and chicken.

THYME (*Thymus vulgaris* or *T. serpyllum*)

The leaves are rich in volatile oils and are used in cooking, medicinal extracts and infusions. Thyme is a good tonic for the stomach and nerves. It relieves flatulence, prevents indigestion and loosens phlegm. Infusions have a calming effect, relax muscle spasms and alleviate exhaustion.

UVA URSI (*Arctostaphylos Uva-Ursi*)

A newly popular herb in health food stores, sold both on its own and as an ingredient in many herb teas. Generally used for urinary disorders.

Uva ursi is an evergreen shrub producing juicy, insipid flavoured berries, and small oval-shaped bitter leaves, abundant in flavonoids and tannins, which suggest strong antibacterial properties. In fact, it has been used in modern medicine as a urinary tract antiseptic, until it was replaced by sulpha drugs and antibiotics.[56] In the past, it was used to treat excessive menstruation.

Other folk uses of uva ursi's disinfectant properties include a tea as a vaginal douche for vaginitis (when used with eucalyptus leaves) as well as a sitz bath after childbirth.[57]

The function of uva ursi is rather versatile. It can aid urination, and also help correct bed-wetting, depending on the amount used. A large amount of it stimulates kidneys, while a very small amount restricts urination.[58]

VALERIAN (Valeriana officinalis)
The roots and rhizomes contain a strong essential oil, and the tincture is a well-known sedative which calms nervousness and reduces heart palpitations, involuntary muscle spasms and epileptic fits. Valerian was once commonly used to prevent fainting. It can also reduce the urge to smoke and help to cure digestive ulcers. It is claimed to help dissolve gallstones.
CAUTION: Prolonged use can cause depression.

VERVAIN, VERBENA (*Verbena officinalis*)
Infusions stimulate vomiting, loosen phlegm so that it can be coughed up, and relieve indigestion, ulcers and colics. Vervain is also a sedative, promoting sleep and alleviating certain types of migraine.

VINE (Vitis vinifera sativa)
Vine leaves are used in cooking. Fresh grapes contain calcium, magnesium, phosphorus, sodium and potassium, and are rich in glucose, which supplies quick energy. They are stimulating, both physically and mentally, and help to cleanse the kidneys. The Yemenites use a grape regime for kidney stones and gravel. Raisins are a mild laxative.

WORMWOOD (Artemisia absinthium)
Prevalent in the deserts of the Middle East. The leaves contain santonin, which is effective against intestinal worms, and are used to prepare a bitter oil and infusions. Wormwood is highly expectorant and a good digestive. As it is very bitter it is normally added to sweetened tea.

YARROW (Achillea millefolium)
Yarrow is an astringent with an aromatic odour and a bitter taste – this is due to its essential oil and two acids, achilleic

and tannic. Infusions are used to alleviate digestive upsets, and to arrest internal bleeding and heavy menstrual flow. Externally, it is used to bathe wounds, as a gargle in gum inflammations, and as a hair tonic.

CAUTION:Yarrow can cause dermatitis in sensitive persons.

WILD YAM (Dioscorea villosa)

Wild yam roots yield an alkaloid which has a sedative effect on the stomach muscles, and were used by physicians of the Southern Confederate States in the American Civil War to treat abdominal cramps and bilious colics. Wild yam can also be used to regularize menstruation and relieve menstrual cramps and morning sickness. Studies done in the 1940s showed that one particular species of wild yam (*Dioscorea vittata*) contains up to 40 per cent diosgenin, a glycoside which can easily be converted to the hormone progesterone[59] (until the second half of this century progesterone was extracted from horse's urine). In tests with 75 women over a four-year period, wild yam was found to be extremely effective as an oral contraceptive.[60] None of the women suffered from any of the side effects – weight gain, swelling, abdominal cramps, hormonal changes – commonly associated with the birth control pill.

CHAPTER 13

HOW TO SUCCEED IN LOSING WEIGHT

Obesity is reaching epidemic proportions in the developed world. A survey in England shows that almost one in five people are obese. Children as young as three are being referred to dieticians for weight control. But, its great prevalence is not in the least comforting to those who are obese (usually defined as being 20 pounds or more above ideal weight for height, build and sex). Obesity is more than unattractive; it is associated with diabetes, arthritis, hypertension, atherosclerosis, coronary heart disease and cancer[1], in fact with a whole cluster of diseases.

The causes of obesity exclude many people who would give anything to shed their extra pounds for good. Doctors can prescribe appetite suppressants or diet pills (mostly dangerous and with adverse effects)[2] but they do not seem to get at the underlying problem. Dr Jean Mayer, professor of nutrition at Harvard University School of Public Health, writes: 'Doctors feel that treating obese people by changing their diets and increasing their physical activity is a waste of time. Moreover, all this requires knowledge in nutrition, calisthenics, eating habits, and food composition, subjects which are hardly studied in medical school.'[3]

Although obesity is associated with a variety of chronic diseases, many obese people are not fit when they are thin; they simply function better when they are heavy.[4] When they lose weight, they feel tired, depressed and irritable. Others, with emotional problems, eat compulsively to compensate for stress, fear, lack of affection, or a deprived childhood, and they normally start dieting because of a guilt complex or self-hatred. Rather than go on a drastic reducing diet such people would do better to go on a natural, wholesome diet, adequately supplemented, so that their metabolism can reach the optimal function it is capable of.

WHAT CAUSES OBESITY?

The main organic cause for obesity, most experts agree, is overeating, consuming more calories than the body can burn. Empty calories in the form of candies, biscuits, ice cream, soft drinks and breakfast cereals are the main culprits. Obesity begins in infancy, when mothers substitute formula feeds and sweetened cereals for breast milk. Breast-fed babies are rarely overweight.[5] Another frequent contributor to obesity is the birth control pill.[6] Then there are food allergies, which can cause water retention and weight gain. Defective carbohydrate metabolism, as in hypoglycaemia and diabetes, can also be to blame.[7] Less prevalent causes are hormonal imbalances such as thyroid insufficiency[8] and high levels of adrenal cortisone,[9] which impair metabolic efficiency. Hormonal imbalances justify medical care.

Fairly rapid weight gain occurs in many young people as they approach their thirties. Over a period of one or two years, they put on 10-20 pounds, for no obvious reason. This may be due to a fall-off in the brain's release of growth hormone, which normally decreases towards the end of the third decade. Growth hormone not only strengthens the immune system, but also stimulates the body to burn fat and build muscle.[10] Supplemental amino acids arginine or ornithine, which are growth hormone releasers, can help to convert fat to muscle.[11] Another weight control hormone whose level falls off in the thirties is dehydroepiandrosterone (DHEA), now available in most health food shops.

Clearly, therefore, when no organic or mental disorders are present, the cause of obesity is nutritional. So what are people eating today that makes them put on weight so easily in all age groups? Even as long ago as 1958, a group of investigators wrote: 'In the economically developed countries a marked change in nutritional patterns has occurred during the last century. In conjunction with industrialization, urbanization, and increase in per capita national income, "richer" diets have become commonplace, diets containing sizeable quantities of the more expensive high-lipid foods of animal origin plus "elegant" white bread and refined sugar. These foods are now consumed en masse in countries like the United States. As a result, intake en masse of total calories, empty calories, total fats, cholesterol, and saturated fats has tended to increase significantly in these economically developed countries. . . In fact, the calorie intake is frequently in excess of the total required to balance energy expenditure, with consequent widespread obesity . . .'[12]

No wonder that 25 per cent of men over the age of 30 and 40 per cent of women over the age of 40 are obese, i.e., weigh at least 20 pounds more than their ideal weight.[13]

WEIGHT-REDUCING DIETS AND THEIR EFFECTS

Countless diets, including many fad diets, have hit the head-lines in the last decade. The ice cream diet, the grapefruit diet, the sweet tooth diet, the drinking man's diet – these are typical examples of regimes aimed at a massive weight loss in a short time. However, these starvation diets are useless in the long run. The body interprets deprivation as 'famine' and hangs on to its reserves of fat for the next time when food is scarce. This is how the human species has survived dearth and plenty for at least half a million years.

Another approach to dieting is the high protein, low carbohydrate diet (the kind often recommended for hypoglycaemics). In the average diet, carbohydrates (sugars and starches) provide about half the body's energy requirements, while proteins and fats provide the rest. But when the diet lacks carbohydrates for more than two days, the body starts burning its own fats for energy, releasing excessive amounts of ketones (acetone bodies) into the blood. That is why high protein, low carbohydrate diets are called 'ketogenic'. They induce a state of ketosis. Ketone levels in the urine indicate the rate at which fats are being broken down, which in turn indicates that weight is being lost.

High protein, low carbohydrate diets are claimed to prevent hunger pangs and provide energy, obviating the need for willpower to overcome the craving for food. One such diet emphasizes lean meat, poultry, fish and cheese, together with eight glasses of water a day and vitamin supplements. Another allows the dieter to eat all types of proteins but no carbohydrates at first, in order to initiate ketosis. Some carbohydrates are allowed later. This diet also calls for vitamin supplementation but does not force you to drink more than you want.

However, it should be remembered that ketosis is an abnormal state of metabolism. Carbohydrates are needed by the body to regulate protein and fat and to maintain adequate functioning of the brain. Dr Carl Pfeiffer warns that long-term ketogenic diets can cause cellular damage and also increase cholesterol levels and the risk of cardiovascular complications.[14] Dr Paavo Airola admits that high protein diets achieve weight loss but claims that the resulting accumulation of protein wastes is a prime cause of arthritis, heart disease and cancer.[15] Clearly, such diets are not for everyone and should not be persisted with for more than a few weeks. Pregnant women and people suffering from gout or arthritis (associated with high levels of uric acid) should not follow high protein diets.

Another popular diet consists of 1,000 calories a day, supplemented by cider vinegar, lecithin, kelp and vitamin B6. These supplements can improve metabolism of food, but just 1,000 calories a day can cause nutrient deficiencies. Vitamin B6, for example, requires additional supplementation of the whole B complex.

THE APPESTAT AND APPETITE CONTROL

According to Dr Roger Williams,[16] obesity results from a disordered appestat mechanism. This vital regulator, which controls appetite, is located in the midbrain. It tells us to eat when the body requires nourishment and to stop eating when those requirements have been satisfied. Like all body cells, the cells of the appestat require adequate nutrition for optimal functioning. If they receive all the nutrients they need, they will control appetite, responding quickly and appropriately to the body's needs. So instead of calorie counting and grimly exercising our willpower, we should concentrate on the health of our appestat. How can this be done? By supplying optimal nutrition to the body.

Many healthy people scarcely think about dieting. They eat freely and rely on their appestat to control their appetite and take care of their weight. They do not count calories. Their weight remains stable, varying by only a few pounds more or less, over long periods. Some people are born with more effective appestats than others, just as some people are born taller or better-looking than others. Some may even be born with fewer fat cells than others.[17] But through nutrition and exercise it is possible to improve general body function and the function of the appestat.

One condition which greatly upsets appestat function is hypoglycaemia.[18] Low blood sugar levels force hypogly-caemics to indulge in compulsive eating of empty calorie foods. These supply calories, but no nutrients to nourish the cells of the appestat, and as blood sugar levels drop even further, the craving for sweets returns with a vengeance. No wonder high protein, low carbohydrate diets are so effective in treating obese hypoglycaemics. In fact, all obese people should have themselves checked for hypoglycaemia – all it takes is a glucose tolerance test (see Chapter 10). Replacing sugary foods with natural wholesome foods will improve nourishment to the appestat and also reduce calories.

Another powerful factor influencing the appestat is exercise. Exercise means more than just burning calories. Exercise improves the quality of the blood and releases valuable hormonal substances which improve the cellular environment in which the appestat works.[19] The appestat only works well with at least a moderate amount of physical activity.[20] In other words, moderate exercise will reduce your appetite.

Cigarette smoking can poison the appestat, as well as the

rest of the body.[21] Long-time smokers find that they gain weight easily once they stop smoking. Ex-smokers would do well to improve the quality of their food, substituting wholesome natural foods for empty calories. This is the only way to repair a damaged biological mechanism.

Frequent small meals can help to prevent obesity. Grazing animals and laboratory rats, who nibble continuously all day, do not put on excess weight. In several animal studies, investigators found that limiting laboratory rats to one meal a day made the rats put on weight.[22] What is more, autopsies revealed that the meat of these rats contained 23.6 per cent fat and 17.7 per cent protein, compared with 7.8 per cent fat and 22.4 per cent protein in rats who were allowed to nibble freely. These percentages are very meaningful. They suggest that we too might be able to stay trim by splitting our main meals into smaller meals and spreading them throughout the day.

In a study done in 1963[23] a number of people were instructed to nibble whenever they wanted; their blood triglyceride (fat) levels were then measured and they were found to have fallen considerably. When these same people ate heavy meals spaced at long intervals, their fat levels increased again.

Night eating is another factor which contributes to obesity.[24] Because a nocturnal meal is usually followed by sleep, there is no physical activity to burn up the calories, which are then converted to fat. This leads us to the importance of a good protein breakfast, the calories of which are burned easily to supply energy for morning activities.

Phenylalanine, an amino acid found in meat, milk and spirulina, also plays a part in reducing appetite. In the brain, it is converted to norepinephrine (noradrenaline), a chemical which transmits nerve impulses and which stimulates the appestat to reduce hunger. Increasing numbers of people are finding that phenylalanine is a useful aid to weight loss. As American research scientist Durk Pearson says: 'It is not a matter of willpower at all. You just feel like eating less. You get up from the table having eaten less.' Over-the-counter appetite suppressants, such as phenylpropanolamine, release norepinephrine in the brain but do not provide fresh supplies. They therefore cease to be effective once norepinephrine is depleted, causing a feeling of letdown and depression, precisely the circumstances which bring on another eating binge. Amphetamines and other stimulants have similar but more severe effects. Phenylalanine or spirulina is the natural way to switch off hunger.

CAUTION: Phenylalanine should be started at low dosages of 100 mg a day. People with hypertension should consult a doctor first, since phenylalanine tends to raise blood pressure. Excessive use can cause irritability and insomnia.

Another thing that phenlyalanine does is stimulate the release of a natural hormone called CCK (cholecystokinin). CCK is secreted by the small intestine and is believed to trigger satiety signals in the brain.[25] According to Dr James G. Jibbs, a scientist at Cornell University, CCK can cause an animal to literally starve itself to death in the midst of plenty.

So it seems that while phenylalanine reduces hunger, CCK terminates it. CCK tablets manufactured from edible bovine tissue are now available from some health food shops. They are usually taken, in a 2,000 mg dose, 30 minutes before each main meal and at mid-evening. In a recent clinical weight loss study, participants taking CCK lost an average of 12.05 pounds over a four-week period; a placebo group averaged a loss of 2.15 pounds over the same period.[26]

Another cause of overweight is carnitine deficiency. Carnitine is an amino acid synthesized by the body, and it helps to ensure that fat is burnt for energy. Any shortage of lysine or methionine – the two essential amino acids from which carnitine is formed – or impaired synthesis of carnitine may account for excessive stores of fat. Carnitine supplements may therefore be useful in cases where obesity is biochemical in origin. In people with prostaglandin imbalance evening primrose oil may help to achieve weight loss.

HORMONES AND OBESITY

There is evidence that endocrine hormones – pituitary hormones, thyroid, adrenocortical, pancreatic and sex hormones – are implicated in obesity.[27] We know, for example, that some women who take the pill, which contains oestrogen and progesterone, put on weight while others taking thyroid hormones lose weight because their metabolic functioning improves. High levels of insulin, the pancreatic hormone which lowers blood glucose levels, have been found to contribute to obesity[28] by causing hunger and eating.[29] Another pancreatic hormone, glucagon, which reverses insulin function, has been found to prevent hunger sensations.[30]

The use of hormones, however, is not simple. It is easy to upset hormonal balance but difficult to restore it. The treatment of infertile women with DES (diethylstilbestrol, a synthetic oestrogen) in the 1950s resulted in many cases of cervical and vaginal cancers in the daughters of those who became mothers (and testicular cancer in some of the sons). Malignancy manifested itself as the daughters reached puberty.[31]

The pill, which is taken by so many women, and ACTH (adrenocorticotrophic hormone), which is injected into arthritic children, often cause hormonal imbalances, reflected in visible symptoms such as fat accumulation, hair loss or oedema. We can only guess at the invisible symptoms.

One hormone which has been used to fight obesity is chorionic gonadotrophin (CGT). CGT is present in the urine of pregnant women, and is used to confirm pregnancy in urine tests. At one time, injections of 125 units of CGT daily for 40 days were recommended as part of a weight loss regime; the other part of the regime consisted of eating only 500 calories a day. Criticizing this regime, two American researchers[32] commented: 'No evidence exists that CGT affects weight reduction; any claims to the contrary are misrepresentation of scientific facts.' The regime in question caused weight loss by a semistarvation diet, reinforced by daily visits to a clinic and daily injections of a drug represented to patients as an aid in weight reduction. The safety of such a regime is questionable and can lead to substantial protein loss.

CONTRIBUTING ELEMENTS TO WEIGHT LOSS

Supplementing the diet with various foods and nutrients described elsewhere in this book, can assist weight loss. Among these are, the amino acids arginine and ornithine, coenzyme Q1O (CoQ), chromium picolinate, cider vinegar, kelp, vitamin B6 and lecithin.

THERMOGENESIS

Different people react to food differently. Some people can overeat and hardly gain any weight, while others put on weight easily hardly eating anything. This was explained by thermogenesis, the individual's ability to burn excess food calories to heat. This is closely related to the basal metabolic rate: if calories are not used or burned, they become stored fat. A few aids to increase thermogenesis were found, especially ephedrine or 'Chinese ma huang' (which is a controversial substance), mustard, aspirin and caffeine. However, such thermogenetic capsules have a few drawbacks: they tend to increase blood pressure, and are not safe for hypertensive people, pregnant and lactating women, children, men with enlarged prostate and people with thyroid problems.[33]

HYDROXYCITRIC ACID (HCA)

Labelled as 'nature's best diet ingredient', HCA was found to help curb appetite, reduce food intake, and inhibit the production of fats and cholesterol.[34]

Unlike citric acid which is prevalent in citrus fruits, HCA is highest in the rind of a fruit which grows in south Asia, called Garcinia Cambogia, also known as 'Malabar Tamarind' or 'Goraka'.[35] For centuries, people in southern India have used the rind as a natural food preservative, flavouring agent and digestive aid.[36]

HCA was found to inhibit fat production from carbohydrates. During food digestion, carbohydrates are broken down to glucose for energy, and any excess, is converted to glycogen and stored in the liver and muscles. When glycogen stores become full, its excesses are converted to fat by an enzyme called ATP-citrate-lyase. HCA was found to temporarily inhibit this action of this enzyme.[37] Animal studies have shown that HCA reduces fat synthesis by approximately 40-70 per cent for eight to twelve hours following a meal.[38]

In addition, HCA can also curb appetite and reduce food intake. Since HCA inhibits ATP-citrate-lyase, less fat is formed and instead, more glycogen. This additional glycogen sends a satiety signal to the brain's appetite control in the hypothalamus, suppressing appetite and food intake.[39] Animal studies have shown that HCA can reduce food consumption by about 10 per cent.[40]

In toxicity tests, HCA was found even safer than citric acid.[41] As most appetite suppressants act by stimulating the central nervous system (CNS), this may lead to side effects such as, nervousness, hypertension, depression and palpitations. HCA on the other hand, is not a CNS stimulant and will not cause such side effects.[42] HCA suppresses appetite safely by working with the body's own natural processes.

OBESITY IS NOT A PROBLEM

Millions of overweight people are constantly on the lookout for that magical pill or diet that will make them thinner. They go on diets for a while and then stop. Falling off their diets makes them feel guilty. Therefore they punish themselves, since guilt always seeks punishment.

But being overweight is not the problem. It is only the manifestation of the problem. The real problem is lack of self-love. This can be manifested by various feelings such as fear, insecurity, stress, low self-esteem or even self-hatred. Usually, compulsive eating means an inner need for protection. When you feel frightened or insecure, you pad yourself with extra layers for protection. Thus, food is abused. It is no longer used for nourishment, but for mental support.

What is really required, is a positive mental attitude of self-love. The release of fears, worries, resentments and grudges. Not diets. Crash diets are a form of self-hatred. In a nutshell, that means learning unconditional self-love. Accepting your body the way it is here and now.

Self-acceptance of a fat body may not sound easy at first, since obese people usually hate their bodies. However, resentment is counter-productive. It can lock-in the excess weight even deeper, by increasing food cravings, for example.

What is needed is a change of concept. Remember that you are your own best friend, so decide to act like one. Don't berate your body, support it. Treat it in a friendly way. Once you learn the art of unconditional self-love, it is very gratifying to note how weight takes care of itself.

Assuming responsibility for one's own happiness and fulfillment, is another step in the right direction. Once you are determined to create a slimmer you, say by mental imaging, exercise, getting nutritional advice or by joining a support group, the correct solution will pop up. Positive conceptualization of life is not easy to achieve, but is definitely possible to those who are willing to invest the mental work required. You may decide to get help from a psychotherapist or such growth classes like the Silva Mind Control. Love is a great healing energy. And with a renewed concept of self-love, food no longer needs to be abused. Recommended reading are *You Can Heal Your Life,* by Louise Hay, and Dr Doreen, Virtue books, *Constant Craving: What Your Food Cravings Mean and How to Overcome Them* and *Losing Your Pounds of Pain: Breaking the Link Between Abuse, Stress and Overeating.*

CALORIE COUNTING AND DAILY WEIGHING

Calorie counting is seldom effective. It is simply not accurate enough and not human enough. People are creatures of emotion. It is unrealistic to expect an obese person to follow a preset calorie plan consistently. However, by sticking to natural, wholesome, high protein foods, excluding empty calorie foods, and fortifying the diet with appropriate supplements, the obese person stands a very good chance of adjusting his or her appestat and losing weight.

Variations in the water content of the body can make

daily weighing a confusing experience. Water content varies from 45.6–70.2 per cent, and the average man contains 10 per cent more water than the average woman.[43]

TWELVE TIPS FOR SUCCESSFUL WEIGHT LOSS

1 Do not eat other people's leftovers.

2 If you must nibble when socializing or when you are on your own, munch carrots or sticks of celery, not sugary snacks.

3 It is preferable to eat a high protein breakfast. Proteins convert slowly to energy and the feeling of satiety lasts much longer. Make breakfast the largest meal of the day, lunch the medium, and dinner the smallest. If you find it hard to begin with, try to eat at least some protein in the morning. Breakfast calories are more easily burned up. Nutritionist Lelord Kordel used to say: 'Eat in the morning like a king, at noon like a prince and in the evening as a pauper.'

4 Do not continue eating until you feel full. Eat until hunger has subsided to a feeling of reasonable well-being. Get used to eating this way for a few days until the volume of your stomach has decreased. Then you will find you require less food than before. Frequent small meals are best.

5 If you tend to overeat in the evening, go to bed before a new craving develops and rise the next morning with an appetite for breakfast.

6 Check that you are not allergic to any of the foods you normally eat, especially to the foods you crave most. Get a skin or pulse test done.

7 When you are hungry and in a hurry, beware of fast food. It may fill you up, but it will quickly slow you down, and your body will be the loser.

8 Avoid empty calorie convenience foods which contain white sugar or white flour and you will not have to count calories. In fact, the body does not react to food in terms of calories, but in terms of protein quality, fat quality and carbohydrate quality. The calories in each of these nutrients are metabolized differently by the body. For dieters, it makes more sense to classify foods according to 'flab units' or fattening potential. Although a chocolate bar has 150 calories, the same as three slices of Swiss cheese, chocolate is nearly 70 per cent more fattening than cheese.[44] Not all calories were created equal.

9 Do not avoid fats altogether and do not be alarmed by their calorie levels. When people on low carbohydrate diets are allowed to eat fat freely, they do not eat any more fat than previously and sometimes a little less.[45]

10 Chew your food more thoroughly and you will get more benefit from it. Digestion will be more efficient, food will be less fattening, and you will eat less. Practitioners of yoga recommend chewing food until it has lost its taste.

11 Experiment with the weight control aids described in this chapter – growth hormone releasers, phenylalanine and HCA. These should help you to control your eating, for good. However, do not neglect nutritional supplementation, because although you may eat less, your nutritional requirements remain the same. Also, dietary stresses may increase these requirements. Vitamin C and B complex can help to reduce emotional stresses, acidophilus tablets and bran will keep your colon healthy, and multivitamin and multimineral supplementation will take care of the rest of your requirements.[46] Eating plenty of natural high fibre foods, particularly raw vegetables, cannot be overemphasized.

12 Start some form of physical activity – walking, jogging, running, cycling, rowing or swimming – and enrol in a

gym or a tennis club. One of the benefits of regular exercise is that it acts as an appetite suppressant. Anyone over the age of 30 should see a physician for a check-up before starting an exercise programme.

CHAPTER 14

NOURISHING THE NEXT GENERATION

Parents are often unaware that many of their children's health problems are a result of poor nutrition and can be avoided. Diets high in processed sugary foods, candies and soft drinks lead to poor resistance to infections, dental problems and obesity.

Our children are our greatest responsibility. Their health is shaped by our own nutrition long before they are born. Parents should start an optimal diet *before conception*[1] in order to build up good nutritional reserves. A balanced, wholesome diet, well supplemented, particularly with vitamin E and iron, is the best possible health assurance for both parents and children.

Many pregnant women do not realize the importance of optimal nutrition in the early stages of pregnancy. They do not realize that the embryo, and later the foetus, has special nutritional requirements. Why should a bud of tissue the size of a pea have special needs, they think. It is no good subsisting on pickles, popcorn and coke in early pregnancy, for it is during the first few months of pregnancy that the baby's organs are being formed. Damage to the foetal brain is often a direct result of poor maternal nutrition.[2] The right nutrients should be present in the mother's diet in adequate amounts and at the right time to ensure proper development. Drugs, diuretics and restricted diets intended to reduce weight during pregnancy create nutritional deficiencies. Morning sickness, for example, is a typical symptom of vitamin B6 deficiency and disappears quickly once this nutrient is supplemented.[3]

NUTRITION IN PREGNANCY

It is generally accepted that nutritional requirements during pregnancy are much higher than usual. Supplemental iron, for example, is almost mandatory. High protein diets are important too. Pregnancy diets lacking in protein have been found to impair the health and development of the newborn.[4]

Dr Roger Williams writes: 'If all prospective human mothers could be fed as expertly as prospective animal mothers in the laboratory, most sterility, abortions and premature births would disappear. Deformed and mentally retarded babies would be largely a thing of the past.'[5] Many studies have been done with laboratory animals with the aim of discovering the connection between nutrition and reproduction. A French study[6] found that a group of female rats fed a low pantothenic acid diet all lost their pregnancies. All the foetuses that had begun to develop were resorbed. But when a little pantothenic acid was added to the diet, pregnancy was maintained. The more pantothenic acid, the greater the number of pregnancies carried to term. Pantothenic acid is found plentifully, by the way, in 'royal jelly,'[7] the food that converts a regular 'worker' bee to a queen bee, who is able to lay eggs and reproduce. Another rich source is codfish ovaries (cod's roe), again a source closely connected with reproduction.

Pantothenic acid, however, is only one link in the nutritional chain. Vitamin A was one of the first vitamins found to be important for healthy reproduction. Its deficiency has been shown to cause birth defects. In an article published in 1933,[7] it was reported that when laboratory sows were fed a low vitamin A diet during early pregnancy, their litters were born with harelips, cleft palates and other malformations, and without eyeballs. Many later studies showed that deficiencies of such nutrients as vitamin E, C, B complex, iodine and zinc during animal pregnancies can also impair foetal development.[8]

Zinc and vitamin B6 are especially important for foetal growth. B6 is also effective against morning sickness. Rats born to mothers deficient in zinc are mentally retarded and have low learning ability (finding food in water maze).[9] Zinc is also required for proper growth in children. A study conducted by Dr Ananda Prasad in Iran, with a group of 20-year-old Iranian dwarfs, revealed that their diets, long deficient in zinc, caused stunted growth, immature sex organs and lack of mental acuity.[10] If we remember that white flour and white sugar are foods denuded of their natural zinc, it is not difficult to imagine the devastating influence such processed foods can have on youngsters in the long run.

Folic acid requirements increase sharply during pregnancy, often causing widespread deficiencies in pregnant women.[11] In fact, it is estimated that pregnant women need four times as much folic acid as non-pregnant women.[12] That is why it is now commonly supplemented during pregnancy.

Folic acid deficiencies during pregnancy not only join iron deficiencies in causing anaemia, but are also known to cause ravaging birth defects such as spina bifida (imperfect closure of the spinal column leaving part of the spinal cord exposed), hydrocephalus (enlargement of the skull due to excess fluid around the brain) and cleft palate (interferes with eating and speech development).[13] Deficiencies of folic acid are aggravated by the previous use of birth control pills, antibiotics, alcohol and a diet low in leafy green vegetables. However, a balanced diet, adequately supplemented, can replenish body stores, promote the health of the newborn and also prevent toxic conditions in late pregnancy (pre-eclampsia, eclampsia).

The ideal diet for one pregnant woman will not be the ideal diet for another. Each woman requires a diet precisely tailored to her specific needs. As a rule, pre-conception diets should be high in proteins and low in empty calories, with plenty of fresh fruit and vegetables, legumes, whole grains, nuts, seeds, buttermilk, yogurt, cheese and milk. Meat eaters should emphasize organ meats such as liver, kidneys, heart, sweetbreads or brains. White flour and white sugar products are out of the question for a mother before, during and after pregnancy, as are alcohol and smoking. Supplementation should include multiple vitamin-mineral tablets, brewer's yeast, raw wheat germ, wheat germ oil, kelp and lecithin. Two very important minerals are iron and calcium.

BREAST-FEEDING

In the early years of this century almost all babies were breast-fed, but today only a minority are that lucky. In many Western countries the breast has been transmogrified from its nutritional role into a sexual symbol. Mother's milk, the most suitable food for a human baby, has been replaced by pasteurized cow's milk and commercial milk formulas.

Breast-feeding is most important. It largely determines

the baby's health in his or her first months and also for many years to come. The flight from nipple to nozzle, especially in poor families, can have disastrous effects. Giving cow's milk to babies has been correlated with later obesity and heart disease.[14] In fact, a study conducted by two leading research biochemists at Texas A & M University has established that the high amount of cholesterol in mother's milk (as opposed to the low amounts of cholesterol in commercial milk formulas) serves to establish *lower* cholesterol levels in adulthood.[15] The cholesterol in breast milk is thought to initiate a feedback control of cholesterol by the liver. Human milk fat is made up of finer globules than the fat in cow's milk, and also contains double the amount of essential fatty acids, in addition to many unknown factors not present in pasteurized cow's milk. Indeed, considerable differences have been found between human and cow's milk. Human milk contains ten times more vitamin E than cow's milk, more lactose (milk sugar), less protein and smaller quantities of minerals.

These differences are not accidental. They suit perfectly the specific growth requirements of the human baby. The extra lactose in human milk helps to maintain healthy flora in the baby's intestines and also contributes to brain development.[16] The additional protein in cow's milk is needed for developing the larger body of the calf. Furthermore, mother's milk is perfectly natural and raw, while cow's milk is processed and pasteurized. Even calves cannot subsist on pasteurized cow's milk! When given pasteurized milk, they die within six weeks.[17]

The advantages of breast-feeding are many. The first milk (colostrum) is rich in white blood cells which increase the baby's immunity to disease.[18] As a result, breast-fed babies are much healthier than bottle-fed babies. Bottle-fed babies suffer more from rash, respiratory disorders and colic.[19]

Breast-feeding is good for the mother too. Figures show that mothers who nurse their babies are less likely to get breast cancer later.[20] Breast-feeding also has a contraceptive effect, although this is not entirely reliable. In Rwanda, lactation was found to prevent conception for an average of 15 months.[21] A lactation period of between six months and a year is generally advocated.

GIVING CHILDREN A CHANCE

Children cannot be expected to grow into healthy grown-ups if their daily diet lacks the nutrients essential for growth. So let's give them a chance, their rightful chance to health, by emphasizing whole foods, healthy snacks and proper supplementation, and skipping sugary foods as much as possible.

It is important to help children develop a taste for fresh fruit and vegetables. They must get used to wholewheat bread, brown rice, eggs, cheese, yogurt, brewer's yeast, organ meats, raw seeds and nuts. They should be educated to satisfy their craving for sweets with dried fruits such as raisins, dates, apricots, prunes and figs.

It is possible and advisable to find substitutes for foods containing refined sugar. Parents have a great ally in the fight against the candy and soft drink problem: the kitchen. Most commercial candy can be duplicated at home, using natural, wholesome ingredients and less or no sugar. A good substitute for cake could be a buttered slice of wholewheat bread with molasses, malt extract, honey or raw maple syrup sprinkled with cinnamon and ginger. Fresh fruit juices can be substituted for soft drinks. Natural snacks can be prepared at home by mixing raw almonds and other nuts and seeds with raisins, carob chips or date cubes. Tasty milk porridges cooked with oatmeal and raw wheat germ, and sweetened with sorbitol or maple syrup, can be prepared for dinner. Pancakes can be made with wholewheat flour and raw honey. Homemade ice cream, using real cream or yogurt and fresh fruit purées, can be even more delicious than commercial ice cream, even without the use of sugar. The possibilities are limitless and so are the benefits. Truly caring parents would do well to invest every every ounce of energy and ingenuity trying to lower the sugar consumption and improve the nutrition of their children.

Proteins are most important in children's nutrition. Unlike adults, children need protein not only for maintenance and repair, but also for growth. Some protein powders, usually made from brewer's yeast, milk solids and soy extracts, to which enzymes are added to help digestion, make ideal supplements and can be used to bring the protein value of other foods up to scratch. They are usually prepared as drinks, which is especially helpful when dealing with picky eaters. Just one or two cups a day will provide a child with all he or she needs.

TONSILLITIS

Why are enlarged and inflamed tonsils (and adenoids) so prevalent among children today? Often because there is a food allergy, usually to cow's milk,[22] chocolate or some other potent allergen. Often because the lymphatic system, of which the tonsils are an integral part, is overburdened by having to produce lymphocytes to engulf the toxins created by junk foods.

Doctors prescribe antibiotics which kill the bacteria causing the inflammation. But antibiotics do nothing to strengthen the child's resistance to disease, and even weaken it, and so a vicious circle is established. Whenever the child is stressed or run down, he or she gets tonsillitis.

Most parents and paediatricians don't ask themselves why the child's tonsils become enlarged and inflamed. If the real causes of tonsillitis were recognized, however, the child would be put on a fruit diet, with herb teas and a few grams of vitamin C a day, and his or her body would purify itself and become more efficient at dealing with hostile organisms of every kind, not just those that cause tonsillitis.

More often, if bouts of tonsillitis are severe and frequent enough, the tonsils are removed as if they were somehow a redundant organ for which nature had no purpose. In reality they serve as the first defence line of the immune system by producing antibodies. Tonsillectomy weakens immunity and reduces resistance. Not only is the system already weak, but part of its cleaning gear is also taken away. In many cases, tonsillectomies do not even prevent the recurrence of sore throats.

Tonsillitis can be quite dangerous, however. Untreated, it can lead to complications such as kidney inflammation, rheumatic fever, abscesses, blood poisoning (septicaemia) and pneumonia.[23] Things should not be allowed to deteriorate to this extent. At all events, a caring parent should always consult a nutrition-oriented doctor or a naturopath before permitting tonsillectomy. Proper nutritional guidance can cause tonsils to heal and shrink, preventing recurrence and fortifying the child's resistance to future infections.

THE CANDY SHOP SYNDROME

Candies and soft drinks are practically a symbol of our culture. They come in innumerable shapes, colours and flavours, and are available everywhere, in dazzling wrappers, waiting to be picked up by eager children. Logical explanations about the health risks of refined sugar fall on deaf ears with a child who is face to face with a shelf full of 'goodies'. Children respond to emotion, not to logic. Grannies and aunts, unconsciously competing for the child's love, contribute their share of sweet, colourful junk. Few people ask themselves: Is this going to distort Tom's taste buds? Is this going to addict him to sugar? ruin his teeth? hamper his scholastic achievement? predispose him to a whole cluster of diseases in later life?

A well-known paediatrician once wrote: 'If school authorities want to stop discipline problems and vandalism in the classroom, they must . . . close the candy stores within two miles of the school.'[24] Unfortunately, the chances of this happening are rather slim. There is no way of imposing restrictions on the huge candy industry. Their lobby is influential. However, within the home, this powerful lobby can be rendered powerless by intelligent, patient and caring parents who set a personal example by avoiding naked calorie foods

Two nutrients which have been found extremely effective in reducing a sweet tooth are zinc and vitamin B1.[25] Glutamic acid, or in its more usable form, glutamine, has also been reported as very effective in reducing the craving for sugar. No effort should be spared in the fight for health.

Nutritional supplementation should begin around the age of four or five, the first school years. During the growing years, when nutritional requirements are at their peak, the body needs to be safeguarded against deficiencies. A recent study with 90 English schoolchildren aged twelve and thirteen showed that a daily multivitamin and mineral supplement has a remarkably beneficial effect on physiological function, and significantly boosts non-verbal intelligence and learning ability.[26]

CHAPTER 15

ADDING YEARS TO YOUR LIFE
AND LIFE TO YOUR YEARS

The prolongation of life is a subject that has fascinated people since the dawn of history, and it is still being enthusiastically studied in many research institutes throughout the world. The main obstacle is, of course, aging and the degenerative diseases associated with it. In the long run, nobody can escape the consequences of age. But by the same token, there is no need to feel old, look old, and act old prematurely. Even if a few signs of aging – like face wrinkles, stiff joints, forgetfulness and fatigue – have already made their debut, do not worry. A great deal can be done to reverse the process. Chronological age is not always the same as biological age. The difference between the two depends, to a great extent, on the constitution and the personality of the individual.

Dr David Stonecypher, a Boston specialist in aging, writes: 'Most people expect their bodies to degenerate automatically with age and develop such frightening diseases as arthritis, cataracts and heart attacks. But these diseases are not caused by growing old. The damage is caused by persistent strain to an organ, or bad nutrition. There are probably no diseases caused by growing old. Diseases associated with old age are simply ones which require decades of poor nutrition to develop and don't usually show up in young people.'[1]

It is most important to realize the role of optimal nutrition, supplementation, physical activity, and a positive self-image in living life to its fullest natural extent and preventing premature aging. Anybody, at any age, can do a lot to improve his or her state of health, both physically and mentally. However, the best results are achieved when proper attention is paid to nutrition from a very young age.

WHAT CAUSES AGING?

For every species, there is a correlation between the life span and the number of times cells can reproduce themselves by division.[2] So to prolong life, we must either seek to prevent the causes of impaired cell division or, better still, attempt to increase the number of times cells divide. Much nutritional study has been done in this field. When cultured human cells are treated with vitamin E, for example, they become capable of 100 or more divisions rather than the usual 50 or so.[3] It is also possible to take laboratory animals from the same mother and produce radiant health in some and signs of premature aging in the others just by changing their diets.[4]

The symptoms of aging, it seems, are ultimately due to poor blood supply. Blood supply can be poor in quantity because atherosclerosis has narrowed vital blood vessels, or poor in quality because of poor nutrition.[5]

However, nutrition is not the only factor in aging. Many other factors influence cell division as well – quality of life, the will to live, state of mind, exercise, stress levels, chronic disease, living and working conditions, heredity, alcohol, smoking, environmental pollution. . . Mental attitude, for example, can stimulate an 'aging control centre' in the brain to send 'youth signals' to those parts of the body which produce hormones, with revitalizing effects.[6]

However, as we have seen in other chapters of this book, the right nutrients can improve our thinking, increase our ability to cope with stress, wean us from alcohol, reduce our susceptibility to disease and neutralize pollutants in our bodies. Nutrition can help each one of us, directly and indirectly, to live longer.

BALANCED NATURAL NUTRITION FOR LONGEVITY

The fact that wounds heal, bones mend, nails grow and colds wear off is proof that the body is in a constant state of repair and regeneration. As Dr Paul Aebersold, former head of the U.S. Atomic Energy Committee, once put it: 'Your body may seem to you much the same as it was a year ago . . . but in a single year, 98 per cent of the old atoms will be replaced by new atoms. . .' [7] To achieve this constant turnover, the body must be supplied with all the raw materials it needs. If turnover is low, regeneration is impaired and the result is premature aging.

There have been many studies of the outstanding longevity of small, isolated ethnic groups such as the Hunza of the Himalayas, the Vilcabamba of Ecuador and the Mayan Indians of Yucatan, many of whom are believed to live to more than 100 years old. Such groups are free of the major afflictions of industrial societies – cancer, heart disease, indigestion, ulcers, and so on.

Dr Robert McCarrison, a British physician who spent seven years living among the Hunzas, attributed their excellent health to three simple facts: they eat natural foods, they grow their food in fertile soil, and they eat their food fresh.[8]

Anthropologist Leon Abrams, who observed the Mayan Indians of Yucatan, discovered that they were free of tooth decay, sterility and senility.[9] Their food consisted mostly of complex carbohydrates – corn, beans, squash – and a little fruit and honey. Meat (especially organ meat) was consumed only occasionally. In another study it was shown that primitive tribes all over the world remain strong and healthy as long as they adhere to their native diet.[10] In short, good eating habits both improve health and slow down the aging process. And good eating habits are something most of us are capable of acquiring.

Many orthodox doctors like to claim that nutritional deficiencies are non-existent in our affluent society. They intimate that almost any diet will supply our nutritional requirements. In view of the evidence presented above, it is clear that such claims fly in the face of modern biochemical research. We know that as soon as isolated ethnic groups adopt the eating habits of our society, their health deteriorates. Young Hunza men drafted into the army and then discharged took 'civilized' foods, infections and tooth decay back to their isolated mountain valleys.[11]

The root of the problem is a lack of public nutritional consciousness. People who suffer from vague pains, exhaustion, infections, frequent colds, brittle nails, headaches and depression never relate these conditions to nutritional deficiencies. They consider themselves healthy. Ironically, dogs in our society fare better than most people. They stand a much better chance of completing their life span. Check the ingredients of common dog food and you will see that it contains such nutritional bonanzas as fish liver oil, barley, soy grits, brewer's yeast and bonemeal.

To any person, even in advanced age, nutrition can offer real improvement in mental and physical functioning. It needs only fresh, natural wholesome foods for basic bodily requirements to begin to be met. Newly supplied vitamins, minerals, enzymes, trace elements and many other factors will stimulate the production of healthy new cells. An enthusiastic, active interest in nutrition and its application is a small investment for a huge dividend in health and a few extra active years.

THE NEED FOR SUPPLEMENTS

Nutritional supplementation, particularly for adults, is of special importance because the efficiency of metabolism and absorption decreases with age, as less stomach acid and other digestive secretions and enzymes are formed. On top of that, many life habits – smoking, alcohol, antibiotics, laxatives and stress – deplete nutrients and contribute to nutritional deficiencies. Yet many people still question the usefulness of supplementation. Let's answer them with the words of a physician member of the New York Academy of Medicine: 'Today we ride so much and sit so much that we can use only about 1,800 calories [a day] without getting fat. Thus we are eating only half the amount of vitamins and minerals consumed by our forefathers (who consumed twice as many calories). What we do eat is of poorer quality due to worn out soil and over-refined foods. The only way to get the necessary nutrients and still maintain a proper weight is to take some of them in a supplemental form.'[12]

All the vitamins, minerals and trace elements are required. However, special emphasis should be put on vitamin E, which is thought to be of major importance in protecting the body from the ravages of free radicals, peroxides and radiation.[13] Without adequate protection against the products of peroxidation, cells become damaged, and damaged cells are a symptom of aging. Other potent antioxidants are vitamins A, C, B1, B5 and B6, PABA, the trace elements zinc and selenium, and the amino acid cysteine. A visible sign of excess peroxidation in many adults is the occurrence of brown 'age spots'. These appear externally on the forehead and the arms. They also occur internally in the brain and heart.[14] They consist of accumulations of a pigment called lipofuscin, a cellular waste which slowly poisons body and mind.

Calcium, magnesium and zinc are among the most common deficient minerals in the elderly. Porous bones and fractures are very common in advanced age due to calcium and magnesium deficiencies, but all of these minerals are vitally important for proper functioning of the endocrine glands which control body chemistry. Enlargement of the prostate gland, for example, so common now in middle-aged and elderly men, was shown by the late J.I. Rodale to be caused by deficiencies in magnesium and zinc, the antioxidant vitamins, and particularly by a deficiency of vitamin E.[15] Good natural sources of calcium, magnesium and zinc are dolomite, pollen, brewer's yeast, molasses, kelp, cider vinegar and spirulina.

GROWTH HORMONE RELEASERS

A few amino acids, particularly arginine, ornithine and phenylalanine, possess the ability to release growth hormone from the pituitary gland in the brain.[16] Growth hormone (GH) is not only vital for growing children but for adults too.

First of all, GH stimulates tissue repair. Wounds heal because GH directs cells in the injured area to repair the damage.[17] Second, GH greatly improves the body's resistance to disease by strengthening the immune system. GH acts on the thymus gland (located behind the breastbone), stimulating it to 'grow' immune cells (T-cells and B-cells) which identify, engulf and destroy invading viruses, bacteria and carcinogens.

Normally, GH ceases to be released in meaningful amounts around the age of 30, when we do not need to grow any more, but it is still stored in the pituitary gland at the base of the brain. As a result, our immune system becomes less effective at combating disease because fewer T-cells are in circulation. We are all aware that a child with a cut finger heals more quickly than an adult with a similar wound. This is because the child has higher levels of GH circulating in his or her bloodstream. When the immune system is less effective, carcinogens and substances which lead to atherosclerosis and heart attack are less efficiently neutralized and eliminated. Antibodies get out of control (due to a lack of T-suppressor cells which supervise their actions) and attack joint tissue, causing arthritis.

GH also helps to burn excess fat while putting on muscle.[18] Most teenagers who have ravenous appetites do not become overweight, even if they are not physically active. After adolescence, the ability of GH to convert fat to muscle is a great asset.

So how can we release GH after adolescence and enjoy the benefits of an efficient immune system, a trimmer body and a longer life span? Studies have shown that GH is released in response to sleep,[19] peak effort exercise (sustained moderate exercise does not trigger the release of GH),[20] fasting and several other factors. Amino acids such as arginine and ornithine (now available in health food shops) are effective GH releasers in adults, particularly when taken on an empty stomach at bedtime or, if this causes insomnia, one hour before vigorous exercise. Arginine is usually taken in doses of 2-5 grams a day, ornithine in doses of 1-2.5 grams a day.

WARNING: Arginine and ornithine are intended for adults only, and must not be used by infants, children or teenagers. They should not be taken by pregnant or lactating women either. Excessive use in adults (over 20 grams a day) may cause thickening and coarsening of the skin, although this is reversible.

THE FREE RADICAL THEORY OF AGING

The theory that free radical pathology lies at the root of the aging process – originated by Dr Denham Harman,[21] a medical researcher at the University of Nebraska Medical Center – is now accepted by most gerontologists. It has also aroused enormous interest in the popular media.

Free radicals are atoms or molecules that are electronically unbalanced and therefore highly reactive. Unlike normal stable atoms which have paired electrons, free radicals are characterized by an uneven number of electrons – either they have a missing electron or they have an extra one. As a result, they readily react with other atoms, grabbing or donating an electron in order to achieve stability. Until they are neutralized, they attack and damage DNA molecules in cell nuclei, distorting the genetic blueprints that control cell division, causing mutations and cancer;[22] they attack blood vessels, cause blood platelets to clump together, and initiate atherosclerosis and coronary heart disease;[23] they attack brain cells, causing memory loss and senility;[24] they attack the skin, causing brown age spots;[25] they attack immune cells and depress the immune system, making us vulnerable to autoimmune diseases such as rheumatoid arthritis and multiple sclerosis

(MS),[26] and they attack large protein molecules and cause cross-linking (abnormal chemical bonds between them).[27] Cross-linked molecules are the main cause of wrinkled skin,[28] stiff joints, hardening of the arteries and cataracts.[29] Over time, these tiny damages add up. We call this damage aging.

Free radicals can be neutralized, eventually, through the mitochondrial electron transfer chain in our mitochondria, the little power plants in our cells that burn sugar and fat into energy. Once in the mitochondria, free radicals cancel each other out.

Free radical pathology seems to be at the root of most aging processes. Dr Harry Demopoulos, a medical researcher from New York University who has conducted over a hundred studies in this field, contends that free radical pathology is as important an advance in medicine as Pasteur's germ theory of disease.[30] By showing that microbes cause disease, Pasteur enabled doctors to understand the mechanism by which diseases are communicable and to intervene in the process. And indeed, in less than a century, most infectious diseases have become a minor problem. Modern medicine has completely wiped out such dreadful diseases as smallpox, for example. However, in spite of its great achievements, medical science is not yet able to combat the degenerative diseases associated with aging. This is because they are not caused by communicable entities but by free radicals.

Free radicals are not complete villains, however. They are needed (in very small amounts) by the T-cells of the immune system for such constructive roles as destroying cancer cells and disease-causing bacteria. It is when they accumulate excessively in the body that they have such devastating effects. They can escape from cell mitochondria, if the diet is high in fat and low in antioxidant vitamins E and C; they can also be generated in the body by exposure to radiation (X-rays, sunlight, ultraviolet light, colour TV screens); and they can be formed from the waste products of smoking and drinking. Alcohol is converted in the body to acetaldehydes,[31] toxic compounds that break down into free radicals. Aldehydes are also found in cigarette smoke,[32] which explains why smokers are often advised to increase their intake of vitamin C, which has potent antioxidant effects.

COMBATING FREE RADICALS

Free radicals are the inescapable intermediates of metabolism, and so human beings (and in fact all organisms) have developed protective enzyme systems to neutralize them. The enzyme catalase, for example, breaks down hydrogen peroxide. Superoxide dismutase (SOD), a very prevalent enzyme in the body, increases life span[33] and alleviates arthritis by protecting joint membranes and other tissues from superoxide free radicals.[34] Glutathione peroxidase also neutralizes peroxides.[35]

To help protect the the body even further against the devastating effects of free radicals, natural foods also provide an abundance of free radical scavenger nutrients, popularly known now collectively, as antioxidants. The natural antioxidant nutrients, which defend the body by cancelling out peroxides and superoxides, include vitamins A, C, E, B1, B5, B6, niacin, PABA, the amino acid cysteine (found in eggs), catechols (found in bananas and potatoes), phenolics (found in grapes and other fruits), bioflavonoids (found in citrus fruits), and minerals zinc and selenium.[36]

But there are many others. We now know that specific fruits, vegetables and herbs carry hundreds of protective antioxidant compounds called phytonutrients. Extensive studies have shown, for example, that catechin polyphenols, components of green tea, are potent antioxidants, which protect blood cholesterols from oxidative damage, thereby protecting artery walls.[37] Lycopene is the red pigment found in tomatoes. Research has shown that it is a more potent antioxidant than beta-carotene.[38]

Most free radicals in the body are formed when unsaturated fats auto-oxidize. The process is very similar to what happens when oily rags, or rags used to clean oil-based paint from brushes, spontaneously catch fire. The unsaturated fatty acids (linoleic and linolenic) in the oil or paint readily react with the oxygen in the air, the reaction releases energy as heat, and the temperature of the rags eventually reaches ignition point.

The same type of reaction takes place in the human body. It takes just one free radical to oxidize one molecule of unsaturated fat for a chain reaction to start. As each molecule of fat is oxidized another free radical is released which oxidizes another molecule of fat, and so on. Just one free radical can oxidize thousands and millions of fat molecules. The body does not ignite, like the pile of rags, because it contains so much water, but that does not mean that it is not being damaged. Free radicals do the same kind of damage as massive doses of X-rays, which generate hydroxyl radicals, the most dangerous of all free radicals. Hydroxyl radicals attack and damage cells as well as the enzymes which protect and repair cells, causing a plethora of afflictions.

The more unsaturated a fat is, the more susceptible it is to free radical attack. The brain and the spinal cord are the most unsaturated fatty organs in the body, and as such are extremely vulnerable to free radical damage. In one laboratory experiment senility was produced in a group of rats in a matter of weeks just by feeding them with unsaturated safflower oil instead of saturated butter.[39] This was due to free radical damage in the brain.

How is it, then, that our brains last, more or less intact, into old age? This mystery was solved only recently. The cerebrospinal fluid (CSF), the fluid that surrounds the brain and spinal cord, was found to contain ten times as much vitamin C as the blood. There are little pumps in the selective membranes surrounding the brain and spinal cord which draw vitamin C from the blood into the CSF, with the result that vitamin C concentration in the CSF is ten times greater than in the blood. The membranes around each nerve cell (continuous with those around the brain and spinal cord) draw vitamin C from the CSF, with the result that vitamin C concentration inside nerve cells is ten times greater than in the CSF. So vitamin C is 100 times more concentrated in nerve cells than in the blood.[40] Large amounts of energy are required for all this pumping and maintaining of different vitamin C concentrations, but without it our brains would literally burn themselves out.

Hypoxia (lack of oxygen) is a condition known to promote free radical activity.[41] An inadequate blood supply, as well as causing strokes and heart attacks, also accelerates the activities of free radicals. In many cases, free radicals are the true cause of death, not impaired circulation. The moral, of course, is to keep vitamin C levels in the body as high as possible, as insurance against heart attacks and strokes.

It is in our best interest to neutralize free radicals as soon as possible, before they do any damage. However, this process takes time and can only be done gradually, since free radicals are highly reactive particles and very difficult to control. The first step is to reduce their energy, make them less chemically reactive. Only then will they combine with other free radicals and cancel themselves out. This is done with the help of scavenger (antioxidant) nutrients.

Let us suppose that a heart attack has impaired blood flow to the brain. The brain is running short of oxygen. Hydroxyl radicals are starting to form and damage the brain membranes. Vitamin E (tocopherol) molecules in the brain bump into some of these hydroxyl radicals, sticking to them and converting them into tocopherol radicals. The new radicals, although very dangerous, are less reactive than the hydroxyl radicals. Vitamin C (ascorbate) ions now bump into the tocopherol radicals and grab their free electrons, regenerating the original vitamin E molecules (which resume their scavenging duties) and forming ascorbyl radicals. These radicals now collide with molecules of glutathione peroxidase, a selenium- and cysteine-containing enzyme. Glutathione peroxidase reduces the ascorbyl radicals back to ascorbate ions (regular vitamin C), but now the glutathione peroxidase is oxidized. In this state it is not as reactive as the ascorbyl radicals, but still reactive and still dangerous. Oxidized glutathione peroxidase is reduced by reduced glutathione, a tripeptide protein which contains cysteine. The reduced glutathione recycles the glutathione peroxidase to its original form, but is now oxidized. Oxidized glutathione is a lot less reactive than the initial hydroxyl radicals we started with, but still undesirable (it will not burn the brain as hydroxyl radicals can do in 15 minutes, but it can cause red, itchy eyes). Oxidized glutathione is turned back into reduced glutathione by another enzyme, glutathione reductase, which is vitamin B2 dependent.[42] This is why many people with red itchy eyes (allergic conjunctivitis), that aren't due to an infection, often respond to a few hundred milligrams a day of vitamin B2.

Finally, the free radicals, now much reduced in their reactivity, are neutralized in the mitochondria of brain cells. Here, free radicals cease to be free. They meet and cancel each other out.

So generous supplementation of antioxidant nutrients – vitamin C, vitamin E, vitamin A, vitamins B1, B2, B3 and B6, selenium, zinc and cysteine – can be of great help in neutralizing free radicals and preventing the damage they do.

IMPROVING T-CELL PERFORMANCE

The mechanism by which free radicals cause coronary thrombosis was only recently revealed. Blood clots do not normally occur in healthy arteries, although plenty of platelets, which normally initiate clotting, are present. Clotting occurs only in abraded or damaged arteries. The factor that prevents abnormal clotting in healthy arteries was found to be a natural hormone called prostacyclin, or PGI2,[43] whose precursor, prostacyclin synthetase, is very easily destroyed by free radicals. Vitamin E in high doses helps to prevent the destruction of prostacyclin synthetase and therefore protects the anticoagulant role of PGI2.

The T-cells of a healthy immune system not only eat up cancer cells and bacteria but also the fatty, hardened 'plaques' which form in the walls of atherosclerotic arteries. When the T-cells are damaged by free radicals (especially superoxides), their ability to dispel plaque is reduced and the danger of atherosclerosis (literally meaning 'hardening of the arteries') is greatly aggravated. This applies particularly in advanced age, since the older we get, the less effective our immune system becomes. By age 60 our immune system is probably only a fifth as effective as it was in our teens. The importance of the antioxidant nutrients to improve T-cell performance and increase resistance to heart disease and other diseases of aging is undeniable. Vitamin E, for example, will double or triple T-cell function when taken in daily amounts of 200 to 2,000 IU.[44]

Autoimmune diseases like rheumatoid arthritis and multiple sclerosis are also caused by a faulty immune system. The T-suppressor cells processed in the thymus control and supervise the function of other antibodies, like the B-cells. When free radicals impair or destroy T-suppressor cells, the antibodies they supervise get out of control and act wild, attacking the joint membranes and other tissues as if they were foreign and hostile. In a good immune system, with abundant T-cells, this does not happen, since T-suppressor cells annihilate or suppress any B-cells which attack our own tissues. Here again, a massive supply of antioxidant nutrients, together with growth hormone releasers such as arginine or ornithine may be of great help, boosting T-cell performance and therefore reducing the scale of attacks on joints and other tissues.

There is much more to be learned about free radical pathology and the function of growth hormone in adults, but judging from present animal experiments, it seems that people who use high doses of antioxidant nutrients can expect to extend their healthy middle years by some 10 years and more.

GINKGO VERSUS SENILITY

The *Ginkgo biloba* tree, which early Buddhist monks considered holy, has recently been found to contain substances capable of reversing aging of the brain. The ginkgo has been in existence for at least 200 million years, surviving parasites, browsing animals, climate changes, moulds, pollution and disease. It is truly called 'a living fossil'. Scientists now believe that unique substances in its fan-shaped leaves are the reason for its exceptional survival. It was 'discovered' by the German botanist Engelbert Kaempfer in 1690 whilst he was working in Japan for a Dutch company, and the first ginkgos were imported into Holland, from where they spread throughout Europe. The first mention of the ginkgo in England, where it is also known as the maidenhair tree, dates from 1760.

Ginkgo's ability to reverse aging of the brain is of particular interest, since pharmaceutical research has not come up yet with a safe drug that can reverse senility. In a recent study done in Munich, 112 patients aged 55-94, all suffering from chronic cerebral insufficiency, were given 120 mg of ginkgo extract a day (40 mg three times a day). All were monitored for one year, and by the end of that time debilitating symptoms such as short-term memory loss, mood disturbances, headaches, insomnia, tinnitus and vertigo were significantly reduced.[45] Other studies have corroborated these results. A French medical journal devoted an entire issue to ginkgo, in which scientists gave details of many clinical trials.[46] Other conditions such as leg ulcers, macular degeneration of the eye and disturbances of equilibrium have also shown improvement with ginkgo extract.

These findings have been supported by EEG (electroencephalography) monitoring. In one double-blind study of cerebral aging, positive results were achieved after only three months.[47]

Test tube research has shown that ginkgoheterosides and proanthocyanidines, the two substances that make up 47 per cent of ginkgo extract, are effective free radical quenchers, halting lipid peroxidation and protecting cell membranes.[48] Studies involving diabetic retinopathy in rats have also demonstrated the anti-free radical activity of ginkgo extract.[49]

In short, scientific research into ginkgo is now in full swing. Both animal and clinical studies are showing its effectiveness in retarding aging processes, particularly in the brain. Capsules of ginkgo extract have recently been made available in health food shops and demand is soaring.

CoQ: A LIFE-EXTENSION NUTRIENT

Coenzyme Q_{10} (CoQ for short) has recently been extolled as a 'breakthrough'. It is, it seems, a heart-strengthener, a high blood pressure reducer, a weight loss aid and a life-extender all rolled into one. What is it? It is a substance present everywhere in the body, ubiquitous in fact, which is why it is also known as ubiquinone. It is not manufactured by the body, so has to be supplied by the food we eat. It is as essential a nutrient as any of the bulk minerals.

As the name 'coenzyme' implies, CoQ is a vital catalyst. Its function is to enable the mitochrondria, the tiny power plants in each cell, to release energy, 95 per cent of the energy required for life in fact. CoQ is so essential that when its levels in the body drop by more than 25 per cent degenerative conditions such as hypertension and heart disease start to flourish. If levels drop by 75 per cent, life cannot be sustained.[50]

CoQ was first discovered in 1957 by the American scientist F. L. Crane, who extracted it from the mitochondria of beef heart, where it is most abundant. This is not surprising. As an energy provider, CoQ is highly concentrated in active organs which have the highest energy requirements, such as heart, liver and immune cells.

Apart from the role it plays in energy production, CoQ has also been found to be a powerful antioxidant, similar in its action to vitamin E.[51] It protects lipids against the peroxidation which damages cell membranes and creates age spots.

From early studies biochemists assumed that CoQ concentration should affect the health of the heart muscle. And, indeed, healthy hearts were found to contain higher levels of

CoQ than failing hearts. Several studies with heart patients have shown that the administration of CoQ increases resistance to heart failure, acting in many cases as a life saver.[52] CoQ has repeatedly demonstrated its ability to reduce heartbeat irregularities (arrhythmias) in heart patients,[53] lower high blood pressure,[54] and bring relief in cases of angina pectoris.[55] In one study performed at Kitasato University, Japan, 20 heart patients were put on a low daily dose of 30mg CoQ. After two months, half of the group found that their breathing had improved remarkably, while the other half were noticeably less short of breath and were reclassified in a lower risk group. Six patients showed a significant decrease in heart congestion and six displayed reduced liver enlargement.[56] The Japanese researchers concluded that optimal levels of CoQ appear to be necessary to maintain normal heart function, although the mechanism by which CoQ exerts these effects is not clear yet.

CoQ was also studied in a variety of other conditions as well. It effectively halted the spread of gum disease, for example, responsible for 70 per cent of all lost teeth.[57] Severely diseased and receding gums that did not respond to brushing and flossing were revitalized by CoQ. Dr E.G. Wilkinson, a U.S. army dentist who conducted some of these studies, commented that CoQ was 'not just a therapeutic treatment to alleviate symptoms,' but achieved 'a reversal of the disease state in some cases and a regrowth of healthy tissue . . .' It appears that most people have an adequate supply of CoQ_{10}, but some people don't seem to be able to assimilate it as well as others. Periodontal tissues are deficient in CoQ_{10} when they are diseased, and appear to require more CoQ_{10} to heal.[58]

A study done in Belgium by Dr Van Gaal revealed low levels of CoQ in obese individuals.[59] Supplemental CoQ caused weight loss in a group of overweight subjects in a trial that lasted nine weeks. Dr Van Gaal commented: 'It looks possible that correcting significant deficiencies of Q_{10} in obese patients might improve lipid metabolism and contribute to the metabolic or cellular control of body weight.' Although CoQ is not a solution for all weight problems, it certainly holds out new hope in cases where there is no obvious reason for accumulating pounds.

CoQ also improves immune response, and hence contributes to life-extension, by enhancing the disease-fighting activities of white blood cells.[60] In fact it plays a crucial role in aging. In animal studies with CoQ, life span has been extended by 50 per cent. More exciting even than that, animals treated with CoQ retain a more youthful appearance right up to the end of their lives.[61] These findings are corroborated by the accumulating evidence that CoQ is a potent antioxidant.[62]

These are but a few of the findings relating to CoQ. Future studies will no doubt elicit additional health benefits, but for many scientists and lay people alike, CoQ is already a daily supplement.

The richest sources of dietary CoQ are beef heart and other organ meats, such as liver and kidney. Smaller amounts are contained in plants, particularly spinach, alfalfa, potatoes, yams, soybeans and wheat seeds. Supplements are now available in most health food stores.

THE WILL TO LIVE

The will to live is deeply embedded in the soul of all living creatures. But it is astonishing the extent to which many people suppress or weaken that natural instinct. In his book *The Will to Live*[63] Dr Arnold A. Hutschenecker writes: '. . . we pick our illnesses, we choose our time to die.' As proof, he cites many cases from his own practice. One man who has been suffering from an ulcer for 30 years told him he wanted to get well. When asked what he would do with his life without the ulcer, the man had no convincing answer. Dr Hutschenecker concluded that he had constructed his life around his illness. His illness provided him with consideration, care, and the attention of people around him. He needed his ulcer. Many ill people show a lack of will, or no will, to get well, even though they say they want to. They either accept their illness as something they 'deserve' or rebel, ineffectually, with a 'Why me?' attitude. Many 'reasons' are given for these negative states of mind, such as family problems and economic failure, but at the root of these is self-pity, a lack of faith in the body's astonishing powers of recuperation and a low threshold of stress. As readers will realize by now, vulnerability to stress is something that can be overcome by improved nutrition.

A distinguished doctor once remarked: 'Dying is 90 per cent habit.'[64] A simple example reported by Ben Sweetland in his book *Grow Rich While You Sleep*[65] will serve to demonstrate the truth of this. He tells the story of an old, illiterate labourer who had worked hard all his life. Suddenly, in his early sixties, he began to manifest signs of aging. He got tired easily and found it difficult to get through a day's work. He was growing old because he *thought* a man of his age *should* act old. To help him out, his family falsely 'proved' to him that he had mistaken his birth date; he was, they said, ten years younger than he thought he was. In a matter of days, he looked and acted younger, and started doing a full day's work again, with not a sign of tiredness. Nothing physically changed, just his thoughts and his faith in his younger self. Awareness, which determines attitudes and reactions, has the power to reverse aging. The classic work on the subject is

Dr Deepak Chopra's *Ageless Body, Timeless Mind*.

Linda Clark, in her book *Stay Young Longer*,[66] cites the findings of various researchers on the great influence emotions have on health and aging. She reports Dr D. M. Kissen's claim that unhappiness and lack of love can contribute to tuberculosis. According to Dr Desmond Caaren, nagging can produce illness. Resentment is believed to play a role in the development of arthritis. Emotions, therefore, are directly related to health and longevity or to sickness and death

THE MIND AS AN IMMUNE SYSTEM BOOSTER

More than ever, scientific research is now focused on boosting the immune system. The appearance of new diseases like AIDS, Ebola virus, drug-resistant pneumonia, drug-resistant tuberculosis and flesh-eating bacteria, struck horror into both scientists and lay people alike. And for good reasons. They are lethal and mostly incurable. Increasing our immunity to diseases, seems now a more promising approach than searching for cures.

Until 30 years ago, the immune system was conceived as a large collection of immune cells, with a few immune organs such as bone marrow, lymph nodes, spleen and thymus. It was regarded as a mostly autonomous system. Very little was then known about the interaction of the immune system with other systems, such as the hormonal system and the nervous system.

Recently, scientists have paid more attention to the relationship between mind and body, or in medical terms, the interaction between the nervous system and the immune system. Studies have shown that health can positively be enhanced by such practices as meditation, visualization, deep faith and positive thinking.[67]

On the other hand, negative thinking and feelings were found to have a detrimental effect on health. Studies have shown, that depression can weaken the immune system, by reducing the number of 'natural killer cells'. These are a type of immune cells that protect the body against cancer and viruses.[68] Another study revealed that psychological stress can cause vulnerability to disease by suppressing the immune system.[69]

It is not fully understood how thoughts, emotions and feelings affect immune cells. We know, however, that stress hormones can weaken the immune response. Mental stress is known to increase secretion of a hormone called cortisol, and cortisol can link with immune cells, slowing down their rate of division and creating deficiencies in B-cells, T-cells and natural killer cells.[70] Neurotransmitters are brain chemicals that transmit impulses between nerve cells and affect our state of mind. During emotional stress, a deficiency of neurotransmitters impairs the flow of brain messages, and in one way or another, depresses the immune system as well.

EAT LESS LIVE LONGER

There is an anecdotal story about Buddha teaching his disciples, that when each person is born, God allocates a lump of food for his life time. The quicker he finishes this lump the quicker he dies.

This story is now getting scientific back up. While researching for life-extension strategies, the calorie restriction strategy was found most effective. Young animals limited to 60 per cent of their normal food intake, lived up to 50 per cent longer than animals with no food limits. In addition, the animals that were eating less were much healthier and looked youthful into their old age.

The anti-aging effects of calorie restriction were discovered as early as 1934, but no one has come up with an explanation of how this works. Scientists found however, that food restriction retards the aging of the pineal gland, the gland that produces melatonin.[71] Research along these lines is still speculative, but isn't it worth trying to eat less to live longer and healthier?

DOWN WITH STRESS

Emotionally free people enjoy life more and often live longer than introverted, inhibited and negative-minded people. A person who cannot learn to relax mentally destroys his or her chances of longevity. Stress and negative emotions such as resentment, nervousness and hatred are all causes of deteriorating health.

What are the physiological effects of stress? Nature has equipped us to cope with emergencies. When we feel tense, afraid, or under mental pressure, our adrenal glands pump extra adrenalin into the bloodstream. Adrenalin accelerates heartbeat and respiration, causes blood pressure to rise and releases glucose from the liver, all of which enable us to react appropriately to the threat of the moment. Adrenalin enabled our ancestors to run faster to escape from predators; it also enables a person to lift a car when a child is trapped under it. However, in our society, few of our feelings of stress come from real emergencies. We sit in our cars, offices or homes and let our anxieties and grudges stress us physiologically and stimulate our adrenal glands. Persistent excess of adrenalin in circulation shortens life by increasing the load on the heart and blood vessels. This triggers a vicious cycle of disorders, including stomach and duodenal ulcers, hypertension, heart attacks and strokes.

In nature, the lion is used to fighting for food. In the zoo cage, he is assured of his meals, but he cannot free himself from his heritage. He paces back and forth, restless, apprehensive and frustrated. When he reaches the age of 25, he looks older and much worse for wear than his wild counterparts. The alligator, on the other hand, lies peacefully most of the time, hardly moving. No wonder he outlives the lion in captivity. Why the difference? Dr George Krila answered this question for a group of physicians visiting the clinical museum in Cleveland[72] (this museum exhibits mummified animals and their organs). The lion's adrenal glands were very large, because his emotions constantly stimulated them to secrete adrenalin. The alligator's adrenal glands, on the other hand, were very small.

Some nutrients really can help us to handle stress. Pantothenic acid, for example, is needed for the synthesis of adrenalin.[73] It is often called the 'stress vitamin' for this reason. Vitamin C and vitamin B1 have been found to have appreciable anti-anxiety effects.[74] Inositol and vitamin B6, often called 'sleep vitamins',[75] can help to ensure a good night's rest, while calcium can help to relieve depression.[76] It is also worth remembering that vitamin B3 (naicin) deficiency can cause a sense of humour deficiency!

CREATIVITY

Creativity influences our well-being, particularly after retirement. It is not by accident that Norman Cousins included a chapter entitled 'Creativity and Longevity' in his book *Anatomy of an Illness*. According to Professor Paul Torrance, a sociologist at the University of Georgia, creativity is 'a process of becoming sensitive to problems . . . gaps in knowledge,

missing elements, disharmonies and so on; identifying difficulties, searching for solutions, making guesses or formulating
hypotheses . . .' All moderately functioning persons have
this ability. The important thing is to learn to manage it.[77]

Between 1977 and 1978, Professor Torrance studied 200
men and women aged between 65 and 85 to find out how
art classes would affect them. After a year of painting and
drawing, they were asked to answer a questionnaire. Ninety-
six per cent reported feeling more active and fresh after art
classes; 71 per cent said they were more active than before; 93
per cent said time passed faster, and 59 per cent said they were
not ill as often as they had been the year before.

An earlier study in Nebraska showed similar findings. In
1960 a group of elderly people took an 18-week course in oil
painting. A follow-up survey eleven years later, revealed that
67 per cent of the participants were still living, compared
with only 38 per cent of a matched control group. All of the
surviving participants were alert and active, while only 62 per
cent of the surviving controls were mentally alert.[78]

As Dr Erwin Dicyan, author of *Creativity – Road to Self
Discovery,* says: 'You have to let your mind go. You do not start
fermenting creativity. You just don't suppress it . . . Creativity
is not limited to composing music or painting a masterpiece
. . . Creativity is a mental attitude, a willingness to be interested and a preparedness to follow wherever that interest
leads.'

Here are a few suggestions from experts on how to take
the first steps toward being more creative: start a neighbour-
hood newsletter; learn to relax by such methods as transcendental meditation, prayer, yoga or tai chi; try to do something
you've never done before, like learning to play a musical
instrument or joining a local drama group; find out what
you really want to do with your time. Remember, there is

creativity in every task that is done fully and with love.

Many artists and scientists keep their creative vitality into their eighties – one has only to think of cellist Pablo Casals, pianist Artur Rubinstein and Dr Albert Schweitzer. However, creativity is something within each of us, not something reserved for professional artists. We all have it and we can all use it to give more life to our years and more years to our life.

CHAPTER 16

THE HEALING MIND

For years we have heard about the constructiveness of positive thinking as opposed to the misery and destructiveness of negative thinking, that you are what you think you are, and that life is not good or bad, just what you make it. The general message is that all achievements in life, from a better- paying job to greater family harmony, come to those capable of thinking optimistically. Indeed, in recent years medicine has gradually expanded its definition of 'psychosomatic disorders' to include arthritis, migraine, ulcers, and many other ailments with a strong psychological component. According to Dr Franklin Ebaugh of the University of Colorado Medical school, one third of all illnesses seen in hospitals have an organic source, one third have emotional and organic sources, and one third clearly emotional.[1] Some physicians estimate that as many as 90 per cent of all diseases have an emotional basis.[2] So, as Dr Flanders Dunbar, author of *Mind and Body,* says: 'It is not a question of whether an illness is physical or emotional, but how much of each.'

EMOTIONALLY INDUCED ILLNESS

In an article entitled 'Heart to Heart Advice about Heart Trouble' Dr Charles Miner Cooper, a San Francisco physician, wrote: 'When I tell you that I have known a patient's blood pressure to jump sixty points almost instantaneously in response to an outburst of anger, you can understand what strains such reactions can throw upon the heart . . . whenever a business problem starts to vex you, let yourself go limp all over. This will dissipate your mounting inner turmoil. Your heart asks that it be permanently housed in a lean, cheerful, placid man.'[3] It *is* possible to make yourself ill by feeling resentment, a sense of guilt, fear or anxiety.[4]

Among emotionally induced illnesses, arthritis is perhaps the one that has been most studied. It has long been linked to prolonged and repressed feelings of frustration and depression.[5] Crippling arthritis, for example, is now accepted by many to be an illness of psychosomatic origin, resulting from an unconscious build-up of anger.[6] Now there is growing evidence that long-standing emotions, such as repressed resentment and grief, can open the door to cancer. Despite existing controversy, scores of studies now suggest that recent personal loss, plus a personality pattern characterized as 'helpless and hopeless' may predate the onset of cancer.[7]

Emotions such as fear, sorrow, jealousy, resentment and hatred can cause high blood pressure, hyperthyroidism, migraines, arthritis, strokes, heart disorders and ulcers.[8] Doctors can prescribe drugs to counteract the symptoms of these conditions, but they cannot do much against their underlying emotional causes. As Dr S.I. McMillen says in his book *None of These Diseases*: 'It is not so important what you eat, as what is eating you.'

Most visits to the doctor end up with the familiar suggestion 'You must try to relax more.' But how is this to be done? Cardiologist Herbert Benson says that a psychophysiological state which he calls a 'relaxation response' can be an antidote to stress.[9] But people find it hard to relax because their stressed consciousness does not seem to respond to their direct wishes; it seems to be detached from their voluntary mind. This is objective as well as subjective fact. The stress-relaxation response is dominated by the autonomic nervous system, over which we do not have direct control. The autonomic nervous system has two operating programmes, the sympathetic and the parasympathetic; the sympathetic deals with alarm, arousal, readiness to fight, and getting stirred up generally, while the parasympathetic mediates rest, relaxation, repair and regeneration. It is the parasympathetic part of the system which makes us feel calm and makes our muscles relax. This is the state which is normally achieved by practising various types of meditation.[10]

Valium, the West's number one prescription drug, is not the answer. This minor tranquillizer, prescribed mainly by family physicians to treat daily stress, anger, agitation or anxiety, has become very controversial among clinicians, and there is now a tendency to prescribe it for short-lived stresses only and discourage its use beyond a number of weeks in order to prevent dependency, side effects and, most important, the temptation to rely on drugs as the principle mode of coping.[11] Valium has no effect on the autonomic nervous system, the system that mounts the body's tension responses. It is only a masking drug. The improvement is always temporary unless the environmental conditions causing the stress are removed.

Physical exercise can provide some relief from stress, but meditation, self-hypnosis and psychic visualization can have a greater stress-relieving effect. More and more relaxation training classes are now available.

THE HEALING POWER OF POSITIVE THINKING

Can faith in God be considered a healing factor? Yes, indeed it can. When no satisfactory scientific or medical explanation can be found for cures and remissions, divine healing must be a possibility. In his book *The Power of Positive Thinking*, Dr N.V. Peale tells of the famous Viennese surgeon, Dr Hans Finsterer, who performed 8,000 gastric resections (removal of part or all of the stomach) using local anaesthesia only. Dr Finsterer, who believed that the unseen hand of God helps to make an operation successful, was cited as Master of Surgery for his achievements in abdominal surgery. It was his opinion that not all the advances in medicine and surgery can ensure that every operation has a happy outcome. 'In many instances,' he said, 'in what appears to be a simple surgical procedure, the patient dies, and in some cases where the surgeon despaired of a patient, there was recovery. Some of our colleagues attribute these things to unpredictable chance while others are convinced that their work has been aided by the unseen hand of God. When we are once again convinced of the importance of God's help in our activities, especially in the treatment of our patients, then true progress will have been accomplished in restoring the sick to health.'[12]

An ex-military physician told Dr Peale that when he returned to private practice he noticed a change in his patients' troubles: 'I found that a high percentage do not need medicines but better thought patterns. They are not sick in their bodies so much as they are sick in their thoughts and emotions. They are all mixed up with fear thoughts, inferiority feelings, guilt and resentment. I found that in treating them I needed to be as much a psychiatrist as a physician, and then I discovered that not even these therapies helped me fully do my job. I became aware that in many cases the basic trouble with people was spiritual.'[13]

Another physician quoted by Dr Peale said: 'We have discovered the psychosomatic cause of high blood pressure as some form of subtle, repressed fear – a fear of things that might happen, not of things that are . . . In the case of diabetes, it is grief or disappointment which we found uses up more energy than other emotions, thereby exhausting the insulin which is manufactured by the pancreas cells until they are worn out.'[14]

The question is, what can we do if we are already sick? Can certain thoughts and emotions help us? Can a better self-image and a greater sense of the divine cure or prevent disease? Faith has been the major ingredient in almost all forms of medical treatment throughout history. In fact, few of the medicines used before this century had any appreciable physical effect on acute diseases. Healers relied heavily on suggestion or make-believe, what scientific medicine now calls the placebo effect. Psychiatrist Jerome Frank calls this 'the power of expectant faith'[15] and he regards it as a major stimulus to the patient's own recuperative powers. Research studies show that placebos have some positive effect in at least one third of all cases. But the placebo effect is not taken as seriously as it should be by today's medical establishment even though it can reduce pain, accelerate recovery, heal tissue and mimic the action of drugs[16] all of which are held to be highly desirable if achieved by means better understood.

A man with severe cancer, who needed an oxygen mask to breathe, asked his doctor for an experimental drug called Krebiozen, at the time being touted as a miracle 'cure' for cancer. After only one dose of the drug, the man's tumours 'melted like snowballs on a hot stove'. He soon regained his health and became so active that he even began piloting his own plane. Shortly afterwards, he chanced to read about a study indicating that Krebiozen was ineffective. Immediately his tumours reappeared and started spreading again, and he was hospitalized. His doctor, following a hunch, told him not to believe the study and promised that he would be treated with more potent Krebiozen. In fact, the man was given only water, but his condition improved significantly. His improvement continued until he read an article in which it was reported that the American Medical Association and the Food and Drug Administration had finally concluded that Krebiozen was worthless. A few days later, the man died.[17]

In February 1977, a seminar was held in Los Angeles entitled 'The Soul in Health and Disease' at which Dr Kenneth Pelletier from the Neuropsychiatric Institute of San Francisco gave a paper. He said: 'In recent years the word psychosomatic has been abused by doctors, who use it to point out that the patient's symptoms are imaginary. But now we are progressively realizing that physical disorders are mostly psychosomatic, in that the body and mind created them, and mind and body can eliminate them.' Talking about the influence of the mind over the body, he continued: 'will power is a vital factor. It derives from this gentle emotion which makes us feel that our lives have meaning. The nature of this emotion is not clear. Something internal, deep in the soul of each of us that cannot be seen through a microscope nor be identified; our connection with the creator.'[18]

THE WILL TO CHANGE

Dr Pelletier's comments were based on observations of or interviews with the few who, for apparently inexplicable reasons, have recovered from cancer and other terminal conditions. The common factors found in all these people were:

• A major mental change. Their thought patterns and view of life were changed by prayer, meditation or some deep spiritual experience. They felt a dramatic shift in awareness. In the words of Dr Deepak Chopra , 'a leap in consciousness'.

• A change in human relations. Their ties with other people were greatly strengthened.

• Dietary changes. They no longer accepted just any food, but began to choose their food carefully and develop healthier eating habits. Many used herbs and folk medicine, as in Ayurvedic medicine or macrobiotics

• They developed a deeper sense of their own spirituality, a stronger sense of the divine.

However, all these people had something else in common: they did not regard their recovery as something that happened to them by mere chance, or by surprise, but as a victory they had won after a difficult inner struggle.

Another common factor in these people involved inner change. Change in their concepts and patterns of thinking. Change in the way they relate to themselves and to other people. According to Louise Hay, author of *You Can Heal Your Life,* the main keys to positive changes are self-approval, self-acceptance and self-love. Unconditional self-love. An important pre-requisite is practising forgiveness. The book *A Course in Miracles* says that 'All disease comes from a state of unforgiveness'. There is a large variety of self-help books, which teach various ways of spiritual growth and improved health, like meditations, affirmations and visualizations. Books by authors like Louise Hay, Shakti Gawain and Sanaya Roman, are amongst the most popular.

Daily stresses at work or at home are unavoidable. Even a simple thing like driving a car in congested traffic can cause the symptoms of stress − release of adrenalin, accelerated heartbeat, higher blood pressure and so on. Many people do not know how to discharge the cumulative effects of stress, so when all the small daily stresses are added to bigger stresses such as weddings, divorces, bereavements, new jobs, losing jobs or moving house, the body becomes overloaded. When the load hits a certain level, disease manifests itself. Relaxation training, spiritual practices, changing one's thought patterns, eating more sensibly and taking regular exercise can all help to dissipate physical, mental and emotional tension and allow the natural healing powers of the body to restore a healthy balance.

Happiness has always been regarded as an antidote against disease. Laughter really is the best medicine, as many spiritual healers, psychotherapists and physicians will tell you. Happiness, and making others happy by relinquishing selfishness, is a great mood-elevator and health-promoter, and should be practised daily through mind-conditioning. Happy feelings release brain chemicals that soothe the nerves and increase immunity against disease.

In a book published in 1905 called *Pleasures of Life* by Lord Avebury we read: '. . . we should all endeavour to contribute as far as we may to the happiness of others. There are many, however, who seem to doubt whether it is right that we should try to be happy ourselves. . .I cannot, however, but think that the world would be better and brighter if our teachers would dwell on the Duty of Happiness as well as on the Happiness of Duty; for we ought to be as bright and genial as we can, if only because to be cheerful ourselves is most effectual contribution to the happiness of others.'

CHAPTER 17

VEGETARIANISM IN PERSPECTIVE

The many vegetarian cookbooks available today testify to the fact that vegetarianism is becoming better understood and more popular. Some people become vegetarian because of the hazards associated with eating meat, or because they find meat indigestible or repulsive. Some dislike the idea of eating slaughtered animals, while others are allergic to certain types of meat. An increasing number of people become enthusiastic about vegetarianism after hearing that it can cure severe diseases. Then there are people who would like to become vegetarians but are inhibited by the unknown. How safe is a vegetarian diet? Is vegetarian cooking difficult, inconvenient, expensive and antisocial? This chapter will help to clarify some of these points.

Modern vegetarianism is based more on science than philosophy. It does not mean subsisting on vegetables alone. There are vegetarians, for example, who eat eggs and/or dairy products. Some people who eat fish still consider themselves vegetarians. What unites them all is the fact that they do not eat the flesh of warm-blooded animals. This is definitely not a deprivation. Let us remember that only a minority of human beings worldwide eat meat. Hundreds of millions of Indians and Chinese do not. Americans eat 30 times as much meat as the Japanese and 66 per cent more than the average Asian. In fact the citizens of the United States, although they make up only 7 per cent of the world population, consume 30 per cent of the world's supply of animal protein. In fact they eat over 10 per cent more animal protein than they need.[1]

Being a vegetarian means enjoying a greater variety of foods than people hooked on meat-centered diets. Plant foods come in a variety of flavours, textures, smells and colours to suit every taste. There are 40-50 different kinds of edible vegetables, including 24 different kinds of peas, beans and lentils; 20 different fruits; 12 different nuts; and 9 different grains. There are only 5 or 6 different kinds of meat and poultry.

Some people are afraid that they will lose their strength if they do not eat a large steak or a giant hamburger every day. This fear is unfounded. A correct balance of cereals, legumes and nuts can provide all the muscle power one needs. In fact, certain vegetarian diets can supply even more energy than meat. In comparative fitness studies done at Yale University a group of vegetarians scored higher than a control group of meat-eaters.[2]

However it must be remembered that a vegetarian diet should be carefully balanced. Meat not only provides protein and vitamin B12 in far greater amounts than vegetables, but also essential minerals which are less abundant in plants. All these must be eaten in adequate amounts to prevent deficiencies. However, this is not a problem if eggs, dairy products or fish are included in the diet.

IS VEGETARIANISM RISKY?

Many people think that giving up meat causes protein deficiency, since plants are not as protein-rich as meat. The fact that certain vegetables can be combined to provide even better quality protein than meat is hardly known. A report prepared for the U.S. National Livestock and Meat Board[3] states that 'a person would have to eat four pounds of corn to get the same amount of protein one pound of meat would provide.' This is true, but meaningless. Certainly no one can eat 4 pounds of corn or soybeans at a sitting, but he could easily eat certain specific vegetables which, when combined in certain proportions, would supply enough good quality protein to fill all his needs.

Vitamin B12 is the most important vitamin missing in vegetables. Strict vegetarians (vegans) can develop deficiencies without the benefit of eggs and dairy products.[4] Abrupt converts to strict vegetarianism would do well to take B12 supplements. Deficiencies of this vitamin can cause pernicious anemia and degeneration of the spinal cord and nerves, and vegans who eat plenty of leafy vege-tables are particularly vulnerable. These are high in folic acid, which can mask B12 deficiency symptoms until irreparable nerve damage has been done. The importance of B12 supplementation cannot be overemphasized.[5] Another vitamin little found in plants is vitamin D. This underlines the importance of milk in vegetarian diets.

Mineral deficiencies, particularly of zinc, are one of the lesser known risks of vegetarianism. Such deficiencies can manifest themselves in nervousness, loss of taste, weakness, anaemia, tooth decay, low sexual potency and irregular menstruation. Vegetarians are susceptible because many of them replace zinc-rich meat with increased consumption of raw oats, peanuts, millet and legumes which are high in phytates (salts of phytic acid). Phytates bind with zinc, calcium, magnesium and other minerals and excrete them from the body. However this can be overcome by using live yeast in the leavening of bread, or by sprouting grains, beans and seeds, which then become highly nutritious. In fact sprouts should be a regular item in the diet of vegetarians and meat-eaters alike. Legumes also contain toxins, which are normally neutralized by cooking or sprouting. These toxins, which interfere with protein digestion or block nutrient absorption in the intestines, make cooking mandatory for legumes. Uncooked fava beans, for example, can cause haemolytic anaemia fever, abdominal pain and headaches.[6] Raw kidney beans contain a substance called alpha–amylase inhibitor, which inhibits the digestion of starch.[7] This substance, better known as 'starch-blocker', was used as a diet aid until it was banned by the FDA in November 1982.

Rhubarb and spinach leaves are high in oxalates, salts which combine with calcium and promote the formation of kidney stones. People susceptible to urinary gravel and kidney stones of the calcium oxalate type should avoid rhubarb and spinach, and also chocolate. People suffering from goitre, who take thyroxine, iodine or kelp supplements, should avoid the Brassica family – cabbage, Brussels sprouts, broccoli, watercress, kale, rutabaga, turnips, rape and mustard.[8] These vegetables contain a goitreogenic factor which inhibits uptake of iodine by the thyroid gland.

The main risks of strict vegetarianism are stunted growth, anaemia and cirrhosis of the liver, all of which have been observed in studies with laboratory rats.[9] Vegetarians would do well to include eggs and dairy products in their diet occasionally and emphasize high protein foods such as brewer's yeast, spirulina, raw wheat germ, pollen, soya beans and raw nuts.

THE VIRTUES OF VEGETARIANISM

As we have seen, the toxins in edible plants are readily neutralized by cooking. Yet plant toxins are negligible when compared to the synthetic hormones, antibiotics, tranquillizers and pesticide residues with which slaughtered animal carcases are saturated today, to say nothing of microbial contaminants such as salmonella, trichina and staphylococcus. Moreover, preserved meats are routinely treated with sodium sulphite,[10] nitrites and nitrates to give them an attractive red colour and prevent botulism.[11] Nitrites and nitrates are powerful toxins that not only inactivate haemoglobin but can also become cancer-causing (nitrosamines) when heated above a certain temperature or when exposed to the acid environment of the stomach.[12]

The vegetarianism versus meat-eating debate is an old one. In 1965, a study was done comparing strict vegetarians, vegetarians who eat eggs and dairy products, and regular meat-eaters.[13] Laboratory tests showed only minor differences in things like blood pressure and protein levels in the blood. But a significant finding was that, on average, strict vegetarians weighed 20 pounds less than the others, all of whom were 12 pounds over their ideal weight. Other studies have found a correlation between meat diets and cancer of the colon,[14] and that vegetarians have a lower cholesterol level than meat-eaters[15] and also suffer less from constipation. All this was seen clearly in Denmark during World War I. There was a meat shortage, so the Danish government based the national diet on whole grain and bran bread, barley porridge, potatoes, greens and dairy products. The Danes emerged from the war with improved health. The death rate fell by over 40 per cent in one year.[16] When they returned to their meat-centred diet, mortality rates from circulatory diseases went up again to their pre-war levels. A similar thing happened to the

Norwegians in World War II, when they were forced to give up meat. The common claim that hard-working people need steaks for energy is quite unfounded. Complementary grains and legumes can provide even more energy than meat. Dr Irving Fisher of Yale University found that vegetarians were capable of greater endurance than meat-eaters.[17] The Hunza of Northwest Pakistan, noted for their stamina, live on simple foods like wheat, corn, potatoes, onions, goat products and fruits (mainly apricots). They can climb 30 miles of rough mountain trail in a single day, and their longevity is almost legendary.[18]

Vegetables provide protein much more efficiently and cheaply than animals do. If we take, for example, a steer as a link in a food chain, it seems that the steer eats the grass and the man eats the steak. A seemingly ideal arrangement, but what a waste! An acre of cereals can produce five times more protein than an acre of grazing land. An acre of legumes (beans, peas, lentils) can produce ten times more. Some leafy plants can produce even more than that. An acre of spinach, for example, can produce up to 26 times more protein than if it were used for rearing beef cattle.[19] In fact, only about 10 per cent of the calories consumed by beef manage to arrive to the table. About one third of North America's land is used for grazing, and about half of all agricultural acreage in the U.S. is used to grow feed for livestock. Meat eating also adversely affects our environment. As more meat is exported from central America, the rain forests, the lungs of our world, are alarmingly disappearing. Eating less meat can actually help save the planet!

THE PROTEIN QUESTION

Proteins make up 20 per cent of body weight, more than any other constituent except water. As we saw in Chapter 2, proteins are involved in such vital processes as the growth and maintenance of body cells, the formation of hormones, enzymes, blood and antibodies, maintaining a healthy acid-alkaline balance and preventing water retention (oedema).

In order to be useful to the body proteins must be broken down into their constituent parts, that is into amino acids. There are 22 amino acids, eight of which must come from food because the body cannot synthesize them itself. The essential amino acids are leucine, valine, isoleucine, threonine, methionine, lysine, phenylalanine and tryptophan.

There is, however, a big catch: *all* of the essential amino acids must be present simultaneously in our food, and in the right proportions, or protein utilization will fall to the level of the amino acid present in the smallest quantity.

For example, if you eat a cereal that contains all the essential amino acids in perfect proportions except for lysine, which is contained at only 50 per cent of the required level, then only 50 per cent of all the amino acids will be used by the body. The rest will be wasted. Lysine in this case acts as a 'limiting amino acid' because it limits absorption of all the others. To use a simple analogy, if we have plenty of flour, unlimited water but only a small amount of yeast, we can only make bread until the yeast runs out.

What really counts therefore is not so much protein quantity as protein quality. The term 'net protein utilization' (NPU) is used to indicate the proportion of protein in different foods which is digested and made available to the body. It is not a measure of how much protein it contains. Utilization depends on how closely the pattern of essential amino acids in the food concerned matches the body's requirements. Because egg protein almost perfectly matches the body's requirements, it is used as a standard against which amino acid patterns in other foods are measured. When the match is close, the food is said to contain 'complete protein'. When the match is poor, as it is in most vegetables, the protein is said to be 'incomplete'.

Theoretically, a food with an NPU of 100 will make available 100 per cent of its protein to the body. In reality, even the egg cannot do that. On the next page are NPU values [20] for a few common foods.

NPU values	Per cent
Eggs	94
Cow's milk	82
Fish	80
Cheese	70
Meat	67
Tofu (soya bean curd)	65
Soybeans	63
Corn	52
Peas	48
Peanuts	43
Chickpeas	40
Beans	38
Lentils	30

IS MEAT SO VITAL?

As already explained, the value of any food as a source of protein depends on the quantity of its protein and on its usability. Meat is not at the top of the NPU table, but somewhere in the middle. At the top are eggs, with an NPU of 94, and milk, with an NPU of 82. True, the NPUs of plant proteins are lower than the NPU of meat, nevertheless the protein in some plants – soya beans, tofu, and whole rice – approaches the NPU of meat.

Quantitatively, soya beans contain 40 per cent protein, Parmesan cheese 36 per cent and meat 20 per cent.[21] Beans, peas and lentils also contain around 20 per cent, so belong quantitatively to the same category as meat.

Animal proteins, although not necessarily meat, are most efficient for human nutrition because their amino acid pattern is more suitable for absorption than that of plants. Therefore, only a small quantity of animal protein is necessary to meet protein requirements. Much larger quantities of cereals are needed.

But it is possible to combine different plant foods which complement each other's amino acid patterns, or to add cheese, milk or egg to vegetable dishes. When a vegetarian meal is supplemented with animal proteins, there is no risk of vitamin B12 deficiency. Eggs also prevent zinc and other mineral deficiencies, particularly sulphur.

EATING THE RIGHT PROTEIN COMBINATIONS

As long as the stomach gets the right patterns of amino acids, it does not care whether they are derived from milk products, meat or vegetables. This explains how different nations through- out history have survived on diets of beans and rice, bread and cheese, potatoes and milk. True, the best combination of plant foods will not yield an NPU of 100. Not even an egg does that. But combining different incomplete proteins improves utilization dramatically. Most of us do this naturally by combining several different foods in one meal. Eating a wheat product and beans together can increase the actual available protein by 33 per cent.[22] Other combinations can surpass even that. For example, soy and wheat products have, separately, an approximate NPU of 60. But when one part soy is combined with six parts wheat, the NPU value of the mixture is raised to 80, 13 points above meat. One part beans with four parts cornmeal increases their combined protein availability by 50 per cent.[23] Three parts white bread and and one part of cheddar cheese would have an NPU of 64 eaten separately, but when eaten together their combined NPU is 76.[24]

Combining complementary proteins is easier than many people think. Although there are eight essential amino acids, only four really matter for complementation purposes: lysine, isoleucine, tryptophan and methionine. These are the least abundant amino acids in plants.

It is obviously best to combine protein-containing foods in proportions which allow their missing amino acids to complement each other. But even if the right proportions are not known, the mere fact of combination significantly raises the biologic value of the mixture. If we know, for example, that peas and rice complement each other, but cannot remember the exact proportions, any reasonable proportion of both will yield a higher NPU than peas or rice eaten separately.

A general rule to remember is that grains, nuts and seeds lack lysine and isoleucine, legumes lack tryptophan and methionine, and leafy green vegetables lack methionine.

DAIRY PRODUCTS

Milk and dairy products are complete proteins and do not need to be complemented. However, as they contain excesses of lysine and isoleucine, they can be used to complement cereals, nuts and seeds which are low in these two amino acids. Small amounts of dairy products can sometimes double or even triple the availability of plant proteins. Only two tablespoons of skimmed milk powder will increase the protein value of one cup of wheat or rye flour by 45 per cent.[25] Some good protein mixes are bread and cheese, cheese and rice casseroles, and cereals with milk. Skimmed milk powder can be added to most vegetarian recipes to increase protein value. An even better complementary food is brewer's yeast powder or flakes, which can also be used by people allergic to milk and by strict vegetarians.

GRAINS, NUTS AND SEEDS

Grains include wheat, oats, corn, barley, buckwheat, rye, millet and rice. Nuts and seeds include almonds, brazil nuts, hazel nuts and cashews, and alfalfa, sunflower, sesame and pumpkin seeds. These food groups are low in lysine and isoleucine, so are easily complemented by legumes (beans, peas, chickpeas, lentils, peanuts and soybeans) which contain excesses of lysine and isoleucine. Grains, nuts and seeds combine excellently with milk products and brewer's yeast. Other common combinations are: beans and rice, lentils and rice, peanut butter on wholewheat bread, and corn bread and beans (tortilla).

As for proportions, here are a few tips: use 1 3/4 cups grains to every 1/2 cup beans; 1 cup grains to 1/8 cup soy grits or flour; 1 cup seeds to every 3/4 cup peanuts. Milk products or brewer's yeast can be added to almost all grain or legume dishes.

LEGUMES (PULSES)

Legumes, as they are known in America, or pulses, as they are known in Britain, are low in tryptophan and methionine and are therefore complemented by grains, nuts and seeds which contain excesses of these amino acids. Legumes can be advantageously complemented by milk products and brewer's yeast (a cup of yogurt can be eaten with a portion of baked beans, for example).

VEGETABLES
Vegetables are low in methionine and should therefore be combined with foods rich in these amino acids, such as sesame seeds (Chinese salad), brazil nuts, millet, wheat germ and brewer's yeast. Seeds and nuts can be ground and sprinkled over salads. Millet and wheat germ go well with vegetable soups. Milk products are also recommended (Greek salad, for example, consisting of coarsely cut tomatoes and onions topped by slices of salted white *feta* cheese).

LOW MEAT DIETS AND MEAT SUBSTITUTES
Those who do not wish to give up meat entirely can still benefit from emphasizing vegetarian dishes, as is done in oriental cooking. Chinese cooking combines raw or lightly cooked vegetables, deliciously seasoned, with small portions of fish, seafood or meat served on beansprouts or rice. Chinese cuisine is characterized by various combinations of plant proteins which increase the protein value of the whole meal. As meat is expensive, this makes good financial as well as nutritional sense.

A common staple of Japanese cuisine is tofu, a cheese-like soya bean curd. Many Japanese depend on tofu for their daily protein. Tofu shops are popular and scattered all over Japan. Tofu can be prepared in almost endless ways, and most good health shops sell several varieties. Tofu can provide the partly-vegetarian Westerner with a safe, unpolluted source of fine protein, just as it does the Japanese. More information on tofu-making at home, and recipes, can be obtained from *The Book of Tofu* by William Shurtleff and Akiko Aoyagi.

Those who enjoy the flavour and texture of meat can use vegetarian meat substitutes, or texturized vegetable protein (TVP). This is available in various forms, as chunks for cooking or as frozen spicy chops which only need heating.

Today, vegetarianism is based not only on beliefs of an ecological and philosophical nature but on sound nutritional principles. Vegetarians now have scientific answers to the questions asked by baffled would-be converts. Sensible vegetarianism can offer a wide range of eating pleasures as well as health. Why not take advantage of it ?

CHAPTER 18

ACID FOODS, ALKALINE FOODS, AND FASTING

The acidity or alkalinity of our body tissues plays a large role in determining whether we stay healthy or succumb to disease. In fact, acidosis, excess amounts of acid in the blood and tissues, is regarded as a basic cause of many illnesses.[1] Acidosis can occur in conditions such as uncontrolled diabetes, in respiratory disorders (emphysema, asthma, pneumonia), in renal insufficiency (inflammation of the kidneys) and in conditions which include heavy loss of intestinal fluids (diarrhoea, colitis).[2] Normally our body systems act to preserve a balance between acidity and alkalinity, but in the conditions mentioned above, that balance cannot be maintained.

Alkalosis, a condition of over-alkalinity, is rare but it can occur after vomiting, depleting stomach acid, overuse of antacids,and sometimes in cases of hysterical hyperventilation.

KEEPING AN ACID-ALKALINE BALANCE

The body has various mechanisms which maintain acid-base equilibrium, normally between pH 6.8 and pH 7.8.[3] The lungs, for example, eliminate volatile acids (carbon dioxide and carbonic acid) through respiration, and the kidneys eliminate non-volatile metabolic acids (lactic, pyruvic and uric acid) through urine. There are also chemicals in the blood, known as 'buffers', which keep the pH of the blood within narrow limits.

However, the ability of the body to maintain a proper acid–alkaline balance is limited. When a person overeats acid foods, as in high protein diets, or when he or she is chronically constipated, alkali reserves can be depleted. With a higher than normal acid level, the body's resistance to disease is reduced.

This is why it is important to include generous amounts of alkaline foods (mostly fruits and vegetables) in the daily diet. All digested foods leave a residue of 'ash' in the body which is acid, alkaline or neutral depending on the kind of food eaten. Dr Paavo Airola estimates the natural alkaline-acid ratio in a healthy body to be approximately four to one. When such a ratio is maintained, the body has a strong resistance to disease.[4] According to Swedish nutritionist Dr Ragnar Berg, the ideal diet should include about 80 per cent alkaline foods and 20 per cent acid foods.[5] Some nutritionists recommend half and half.

Adopting a vegetarian diet, rich in highly alkaline fruits and vegetables, is highly therapeutic in many diseases as well as an excellent preventive. Here, in descending order of their ability to form alkaline and acid ash in the body, are some of the commonest foods. Many people have found this information invaluable in developing a balanced diet. Fresh fruits and vegetables are particularly beneficial in correcting overacidity.[6]

ALKALINE FOODS

Figs, soybeans, lima beans, bean sprouts, apricots, prunes, turnips, raisins, almonds, carrots, dates, celery, cucumbers, cantaloupe melons, lettuce, watercress, potatoes, cabbage, grapefruit, tomatoes, peaches, apples, grapes, bananas, millet, brazil nuts, buckwheat.

ACID FOODS

Oysters, fish, all kinds of meat, chicken, eggs, grains, wheat, nuts (except almonds and brazil nuts), cheese, lentils, peanuts.

NEUTRAL FOODS

Milk, butter, vegetable oil, white sugar.

Naturopaths recommend spring water as a partial treatment in many seemingly unrelated disorders such as kidney stones, prostate enlargement, indigestion and fatigue. These have one possible common cause: overacidity. Mineral water, which is rich in alkaline ions, can help to neutralize acidity and purify the body. In Europe, it is common practice to prescribe specific spring waters for specific disorders.

FASTING FOR HEALTH

Nutritionally speaking, the purpose of fasting is to purify the body by stimulating the elimination of waste substances. Water is a most important part of the process. At least 2 quarts (4 pints) a day should be drunk to help detoxification.

Toxic wastes accumulated in the body during years of

careless eating and living impair the functions of cells and tissues and cause various chronic disorders. When they are eliminated, therapeutic and rejuvenating effects are experienced.[7] Animals fast intuitively; whenever they feel sick, they stop eating until they feel better again.

CAUTION: Fasting can be dangerous for people who have a heart or kidney problem, or diabetes. In fact, anyone with a health problem should seek medical clearance before going on a fast. Even without a health problem, fasting for more than three days should only be done under medical supervision.

SOME PROS AND CONS

Weight loss is the immediate result of a fast. Up to 3 pounds can be lost during the first 24 hours, provided only water or non-caloric beverages are taken.[8] If fasting continues, the average loss over the next ten days will be 2 pounds per day. The loss, however, is not all fat. Fat accounts for roughly a third of the loss, water for about half, and lean tissue for the rest.

Apart from being useful for dieters, fasting can rejuvenate the body and also help to break self-destructive habits such as alcoholism and smoking.[9] Fasting also stimulates the release of growth hormone, the hormone which strengthens our immunity to disease[10] (see Chapter 15). Some German and Swedish health clinics use fasting to treat virtually all degenerative diseases, from arthritis and atherosclerosis to digestive disorders and skin condititions.

A distinction should be made between fasting and starvation. 'Hunger pangs' are not a sign of true biologic hunger.[11] They are merely gastric contractions which we interpret as hunger; they are a craving for pleasure, comfort and the relief of boredom and can be largely be alleviated by drinking water.

Appetite and stomach rumblings cease after two to four days.[12] Then follows a period of about three to four weeks when no hunger or fatigue are felt. This is true physiological fasting. However, when appetite returns, it is a natural signal to break the fast, or else starvation will set in and vital tissues will start to be dismantled to provide energy.[13] Why doesn't the body consume itself in fasting? Because as cells break down, they are very efficiently recycled. The products of cellular breakdown are used to build new cells. Protein levels in the blood of a group of people who walked 325 miles in 10 days while on a total fast remained perfectly normal.[14]

However, prolonged fasting on only water has its drawbacks. First, the body has less than 1,000 calories in reserve at any one time; these are stored in the liver as glycogen and are used up in the first two days of fasting. The body then starts to break down fat for energy, converting it into ketone bodies, such as acetone, acetoacetic acid and betahydroxybutyric acid. These ketone bodies replace glucose as a source of energy, supplying 70 per cent of the body's requirements. The rest of the body's energy needs are derived from the breakdown of lean tissue.[15] However, these processes lead to ketosis and acidosis unless some glucose is taken orally or by injection. Ketosis is characterized by slight nausea, a bad taste in the mouth and acetone ('pear drops') breath. Acidosis usually begins a few days after the onset of ketosis and can be very dangerous, especially in people susceptible to kidney malfunction or diabetes. An additional danger is that as fat is broken down, toxic residues are released into the blood. It is not commonly realized that body fat is a dump for toxins which cannot be dealt with by the liver, kidneys, lungs and skin.[16]

Sodium and potassium are largely depleted during

prolonged fasting. Potassium loss can average as much as 1,500 mg a day.[17] This can cause severe deficiencies, which manifest themselves as weakness, lassitude, nausea and kidney problems. Significant amounts of potassium should therefore be taken while fasting.

SHORT FASTS

Fasts of one to three days do not normally require medical supervision, but it is advisable to check with a doctor first if you are in the slightest doubt about your health. If you have never fasted before, start with a one day fast, and see how you feel. What fasts of one to three days achieve is cleansing and quick weight loss of 2 to 6 pounds.

Fasting should not be thought of as deprivation, but as a positive act. It rests the digestive system and is a step towards improved health. On rising, only water should be drunk, preferably pure mineral water. It is permissible to squeeze half a lemon or an orange into the water. To encourage bowel movements and promote elimination of waste substances, do the elimination exercises shown on pp. 249-50

During fasting, symptoms such as slight fever or chilliness, dizziness or headaches, are not uncommon, particularly in people who have never fasted before. These normally disappear after a day or so. Bad breath, sore gums and a 'coated' tongue are signs that wastes are being eliminated.

Breaking a fast properly is of the utmost importance. Eating should be resumed gradually, depending on the duration of the fast. A day's fast can be broken by sipping a little milk, fresh fruit juice or some vegetable soup and then resuming the normal diet at the next meal. A two- or three-day fast should be broken by sipping moderately diluted milk, fruit juice or vegetable soup for at least a day. The next day light meals only should be eaten, preferably of fruit and vegetables (fresh orange juice, grapes or an apple for breakfast; fresh tossed salad, carrot sticks, whole bread and butter, and fruit for lunch; steamed vegetables or dried fruit for dinner).

RAW JUICE FASTING

A safer and easier type of fast, rapidly growing in popularity, is the raw juice fast or juice therapy. In this regimen, only fresh raw juices of fruits and vegetables are allowed; no solid food is eaten at all. Juices provide plenty of natural sugars, vitamins, minerals and trace elements, and alleviate the stress which accompanies water fasting. They supply the basic elements needed for body healing and cell rejuvenation,[18] stimulate cleansing, normalize biological processes and, most importantly, eliminate the risk of ketosis or acidosis.

As Dr Ragnar Berg says: 'During fasting the body burns up and excretes huge amounts of accumulated wastes. We can help this cleansing process by drinking alkaline juices instead of water while fasting. I have supervised many fasts and made extensive examinations and tests of fasting patients, and I am convinced that drinking alkali-forming fruit and vegetable juices, instead of water, during fasting will increase the healing effect of fasting. Elimination of uric acid and other inorganic acids will be accelerated.'[19]

A juice therapy now becoming popular in many clinics is the 'grape cure', used to correct numerous disorders arising from toxic overload. Only fresh grape juice is permitted. However, a juice fast need not be restricted to one type of fruit or vegetable. In many sanatoriums, a cocktail of mixed fresh juices is served to achieve various therapeutic effects. Vegetables and fruits should be juiced just prior to their consumption. They must not be peeled or soaked in water.

Root vegetables should be vigorously scrubbed.

Various types of fruits and vegetables are used in juice fasting, depending on the desired effect. Common ones are apples, celery, carrots, parsley, beets, cabbage, broccoli and kale. Gayelord Hauser, the distinguished nutritionist, has created the 'Gayelord Hauser Cocktail'. This consists of equal amounts of celery, carrot and apple juiced together. It contains a balanced abundance of vitamins, minerals, enzymes and chlorophyll, and is delicious. Three glasses a day can become the best life and health insurance you have ever invested in.[20]

CHAPTER 19

SEXUAL POTENCY

All our bodily functions, including sexual activity, are influenced by our state of health, and general health and mental state influences our willingness to be aroused by sexual feelings. We have to feel good physically and mentally to enjoy sex.

Psychiatrists are fond of saying that the main causes of sexual dysfunction are mental, or as Dr Carlton Fredericks says, 'located above rather than below the collar line'.[1] This is true, but the influence of nutrition and nutritional disorders on libido is considerable and seldom seriously discussed. One study found that 29 per cent of male hypoglycaemics and 44 per cent of female hypoglycaemics were sexually dysfunctional.[2] There are other causes for sexual problems in men and women, such as low histamine levels in the blood (correctable by taking niacin) and pyroluria, a condition which can be rectified by taking extra vitamin B6 and zinc.[3] Incidentally, these last two nutrients also help to regulate menstruation; young women who stop menstruating as a result of crash dieting often regain their periods by taking supplements of vitamin B6 and zinc.

NOURISHING YOUR SEX GLANDS

The endocrine glands and their hormones are essential to sexual potency. Dr Paavo Airola describes hormones as 'spark plugs' that not only trigger and stimulate sexual activity but also dramatically affect general well-being.[4] The sex glands secrete testosterone (male sex hormone) or oestrogen (female sex hormone), indispensable for healthy sexual functioning. But they are not the only hormones involved. All endocrine hormones function in harmony, as an orchestra. Take the thyroid gland, for example. This gland controls metabolism through its hormone thyroxine. When the gland is under-active, metabolic rate slows down, and obesity, a chilly feeling, fatigue and loss of interest in sex are the result. Iodine is necessary for proper thyroid function. It occurs abundantly in seafood and kelp. (However, if you have an underactive thyroid and are on iodine medication or kelp supplementation, remember that the Brassica family of vegetables – cabbage, Brussels sprouts, broccoli, watercress, kale, rutabaga, turnips, rape, mustard – and also peanuts contain substances which combine with iodine and inhibit its absorption.[5])

A high protein diet speeds up the activity of the thyroid by supplying the amino acid tyrosine from which thyroxine is produced.[6] Thyroxine formation also requires choline.[7] However, without vitamins B6 and C thyroxine will not do what it is supposed to do, speed up metabolism.[8] Lack of vitamin B1 lowers thyroid function.[9] To ensure satisfactory thyroid function, the diet should be rich in B vitamins, proteins and vitamin C. Desirable foods are wheat germ, brewer's yeast, liver, whole grains, nuts (not peanuts), beans and brown rice. Kelp is a better source of iodine than sea salt. Since vitamin E has been reported to increase iodine absorption and hormone production, it would be worth drinking a glass of fresh tomato juice blended with 1 or 2 teaspoons of wheat germ oil and sprinkled with kelp powder on a daily basis.[10] This may do more for your sex life than wine and candlelight.

The conductor of the hormonal orchestra is the pituitary gland, located at the base of the brain. Pituitary hormones control the functioning of all the endocrine glands, including the sex and adrenal glands. They stimulate the male testes to produce seminal fluid and the female ovaries to produce ova,[11] and the adrenal glands to maintain a proper blood sugar level for a feeling of well-being, a prerequisite for any sexual activity.

How can we protect the pituitary gland's managerial function? Largely by stepping up vitamin E intake. One study showed that vitamin E is mostly found in the pituitary gland, where it prevents undue oxidation of its hormones.[12] Vitamin E occurs in foods such as raw wheat germ and wheat germ oil, and in other cold pressed oils. For proper adrenal function, several studies emphasize the importance of protein, vitamin E and the B vitamins, particularly B2 (found in milk), choline and pantothenic acid.[13] Pantothenic acid helps the adrenal glands to maintain a proper blood sugar level and therefore promotes energy and stamina. Raw sunflower seeds are a good source of B vitamins and protein as well as vitamin E, and so are sesame seeds. Rare grilled liver with sesame seeds and wheat germ flakes can be a fine aphrodisiac.

The pituitary, adrenal and sex hormones are all based on cholesterol, which is depleted by sexual activity unless pantothenic acid is present to help replace it.[14] Foods rich in pantothenic acid are beans, desiccated liver, nuts and brewer's yeast. Royal jelly, the richest known source of pantothenic acid (after codfish ovaries),[15] deserves a special mention. In the author's practice it has been found to improve sexual functioning when taken in high doses.

Several brain neurotransmitters such as norepinephrine, dopamine and acetylcholine are associated with sex drive. The precursors of norepinephrine and dopamine are the amino acids phenylalanine and tyrosine, which are also effective antidepressants.[16] Phenylalanine can be taken in doses of 100 to 500 mg a day to relieve depression and revive sexual interest.

CAUTION: As phenylalanine tends to raise blood pressure, hypertensive people should take only low doses, – 100 mg a day – to start with. Dosage can be gradually raised provided blood pressure is checked frequently.

ZINC, THE CRUCIAL ELEMENT

Zinc is crucial to a healthy sex life. The whole male reproductive system – prostate gland, seminal fluid and sperm – contains high concentrations of zinc. In fact sperm contain the highest concentration of zinc of any body fluid or tissue.[17] Oysters, a traditional aphrodisiac, are among the richest sources of zinc. The first scientific awareness of the relationship between zinc and the male reproductive system came from the researches of Dr Ananda Prasad during the 1960s. He found that although iron supplementation improved growth in sexually underdeveloped and undernourished boys, only zinc supplementation promoted sexual maturity. Later studies in Iran confirmed these findings and showed that zinc deficiency also caused sexual underdevelopment in young women as well.[18] The most recent studies of zinc and sex show that even a mild zinc deficiency for a few months can cause serious sexual dysfunction and reduced sexual desire.[19] Zinc supplements have been found to raise low sperm counts and increase sexual desire in people who have been living on zinc restricted diets.[20] Dr Prasad recommends 20 to 30 mg of supplemental zinc a day for six months to treat sexual dysfunction.[21]

Why is zinc missing from our diets in the first place? Because food processing (flour refining and rice polishing) removes zinc, and because junk foods and soft drinks contain no zinc. Because cigarette smoke contains toxic cadmium which interferes with zinc metabolism and can accumulate in the testes – heavy smokers are therefore particularly vulnerable.[22] Because alcohol excretes zinc from the body, while high phosphorus diets inhibit zinc absorption.[23] And because contraceptive pills deplete zinc. No wonder impotence and infertility are such common problems. The best food sources of zinc, apart from oysters, are herrings, meat, mushrooms, raw wheat germ, brewer's yeast, pumpkin seeds, eggs, nuts, pollen and molasses.

OTHER VITAL NUTRIENTS

Vitamins A and C also concentrate in the prostate gland.[24] Vitamin C is highly concentrated in prostate fluid and also in the adrenal glands, whose secretions stimulate the testes or ovaries to produce sex hormones.[25] Vitamin A is essential for the production of sperm. One of the reasons why many alcoholics suffer from sterility may be that alcohol interferes with the conversion of vitamin A to its active form in the testes.[26] When vitamin E is inadequate, there is a decrease in both sex hormones and gonadotrophin, the pituitary hormone which directly stimulates the sex glands.[27]

Essential fatty acids are necessary for adrenal and thyroid

activity and have also been found to cure prostate disorders.[28.] Cold-pressed, unrefined oils like wheat germ oil, sunflower or safflower are good sources. Raw sunflower and pumpkin seeds are very beneficial as nibbles between meals.

Histamine release is a prerequisite for orgasm. Men or women who have difficulty reaching orgasm often respond to vitamin B3 (niacin) supplements, because B3 is a well-known histamine releaser. In fact, it is the histamine released during sexual excitation that causes blushing on various parts of the body, such as the face or neck,[29] and mucus secretion by the membranes of the sexual organs. Since vitamin B6 helps to convert the amino acid histidine to histamine, supplements of B6 and adequate histidine-rich foods (meat, cheese) can be beneficial.

Selenium-deficient diets have been reported to increase male impotency even in young men.[30] Magnesium and potassium are also important. Potassium and magnesium aspartates (salts of aspartic acid) can increase sexual responsiveness in middle-aged men and women.[31] Both potassium and magnesium can relieve drowsiness by removing excess ammonia from the body. Potassium is contained in meat, nuts, legumes, lettuce, spinach, oranges and bananas. Magnesium, which accompanies potassium in many foods, is best obtained from dolomite. Pumpkin and sunflower seeds, pollen and cashew nuts are other good sources. Aspartic acid is found in asparagus, soya beans and sugar beet molasses.

Snacking is a convenient way of boosting sexual responses. Make it a habit to snack on mixed seeds, nuts and soy beans. Avoid salt as it depletes potassium.

LIBIDO LOSERS

Frankfurters and preserved meats are loaded with nitrates and nitrites, which are sexual downers. Potassium nitrate, commonly called saltpetre, was once sprinkled on prisoners' food to reduce their sexual desire. Cigarette smoke is another thing that those who care about their sex life should do without. So are alcohol and the contraceptive pill, which deplete zinc.

According to Dr William Masters of the St. Louis Reproductive Biology Research Foundation, the pill is often the cause of loss of libido. Prolonged use may cause secondary dysfunction (failure to reach orgasm) in some women. 'The pill does not always cause loss of libido,' says Dr Masters, 'but it is prevalent enough to make us suspicious when someone develops a lack of responsiveness while taking it.'[32]

It is important to remember that nutrients, unlike drugs, exert their beneficial effects gradually and their action is greatly enhanced when the correct supplements are taken in proper amounts, as a part of a wholesome and balanced diet. In many cases, improved nutrition rather than the psychiatrist's couch is the quickest and cheapest way to solve sexual problems.

CHAPTER 20

EXERCISE:
THE NUTRIENT MONEY CANNOT BUY

It is possible to eat the most wholesome balanced diet, and still fail to be healthy. The complement of a good diet is adequate exercise. To achieve optimal energy level, fitness and health, one needs to exercise the body as well as feed it. Exercise is a kind of nourishment.

WHAT WILL EXERCISE DO FOR ME?

Regular exercise can relieve fatigue, control weight[1] and stimulate elimination. However, recent studies have shown that exercise can also lower cholesterol levels and improve heart function.[2] Exercise is very likely to save you from heart attack.[3] In addition, a number of studies have demonstrated significant increases in HDL cholesterol, the protective type of cholesterol, in groups involved in aerobic exercise programmes.[4] And in spite of previous scientific controversy, there is now general agreement that regular exercise achieves reductions in blood triglycerides, particularly in people whose triglyceride levels are high.[5]

Exercise tones up the heart.[6] At a preset level of effort, exercise-trained individuals can maintain lower heart rate and lower blood pressure than individuals who take little or no exercise. Runners generally have lower blood pressure than non-runners. This is highly significant. An exercise-trained heart is a much more efficient pump and needs less oxygen to perform its duties. It should therefore have greater resistance than an untrained heart to a sudden reduction in oxygen supply, which is what happens during a heart attack. Exercise training has been used successfully in the treatment of angina[7] and mild hypertension.[8]

Many people find that regular exercise helps them to relieve daily stress or depression. This is because exercise stimulates the release of endorphins (natural painkillers) in the brain. Exercise can also help diabetics, by improving tissue sensitivity to insulin; in fact, in juvenile diabetics, regular exercise can reduce insulin requirements.[9] Regular exercise can also reduce joint swelling,[10] alleviate respiratory disorders[11] and even prolong life span.[12] In the author's practice, regular exercise has been found to improve vision in many cases of impaired eyesight.

Exercise does not have to be strenuous to produce good results. At the Veterans Administration Hospital in Lexington, Kentucky, Dr James Anderson demonstrated that diabetics with blood sugar counts three times higher than normal were able to do without drugs just by walking for half an hour directly after every meal.[13]

However, exercise, like diet, is an individual matter. The wrong kind and intensity of exercise can cause trouble, particularly in people who are unfit. It would be worthwhile to consult a doctor and a professional instructor on the type and frequency of exercise you should take, particularly in the beginning. Moderation is important. Whether you are seven years old or 70, you should exercise regularly, and the best time to start is now.

There are basically two kinds of exercise: aerobic and non-aerobic. Aerobic exercises involve intensive breathing. Their main purpose is to get you fit. Into this category come hiking, dancing, running, jogging, swimming, cycling, rope skipping, etc. These are all forms of exercise which improve oxygen circulation, strengthen the heart and improve respiration. Non-aerobic exercises do not involve intensive breathing. Their main purpose is to develop power. Typical examples are weight lifting, weight workouts and isometric exercises, all of which increase muscle tone, strength and endurance.

NON-AEROBIC EXERCISE

Non-aerobic exercises have two immediate benefits. The first is that they increase muscle tone (the ability of muscle to contract) and strengthen bone; this is because they increase the amount of nitrogen in muscles and calcium in bones.[14] Lack of exercise causes bones to lose calcium and become brittle. Astronauts, confined in a spaceship capsule, can lose 200 mg calcium a day due to weightlessness and lack of activity. The second benefit of non-aerobic exercises is that they enable muscles to endure physical stress for longer. For example, they can strengthen back muscles and improve the mechanics of the vertebral column, preventing common conditions such as back pain, slipped discs and sciatica. To strengthen a muscle, it should be worked against progressively greater resistance, or with added weights. To increase muscle endurance, however, repetitions should be increased and weights should be decreased. A lighter barbell can then be used longer for the same exercise. Weight workouts are excellent for women, helping to firm up muscles and get rid of cellulite.

However, non-aerobic exercises do not normally strengthen the heart or increase its fitness. This is the role of aerobic exercises.

AEROBICS

The benefits of aerobic exercises are many and varied. First, they raise general muscle fitness and the fitness of the heart, which is basically a muscular organ. Second, they improve metabolism, contributing to a sense of well-being and helping to rectify digestive and eliminative disorders. Third, they revitalize the capillary networks of the heart and all the muscles,[15] increase lung capacity and improve oxygen supply to every cell in the body. Fourth, they encourage excretion of body toxins through the skin, mouth and nose by increasing perspiration and the discharge of mucus and phlegm. A smoker who starts running will often choke on excess phlegm abruptly discharged through the respiratory system. Fifth, they can reduce blood cholesterol levels.[16]

Two East African tribes, the Masai and the Samburu, live mainly from hunting and cattle herding, and subsist mostly on meat and milk, two foods high in cholesterol. However, there is very little heart disease among them.[17] They are physically very active, spending most of the day hunting or running after their animals. Most of their activities are therefore aerobic, outdoor activities. Their sugar consumption is virtually nil,[18] which also helps to account for their low cholesterol levels.

The benefits of aerobic exercise on the heart depend on the duration and regularity of exercise. To be effective, one should exercise for at least 20 minutes three times a week.

Enthusiastic beginners should not overdo vigorous exercise. Usually the people who get into trouble are those who were physically very active in their youth.

Exercise should be started slowly. The heart, lungs and muscles must be given a chance to adjust to the greater workload. If you wish to run, for example, start by walking, then increase the length of your walks, and walk faster; then begin slow jogging, slowly increasing your pace; after several months, you should be fit enough to start running. If you can, join a health club. This is a good idea because buying your own exercise equipment can be expensive and exercising by yourself can be extremely boring and unsociable. Besides, in a health club you can enjoy the benefit of professional instruction, which could stop you making serious mistakes, particularly at the beginning.

Although sedentary people usually begin to feel better after only a few aerobic sessions, real physical and physiological improvements take somewhat longer, so a little patience is required. With perseverance, results will come. Chronic backaches can disappear, eyesight can improve, migraines can vanish. Fatigue, that great and common obstacle to a happy and useful life, can be sent packing. The best antidote to tiredness is physical activity, *especially when you feel tired*. Physical activity at the end of a trying day creates a feeling of freshness and renewed energy that nothing else can equal.

CHECKING YOUR AEROBIC FITNESS

The pulse is the body's most important index of well-being, stress or illness. Pulse rate, the rate at which the heart beats, can be used to determine maximum exercise load and measure fitness gains. Three pulse measures are used.

RESTING PULSE RATE

This is normally 68-80 beats per minute in adults (children may have higher rates). As fitness goes up, the resting pulse rate comes down. Professional runners, for example, have resting pulse rates lower than 60, sometimes as low as 45-50.

MAXIMAL PULSE RATE

This has to be taken at the peak of vigorous exercise. However, it should not exceed specific values for specific exercises at specific ages. If it does, you may damage your heart. Here are the maximal pulse rates for riding a stationary bicycle:[19]

Age	Maximal pulse rate
Under 30	160
30-34	155
35-39	150
40-44	145
45-49	145
50-54	140
55-59	140
60-64	135
65 and over	130

RELAXATION TIME

This is the time needed for the pulse to return to normal after vigorous exercise, and it gives a clear indication of whether an exercise regime is too strenuous. After a minute, pulse rate should come down by at least 10 counts and after 20 minutes it should be normal again. If not, exercise has been too vigorous. Pulse rate can be measured wherever it can be felt, usually at the wrist (radial artery), but also in the neck (external carotid artery) and at the temple (temporal artery). You can either count the number of heartbeats for 15 seconds and multiply by four, or count for a whole minute.

DOING YOUR HEART A FAVOUR

Any engineer will tell you that the longer a machine works at peak output, the greater the wear on the moving parts and the shorter their working life. Something is bound to break down, sooner or later. Let us imagine two pumps, one next to the other, both working 24 hours a day, one at full load and the other at half load. Clearly the latter will last longer.

The same is true of the heart, the human double pump. The heart draws blood into its right side and forces it out of its left side, just like a mechanical pump, and it does this by contracting about 75 times a minute, on average, when the body is at rest. Higher rates of contraction – of 85-90 beats a minute, say – do not necessarily indicate disease, but obviously a heart which is working at above the normal rate will start to fail before it should. It may not last as long as a heart which contracts only 60-70 times a minute.

The heart has a tremendous job to do. Even in normal conditions it contracts and expands 100,000 times a day, pumping 18,000 litres (3,960 gallons) of blood. Clearly, if we can increase the pumping force (capacity) of the heart and at the same time reduce the number of times it has to beat (load), we will increase its efficiency and endurance. Indeed, the efficiency of heart contraction and expansion (and therefore the volume of blood pumped with each beat) is much greater in athletes than in average individuals. A low pulse rate is a great advantage because it means improved blood flow and increased oxygen supply without the need to exert the heart.

Moreover, by lowering pulse rate, we not only give the heart more time to rest between beats but also more time to repair and maintain itself. We are talking in terms of half seconds, it is true, but this is a lot in cardiac terms. A heart which is beating 60 times a minute is actually resting for half that time. During a whole day, this amounts to 12 hours' resting time, a very meaningful rest period indeed.

HOW TO USE EXERCISE TO CONTROL YOUR WEIGHT

In most people, normal weight is a matter of balancing calories eaten against calories burnt. Calories eaten must be used up through exercise or weight gain will occur. Do you know how many calories you should be consuming every day? If you do, you should be able to balance your daily food intake with your energy output.

To roughly calculate what your daily calorie intake should be, you need to know your basal metabolic rate (BMR). This represents the number of calories your body needs just in order to tick over and maintain normal physiological functions. To work out your BMR, find out what your ideal weight should be in pounds, taking into account your sex, height and build; multiply it by 0.455 if you are a man and by 0.409 if you are a woman; then multiply the answer by 24 to arrive at your basic daily calorie requirement. Men usually need between 1,600 and 1,800 calories a day and women between 1,250 and 1,450 calories a day to satisfy their BMR. On top of that, a certain number of 'activity calories' are needed. The more active you are, the more activity calories you will need over and above your BMR.

If you lead a fairly sedentary life, doing a lot of sitting, reading and writing, with not much walking or standing, you will need your BMR calories plus 30 per cent more. If you lead a moderately active life, exercising up to three times a week, and your job involves rather more walking and standing than sitting, you will need your BMR calories plus 50 per cent more. If you lead a very active life, with lots of strenuous activity, and exercise more than three times a week, you will need your BMR calories plus 80 per cent.

Let us suppose you are a 200-pound man and sit at a desk most days of the week and watch television in the evenings. First of all, 200 is not your ideal weight; you should weigh about 160 pounds, given your height and build. So your true BMR requirement will be 160 x 0.455 x 24 calories, which comes to 1,747 a day. Because you lead a sedentary life you only need 30 per cent more calories than your BMR, which is another 524 calories. So unless you keep your daily intake to 1,747 + 524 calories, or 2,271 calories, you will not achieve your ideal weight.

Let us suppose instead that you are a nurse and weigh 120 pounds, which is about right for your height and build. Just to keep you going you need 120 x 0.409 x 24 calories a day, which comes to 1,178. Because you lead a busy, active life, you need 80 per cent more calories than your BMR, which is another 942 calories. So your total daily requirement is 2,120 calories.

Regular exercise can be used to burn up more calories than you consume, in other words to put your calorie account into overdraft so that you lose weight. Different forms of exercise burn up different amounts of calories.

Sport	Calories used per minute
Horse riding (walking)	3.0
Volleyball	3.5
Walking (2.5 mph)	3.6
Bowling	4.5
Cycling (5.5 mph)	4.5
Golfing	5.0
Swimming (200 yards per minute)	5.0
Rowing (2.5 mph)	5.0
Walking (3.8 mph)	5.6
Skating	6.0
Tennis	7.1
Water skiing	8.0
Aerobic dancing	8.5
Skiing	9.0
Cycling (racing speed)	14.0
Running (10 mph)	15.0

Weight control really is like balancing a bank account, except that most people worry more about the credits than the debits! The credits equal calories eaten and the debits equal calories used in activity and exercise. One pound of body fat contains 3,500 calories, so if you eat 500 excess calories every day, in a week you will gain one pound of fat.

The importance of planning activity debits cannot be overemphasized if you want to keep your weight down or lose weight. Apart from regular sporting activities, here are a few ways of building exercise into your daily schedule.

•Have a good stretch in the mornings when you wake up.
•Take the stairs rather than the elevator/escalator.
•Perform calisthenics while watching television.

•Park your car farther from the office/supermarket.
•Get off the bus/train one stop before you need to.

TEN TIPS FOR SAFE, SUCCESSFUL EXERCISE

1 Exercise regularly. Make exercise a habit at least three times a week, or try to make it a social occasion. Exercise should be enjoyed, not put up with!

2 Warm up before you start – this will prevent muscle strains and cramps.

3 Wind down gradually at the end of your exercise. Do not sit or lie down immediately afterwards.

4 Try to raise your pulse rate during exercises to 160 beats per minute, or to the maximal rate for a person of your age (refer to the table on p. 392). Consult a professional instructor if you are in doubt as to what your maximal pulse rate should be.

5 *Gradually* increase the load on your heart, lungs and muscles. This way, you will lower your pulse rate while strengthening your body.

6 Never hold your breath when straining – the increased pressure in your chest could reduce your blood pressure enough to cause you to black out or faint.[20]

7 Balance your exercises. Include aerobics for fitness and non–aerobic exercises for strength and endurance.

8 Eat a wholesome, balanced diet, carefully supplemented, and do not smoke or drink. The effects of a good diet and
regular exercise are synergistic – the effects of both together
are greater than the effects of either on its own.

9 Get adequate sleep.

10 Don't hurt yourself during exercise. Learn safety rules
from a professional instructor in any specific field of interest.
If you pull a muscle, rest until it stops hurting. If you keep
hurting yourself, your technique may be at fault, or perhaps
your chosen activity is not the right one for you. Try something else – there are dozens of sports to choose from.

CHAPTER 21

HEALTH:
THE PERMANENT CHALLENGE

Everyone has a slightly different conception of what is meant by health. For some, health means never missing a day's work. For others, frequent minor complaints, which do not require hospitalization, are normal health. The medical definition of health is absence of disease. But all of these definitions are a misuse of the term 'health'.

WHO IS HEALTHY?

Today one is considered healthy by life insurance companies even if one suffers from obesity, dandruff, poor vision, migraines, backache, sinusitis, insomnia, heartburn, tooth decay, depression, fatigue, nervousness, low sex drive or painful menstruation. Many of us tend to forget that good health also implies physical and intellectual vigour, an all-pervasive feeling of well-being and freedom from emotional, functional and minor illnesses.[1]

The incidence of diseases such as flu, allergies, emphysema, cirrhosis and hepatitis is rising.[2] These diseases are not part of normal health, but they are often accepted as such. Major problems such as cancer, heart disease and diabetes are tolerated because they are thought to be 'unavoidable'. Few people stop to think how they might prevent them, and fewer still know that nutrition plays a crucial preventive role. Many surgical operations would be unnecessary if we considered our food in terms of nourishment rather than taste appeal and palatability. Tonsillectomies and haemorrhoid and cataract operations are classic examples. Why should the surgeon's scalpel be necessary to eliminate the symptoms of nutritional deficiency?

The increased incidence of minor and major illness in Western societies not only parallels the increased consumption of sugar, refined foods and soft drinks, but also the decreased use of fresh vegetables, whole grain breads and cereals, legumes and potatoes.[3] Surveys show that 75 per cent of teenagers do not even eat the scanty minimum RDAs![4]

Most drugs are intended to alleviate the symptoms of disease, not to treat and abolish its causes. Misunderstanding the role of drugs, too many people come to depend on them. They feel that no matter what happens, their doctor will always come up with the right pill or tablet. They abdicate responsibility for their own body. As a result, their level of health, such as it is, is always dragged down. Drugs cannot counteract the effects of continuing self-abuse in the form of undersleeping, overdrinking, smoking, never exercising and subsisting on a diet of processed convenience foods. They mask them, and do nothing to boost natural immunity.

To a nutritionist, health is a positive state of well-being, a composite of good intellectual and physical functioning, good appetite, digestion and elimination, good muscle tone, resistance to infection and fatigue, and that wonderful feeling of buoyancy which makes each day a new adventure.[5]

HEALTH:
GOD-GIVEN OR MAN-MADE?

The best way to practice health is to regard it as a talent which requires constant development and practice, like singing or dancing. Take singing, for example. Everyone can sing in one way or another, even if tone deaf and occasionally off key! Those who practice regularly improve. The same applies to health. Some people are born with little talent; they have a weak immune system and are often sick, and their entire life is a struggle against debilitating illnesses. Others are born robust, break all the rules and stay healthy to a ripe old age. Most of us hover somewhere between these extremes, but each of us can improve what he or she was born with. In fact, it is quite easy to improve our health once we make our mind up to do it. The rules of basic health are simple. Do everything in moderation. Avoid sugary, processed foods. Get adequate sleep. Exercise every day (the Spartans used to say: 'Work up a sweat once a day.')

Is it really worth living a year less to 'enjoy life' more, when often the expected joy turns into chronic debilitating disease which makes life one long misery, for everyone? At one time the hedonists, the 'have a good time' brigade, were in the majority. The health-conscious minority were laughed at as 'food faddists' or 'health nuts'. But now that morbidity and mortality from heart disease, cancer and strokes have reached epidemic proportions, the 'eat, drink and smoke and devil take the hindmost' philosophy is wearing a bit thin. Chronic diseases such as arthritis, hypertension, atherosclerosis, cataracts, hearing impairment and mental disorders are now so prevalent that people are beginning to heed the message that prevention is better than cure. Sufferers are increasingly willing to consider alternative therapies, not only because they are disillusioned with orthodox medicine but also because they want a say in their treatment and realize that they can do a lot to help themselves. A tremendous health-building trend has started. People are beginning to develop and assert their talent for health.

THE EIGHT SYMPTOMS OF HEALTH

Health is not just the absence of disease. It is far more complex than that. So let us split it into its main ingredients.

ENERGY AND PERSONAL EFFICIENCY

Are you efficient enough in your daily activities? Do you overcome stress easily? Can you work all day and still have enough energy left to enjoy the evening, or do you collapse in front of the TV? These are questions that are intimately related to your state of health yet they are seldom asked in medical examinations. Doctors and specialists are trained to treat only the diseased part of your body. They do not take the holistic view. Alertness, energy, endurance, resistance to daily stresses and the ability to relax easily are all symptoms of good health.

BUOYANT MENTAL STATE

Mental health is part of total health, and nutrition can strongly influence the mind, as we saw in the first three chapters of this book. Megavitamin or orthomolecular therapies can effectively treat various schizophrenias, but much simpler nutrition regimes can still have a beneficial, although gradual, effect on mental efficiency. As we saw in Chapter 10, a low sugar diet can correct hypoglycaemia, and symptoms such as nervousness, irritability, depression and dizziness. Wholesome, natural foods, free from additives, can often minimize behavioural problems in hyperactive children. Our ability to withstand daily stresses is directly related to our food.

SLOW AGING
The rate at which people age depends on their genetic heritage but also on differences in lifestyle. One smoker may be weakened from emphysema, by the time he is 50, while another keeps jogging well into his 80s. Nevertheless, people who eat sensibly, exercise moderately and lead relatively happy, sociable lives are likely to age more slowly and find life more rewarding than people who don't.

PHYSICAL FITNESS
In the previous chapter we saw how regular exercise can benefit health. In fact, physical fitness is an indicator of health. You do not have to be totally dedicated to a sport to be fit; you just have to be physically active in a gentle, regular way.

HIGH RESISTANCE TO INFECTION
This is highly indicative of genuine health. Your resistance to bacteria, viruses and other microorganisms is not something which shows up in a medical examination, yet it is as good an indicator of health status as heart rate and blood pressure. In fact, bacteria and other microbes do not cause diseases. If they did, we would be sick all the time, as they are present everywhere. They carry disease but only invade the bodies of people whose resistance happens to be weak at a particular moment. Our immune system determines our resistance, using proteins and other nutrients to produce T-cell lymphocytes, antibodies and interferon to identify, engulf and destroy hostile microbes. Nutrition, immunity and infection are inextricably related. Nutritional deficiencies increase

our vulnerability to infections, while infections aggravate nutritional deficiencies.[6] That is why nutrient requirements are higher when we are ill. Proteins are of prime importance in boosting resistance to disease. People who are prone to infections are usually found to have protein deficiency or a faulty protein metabolism.[7] Infections of the mucous membranes are related to deficiencies of vitamins A, C, B12 and protein.[8] Other infections are related to deficiencies of vitamin B6 and pantothenic acid.[9]

In spite of medical progress, doctors still cannot prevent infections. They can only treat them after they occur, using powerful antibiotics, but even these have no effect against viruses.

By strengthening our immune system through improved nutrition, we can prove the truth of the old adage: 'An ounce of prevention is better than a pound of cure.'

LOOKING ALIVE

Health and beauty go hand in hand. Of course people with robust health are not necessarily handsome or good looking, but they have a glowing vitality which radiates from within. Whatever looks you have, they will be enhanced by a wholesome, well-supplemented diet. A shapely figure depends on a natural, wholesome diet, free of empty-calorie foods, coupled with regular exercise. The condition of your skin, hair and eyes, all vital ingredients of overall beauty, reflect the quality of your nutrition. Vitamins A, C, E, the B complex, minerals, trace elements and protein, all take part in promoting your natural good looks.

SEXUAL VITALITY

The ability to enjoy sex is another index of health. As we saw in Chapter 19, low sex drive is prevalent even in younger people due to poor nutrition. Many people in the prime of life excuse their lack of sex drive by saying they are tired or busy. Proper nutrition will not necessarily turn you into a sexual athlete, but it will help you to stay sexy or interested in sex to a ripe old age.

Isolated ethnic groups like the Abkhasians in Russia, many of whom live to 100, are known to be sexually active to a very old age. The Hunzas often become parents at advanced ages, as do the Vilcabamba of Ecuador. This is achieved with no other aphrodisiac than a simple, natural unprocessed diet, rich in vitamin E, zinc, and other 'sexual' nutrients. They prepare fresh food for every meal and they eat much less than the average person in the West. They also keep physically active. In other words, they live sensibly and their fantastic health and longevity are the direct results.

A POSITIVE ATTITUDE TO HEALTH

Healthy people like being healthy and take steps to keep themselves healthy. They do not see themselves as being at the mercy of microbes, stress or the whims of others. They are very much in control of their lives, and know when to work and when to play. Often their bid for health has grown out of illness – that is the great virtue of illness, that it makes us rethink our lives – and the intensity of the challenge often determines the rate at which they develop their talent for health. There is always room for improvement. Let us break our personal health records.

REFERENCES

PREFACE

1 Turnau, A. An interview on Israeli television, April 25, 1978
2 *National Enquirer*, August 7, 1984
3 Weir, C.E. "Benefits from Human Nutrition Research," Washington D.C., 1971, U.S. Department of Agriculture, Science and Education Staff.
4 An address to Israeli Health Ministry officials, as reported in *Yediot Aharonot*, June 2, 1982
5 "Ban on Saccharin for Food Additive Use is Seen as Possibility," *Chem. Eng. News*, 50(6):5
6 A survey conducted for the Wheat Industry Council, reported in *National Enquirer*, December 20, 1983

CHAPTER 1

1 Fredericks, C. *Psycho-Nutrition*, New York: Grosset & Dunlap, 1976, p. 167
2 Pfeiffer, C. *Mental and Elemental Nutrients*, New Canaan, Conn.: Keats, 1976, p.42
3 Schroeder, H. *Trace Elements and Man*, Old Greenwich, Conn.: Devin-Adair, 1973, p.83
4 Schauss, G.A. An Address to the South West Health Organization, Fort Worth, Texas, February 1983. Recorded on tape by Audio Recording Services, Las Vegas Nevada
5 Catt, J. "Growth Hormone," *Lancet*, 1970, 1:933-939. Also Maeda F. et al. "Suppression by Thyrotropin-Released Hormone (TRH) of Growth Hormone Release Induced by Arginine and Insulin-Induced Hypoglycemia in Man." *J. Clin. Endocrinol. Metab.*, 1976, 43(2):453-456
6 Yudkin, J. *Sweet and Dangerous*, New York: Bantam, 1972, p. 40
7 Schroeder, H. *The Poisons Around Us*, New Canaan, Conn.: Keats, 1974, p. 124
8 Davis, A. *Let's Eat Right to Keep Fit*, New York: Harcourt Brace Jovanovich, 1970,.p. 63
9 Fredericks, C. *Nutrition Handbook*, Canoga Park, CA: Major Books, 1977, p. 20
10 Herbst, A.L. et al. "Clear-Cell Adenocarcinoma of Vagina and Cervix in Girls: Analysis of 170 Registry Cases," *Amer. J. Obstet. Gynecol.*, 1974, 119:713-724
11 Null, G. *The New Vegetarian*, New York: William Morrow, 1978, p. 117
12 Ibid. p. 72
13 Fredericks, C. *Psycho-Nutrition*, op. cit., p. 21
14 Williams, R. *Nutrition Against Disease*, Huntington Beach, CA: Int'l Ins. Nat. Health Sci., 1976, p. 5
15 Spies, T.D. "Some Recent Advances in Nutrition," *J. Amer. Med. Assn.*, 1958, 167(6):675-690
16 Williams, R. op. cit., p. 11
17 Mindell, E. *Vitamin Bible*, New York: Rawson Wade, 1979, p. 219

18 Brodie, D.A., Tate, C.L. and Hooke, K.F. "Aspirin: Intestinal Damage in Rats," *Science*, 1970, 170: 183-185

19 Fredericks, C. *Psycho-Nutrition*, op. cit., p. 70

20 Pearson, D. and Shaw, S. *Life Extension*, New York: Warner, 1982, p. 134

21 Ibid.

22 Rodale, R. (ed.) *Prevention*, February 1975, p. 9

23 Silva, J. (ed.) *Modern Med.*, 1979, 47(21):37

24 Salaman, M. "Dr. William Crook on Yeast Infections," *Let's Live*, September, 1984, p. 78

CHAPTER 2

1 Kugler, H.J. *Slowing Down the Aging Process*, New York: Jove, 1973, pp. 71, 148, 173

2 Pearson, D. and Shaw, S. *Life Extension*, New York: Warner, 1982, p. 332

3 Donsbach, K. *Positive Nutrition in Action*, Huntington Beach, CA: Int'l. Ins. Nat. Health Sci., 1978, p. 4

4 Holvey, N.D. (ed.) *The Merck Manual of Diagnosis and Therapy*, Rahway, N.J. Merck, Sharp & Dohme Laboratories, 1972

5 Wohl, M.G. et al. *Modern Nutrition in Health and Disease*, Philadelphia, PA: Lea and Febiger, 1955

6 Hauser, G. *New Treasury of Secrets*. Greenwich, Conn.: Fawcett, 1974, p. 24

7 Wooster, Jr. H.A. and Blanck, F.C. *Nutritional Data*, Pittsburgh, Pa: Heinz Nutritional Research Division, Melon Institute, 1949, p. 55

8 Cannon, R.P. *Recent Advances in Nutrition*, University of Kansas Press, 1950, p. 33

9 Griffith, R.S. et al. "A Multi-centered Study of Lysine Therapy in Herpes Simplex Infection," *Dermatologica*, 1978, 156:257-267

10 Chouinard, G. et al. "Tryptophan Critical for its Anti-depressant Effect." *Brit. Med. J.*, 1978, I: 1422.

11 Medsger, T.A., Jr. "Tryptophan-induced Eosinophilia-myalgia Syndrome," *New Engl. J. Med.*, 1990, 322: 926-7.

12 Ehrenpreis, S. et al. "Further Studies on the Analgesic Activity of D-phenylalalnine (DPA) in Mice and Humans," *Endogenous and Exogenous Opiate Agonists and Antagonists*, Way, E. (ed). New York: Pergamon Press, 1978, pp. 379-382. Also Balagot, R. et al. "Analgesia in Mice and Humans by D-phenylalanine: Relation to Inhibition of Enkephalin Degradation and Enkephalin Levels," *Advances in Pain Research and Therapy*, Bonica, J.J. et al. (eds). New York: Raven Press, 5:289-299

13 Fox, A. *DLPA*. New York: Simon & Schuster, 1985

14 Williams, R. *Nutrition Against Disease*, Huntington Beach, CA: Int'l Inst. Nat. Health Sci., 1976, p. 158

15 Merimee, J. et al. "Arginine-initiated Release of Human Growth Hormones," *New Engl. J. Med.*, 1969, 280(26): 1434-1438

16 Barbul et al. "Arginine: A Thymotropic and Wound-Healing Promoting Agent," *Surgical Forum*, 1977, 28:101-103

17 Pearson, D. and Shaw, S. *The Life Extension Weight Loss Program*, New York: Doubleday & Co., 1986, pp. 29-34

18 Pfeiffer, C. *Mental and Elemental Nutrients*, New Canaan, Conn.: Keats, 1976, p. 448

19 Erdmann, R. and Jones, E. *The Amino Revolution*, London: Century Hutchinson, 1987, pp. 41-42

20 Campbell, G. et al. "Effect of Cysteine on the Survival of Mice with Transplanted Malignant Thymoma," *Nature*, 1974, 251:158-159

21 Ryzewski, J. et al. "Studies on the Influence of Cysteine Derivatives on the Cell-mediated Immunity," *Arch. Immunol. Ther. Exp.* (Warsaw), 1981, 29(6): 801-804

22 Pearson, D. and Shaw, S. op. cit., p. 482

23 Ibid. p. 372

24 Erdmann, R. and Jones, E. op. cit., p. 111

25 Maebashi, M. et al. "Lipid Lowering Effect of Carnitine in Patients with Type-IV Hyperlipoproteinaemia," *Lancet II*, 1978, 805

26 Thomsen, J.H. et al. "Improved Stress Tolerance of the Ischemic Human Myocardium after Carnitine Administration, *Amer. J. Cardiol.* 1977, 39:289

27 McCarty, M.F. "Orthomolecular Aids for Dieting," *Med. Hypoth.*, 1982, 8:269

28 Erdmann, R. and Jones, E. op. cit., p. 86

29 Erdmann, R. and Jones E. op. cit., pp. 30,43

30 Whitaker, J. "When You Need to Get a Grip, Think GABA," *Health & Healing*, March 1994, vol. 4, No. 3

31 "Vascular Research Laboratory," A.M.A. News Release, June 21, 1956

32 Visek, W. "Report on Cornell University Research," *Los Angeles Times*, March 29, 1973, p. 12

33 Gerber, A.D. *New York Times*, April 7, 1965, p. 6

34 Donsbach, K. op. cit., p. 7

35 Williams, R.J. "We Abnormal Normals," *Nutrition Today*, 1967, 2:19-23

36 *Protein Requirement*, report of a Joint FAO/WHO Expert Group, Food and Agriculture Organization, Rome, 1965, p. 32

37 Martin, W.M. Mayes, P.A. and Rodwell, V.W. *Harper's Review of Biochemistry*, Los Altos, CA: Lange, 1981, p. 181

38 Pfeiffer, C. op. cit., p. 96

39 Martin, Mayes and Rodwell. op. cit., p. 183

40 Colimore, B. and Colimore, S.S. *Nutrition and Your Body*, Los Angeles, CA: Light Wave, 1974, p. 53

41 Pfeiffer, C. op. cit., p. 387

42 Pearson, D. and Shaw, S. op. cit., p. 315

43 Davis, A. *Let's Eat Right to Keep Fit*, New York: Harcourt Brace Jovanovich, 1970, p. 22

44 Airola, P. *Hypoglycemia - A Better Approach*, Phoenix, AZ: Health Plus, 1977, p. 80

45 Yudkin, J. *Sweet and Dangerous*, New York: Bantam, 1972, p. 5

46 Ishmael, W.K. "Atherosclerotic Vascular Diseases in Familial Gout, Diabetes and Obesity," *Med. Times*, 1966, 94(2):157-162.

47 Heaton, K.W. "Food Fibre as an Obstacle to Energy Intake; *Lancet*, 1973, II:1418

48 Barboriak, J.J. et al. "Influence of High-Fat Diets on Growth and Development of Obesity in the Albino Rat", *J. Nutr.*, 1958, 64: 241

49 "Nutrient Intake and its Association with HDL and LDL Cholesterol in Selected US and USSR Subpopulations. The US-USSR Steering Committee for Problem Area I: The Pathogenesis of Atherosclerosis," *Amer. J. Clin. Nutr.*, 1984, 39(6):942-952

50 Lieber, C.S. and Rubin, E. "Alcoholic Fatty Liver," *New Engl. J. Med.*, 1969, 280:705

51 Moskow, H.A. et al. "Alcohol, Sludge, and Hypoxic Areas of Nervous System, Liver and Heart" *Microvascular Research*, 1968, 1:174

52 "Psychiatric Aspects of Alcoholism," *Amer. J. Psychother.*, 1965, 19(3):408-416

53 Schuckit, E. and Rayses, A. "Ethanol Ingestion: Differences in Blood Acetaldehyde Concentrations in Relatives of Alcoholics and Controls," *Science*, 1979, 203(5):54-55

54 Sprince, H. et al. "Protectants Against Acetaldehyde Toxicity: Sulfhydryl Compounds and Ascorbic Acid," *Fed. Proc.*, 1974, 33(3):1

55 Rogers, L.L. Pelton, R.B. and Williams R.J. "Voluntary Alcohol Consumption by Rats Following Administration of Glutamine," *J. Biol. Chem.*, 1955, 214:503

56 Mendelson, J.H. et al. "Effects of Alcohol Ingestion and Withdrawal on Magnesium States of Alcoholics: Clinical and Experimental Findings," *Ann. New York Acad. Sci.*, 1969, 162:918

57 Fredericks, C. *Nutrition Handbook*, Canoga Park, CA: Major Books, 1977, p. 128

58 Donsbach, K. op. cit. (Fats) p. 1

59 Ibid. p. 3

60 Ibid.

61 Johnston, I.M. and Johnston, J.R. "Flaxseed Oil and the Power of Omega-3," 1990, Keats Publishing, New Canada, Conn., p. 19

62 Dyerberg, J. et al. "Fatty Acid Composition of Plasma Lipids in Greenland Eskimos," *Amer. J. Clin. Nutr.*, 1975, 958-66

63 Colimore B. and Colimore, S.S. op. cit., p. 147

64 Szabo, S. and Rogers, C. "Diet, Ulcer Disease, and Fish Oil," *Lancet*, 1988, 8577 (1):119

65 Mukai, E. and Goldstein, B.D. "Mutagenicity of Malonaldehyde, a Decomposition Product of Peroxidised Polyunsaturated Fatty Acids," *Science*, 1976, 191:868-869

66 Pfeiffer, C. op. cit., p. 193

67 Colimore, B. and Colimore S.S. op. cit., p. 51

68 Davis, A. op. cit., p. 45

69 Pearson, D. "Mechanisms of Aging and Life Extension," an address to the Northern California Food Association, 8th Annual Show, Reno, Nevada. Recorded on tape by Audio Recording Services, Las Vegas, Nevada

70 Horwitt, M.K. et al. "Polyunsaturated Lipids and Tocopherol Requirements," *J. Amer. Diet. Assn.*, 1961, 38:231-235

71 Fredericks, C. op. cit., p. 99

72 Colimore, B. and Colimore, S.S. op. cit., p. 86

73 Martin, Mayes and Rodwell op. cit., p. 237

74 Ibid.

75 Colimore, B. and Colimore, S.S. op. cit., p. 88

76 Ibid. p. 89

77 Ibid.

78 Fredericks, C. op. cit., p. 99

79 Ginter, E. "Cholesterol: Vitamin C Controls its Transformation to Bile Acids," *Science*, 1973, 179:702

80 Martin, Mayes and Rodwell. op. cit., p. 252

81 Thomas, L. "Mortality from Arteriosclerotic Disease and Consumption of Hydrogenated Oils and Fats," *Brit. J. Prev. Soc. Med.*, 1975, 29:82-90

82 Olsson, A.G. and Eklund, B. "Studies in Asymptomatic Primary Hyperlipidemia, Vascular Peripheral

Circulation," *Acta Med. Scand.*, 1975, 198(3):197-206

83 Kavanash, T. et al. "Influence of Exercise and Life-Style Variable Upon High Density Lipoprotein Cholesterol After Myocardial Infarction," *Arteriosclerosis*, 1983, 3(3):249-259

84 Martin, Mayes and Rodwell. op. cit., p. 242

85 "Nutrient Intake and its Association with HDL and LDL Cholesterol in Selected US and USSR Subpopulations. The US-USSR Steering Committee for Problem Area I: The Pathogenesis of Atherosclerosis," *Amer. J. Clin. Nutr.*, 1984, 39(6):942-952

86 Carew, T.E. et al. "A Mechanism by which High-Density Lipoproteins May Slow the Atherosenic Process," *Lancet*, 1976 1:1315-1317

87 Ibid.

88 Rossner, S. et al. "Normal Serum-Cholesterol but Low HDL-Cholesterol Concentrations in Young Patients with Ischaemic Cerebrovascular Disease," *Lancet*, 1978, 1: 577-579

89 Ter Welle, H.F. et al. "The Effect of Soya Lecithin on Serum Lipid Values in Type II Hyperlipoproteinemia," *Acta Med. Scand.*, 1974, 195:267

90 Dyerberg, J. et al. "Eicosapentaenoic Acid and Prevention of Thrombosis and Atherosclerosis," *Lancet*, 1978, II:117

91 Niazi, S.K. "The Omega Connection - Facts about Fish Oils and Human Health", Esquire Books, 1987, pp. 19-23

92 Hay, C.R.M. et al. "Effect of Fish Oil on Platelet Kinetics in Patients with Ischaemic Heart Disease," *Lancet*, 1982, I:1269

93 Bordia, A. "Effects of Essential Oil of Onion and Garlic on Experimental Atherosclerosis in Rabbits," *Atherosclerosis*, 1977, 26(3):379-386

94 Donsbach, K. op. cit., (Fats) p. 7

CHAPTER 3

1 Williams, R. *Nutrition Against Disease*, Huntington Beach, CA: Int'l. Ins. Nat. Health Sci., 1976, p. 40

2 William, R.J. "We Abnormal Normals," *Nutrition Today*, 1967, 2:19-23

3 Schroeder, H. *The Poisons Around Us*, New Canaan, Conn.: Keats, 1974, p. 27

4 Orton, J.H. and Neuhaus, O.W. *Biochemistry*, St. Louis, Mo.: C.V. Mosby, 1970, p. 768

5 Ibid.

6 Giovannucci, E. et al. *Journal of the National Cancer Institute*, 1995, 87:176-177

7 Murakoshi, M. et al. *Journal of the National Cancer Institute*, 1989, 81:1649-52

8 Dr Joanne Curran-Celentano, oral presentation at Henkel Symposium, Pine Mountain, Georgia, June 1996

9 Fredericks, C. *Nutrition Handbook*, Canoga Park, CA: Major Books, 1977, p. 173

10 Modan, B. et al. "Retinol, Carotene, and Cancer," *Int'l. J. Cancer*, 1981, 28:421-424. Also Bjelke, R. "Dietary Vitamin A and Human Lung Cancer," *Int'l J. Cancer*, 1975, 15:561-565

11 Griffin, A.C. "Role of Selenium in the Chemoprevention of Cancer," *Adv. Cancer Res.*, 1979, 29:424

12 Shekelle, J. et al. "Dietary Vitamin A and Risk of Cancer in the

Western Electric Study," *Lancet*, 1981, 2:1185-1190

13 Colimore, B. and Colimore, S.S. *Nutrition and Your Body*, Los Angeles, CA: Light Wave, 1974, p. 142

14 Fredericks, C. op. cit., p. 181

15 Colimore, B. and Colimore, S.S. op. cit., p.66

16 Martin, D.W. Mayes, P.A. and Rodwell, V.W. *Harper's Review of Biochemistry*, Los Altos, CA: Lange, 1981, p. 165

17 Fredericks, C. op. cit., p. 184

18 "Treatment of Hypercholesterolemia with Nicotinic Acid," *Nutrition Reviews*, 1961, 19:325-328

19 Pfeiffer, C. *Mental and Elemental Nutrients* New Canaan, Conn.: Keats, 1976, p. 120

20 Ibid. p. 121

21 Ibid. p. 174

22 Fredericks, C. op. cit., p. 87

23 Hurley, L.S. and Morgan, F.A. "Carbohydrate Metabolism and Adrenal Cortical Function in the Pantothenic Acid-Deficient Rat," *J. Biol. Chem.*, 1952, 195(2): 583-589

24 Pearson, D. and Shaw, S. *Life Extension*, New York: Warner, 1982, p. 187

25 Colimore, B. and Colimore, S.S. op. cit., pp. 93 & 150

26 Miller, L.T. et al. "Vitamin B6 Metabolism in Women Using Oral Contraceptives," *Amer. J. Clin. Nutr.*, 1974, 27:797-805

27 Levodope, M.H. "Carbidopa and Pyridoxine in Parkinson's Disease," *Arch. Neurol*, 1974, 30:443-447

28 Reinken, I. and Gant, H. "Vitamin B6 Nutrition in Women with Hyperemesis Gravidarum During the First Trimester of Pregnancy," *Clinica Chimica Acta*, 1974, 55:101

29 Klieger, J.A. et al. "Abnormal Pyridoxine Metabolism in Toxemia of Pregnancy," *Ann. New York Acad. Sci.*, 1969, 166:288-296

30 Rosenberg, S.J. and Bennett, J.M. "Pyridoxine Responsive Anemia," *New York State J. Med.*, 1969, 91:1430-1433

31 Appleyard, J.G. and Stanley, D.A. "The Evaluation of the Vitamin B6 Status in Children with Convulsions," *Med. Lab. Tech.*, 1972, 29:160-170

32 Pfeiffer, R. and Ebadi, M. "On Mechanisms of Nullification of CNS Effects of L-Dopa by Pyridoxine in Parkinsonian Patients," *J. Neurochem*. 1972, 19:2175-2181. Also Schlesinger, K. and Schreiber R.A. "Interaction of Drugs and Pyridoxine Deficiency on Central Nervous System Excitability," *Ann. New York Acad. Sci.*, 1969, 166:281-287

33 Pfeiffer, C. op. cit., p. 150

34 Ibid. p. 161

35 Ibid.

36 Hanson, Wm. "B12: Basic Action and Associated Physiology," *The Physician's Diet Reference*, CA: Van Nuys, 1961

37 Abramsky, O. "Common and Uncommon Neurological Manifestations as Presenting Symptoms of Vitamin B12 Deficiency," *J. Amer. Geriat. Soc.*, 1972, 20(2):93-96

38 "Laetrile - an Answer to Cancer?" *Prevention*, December 1971, p. 162

39 Kirschmann, J. *Nutrition almanac*, New York: Nutrition Search - McGraw Hill, 1975, p. 35

40 Krebs, E.T. "The Nitrilosides (Vitamin B17)," *Cancer News J.* 1971, 6:1-4

41 Davis, A. *Let's Get well*, New York: Harcourt Brace Jovanovich, 1965, p. 154

42 Chnarin, I. et al. "The Biochemical Lesion in Vitamin B12 Deficiency in Man," *Lancet*, 1974, I:1251-1252

43 Daniel, W.A. et al. "Dietary Intakes and Plasma Concentrations of folate in Healthy Adolescents," *Amer. J. Clin. Nutr.*, 1975, 28: 363-370

44 Pfeiffer, C. op. cit., p. 163

45 Reynolds, E. et al. "Folate Metabolism in Epileptic and Psychiatric patients," *J. Neurol. Neurosurg. Psychiat.*, 1971, 34:726

46 Salmon, W.D. and Copeland, D.H. "Liver Carcinoma and Related Lesions in Chronic Choline Deficiency," *Ann. New York Acad. Sci.*, 1954, 57:664-676

47 Sitaram, L. et al. "Human Serial Learning: Enhancement with Arecholine and Choline and Impairment with Scopolamine Correlate with Performance on Placebo," *Science*, 1978, 201:274-296

48 Jungalwala, F.B. "The Metabolism of Phosphatidylinositol in the Rat Brain," *Int. J. Biochem.*, 1973, 4:145-151

49 Orton, J.H. and Neuhaus, O.W. op. cit., p. 304

50 Hodges, E.R. "Ascorbic Acid," *Present Knowledge in Nutrition*, Washington, D.C.: Nutrition Foundation, 1976, p. 123

51 Ibid.

52 Shute, W. "An Update on Vitamin E," an address to the 1979 annual convention of the national Nutritional Foods Association (NNFA), Las Vegas, Nevada. Recorded on tape by Audio Recording Services, Las Vegas, Nevada.

53 Pauling, L. *Vitamin C and the Common Cold*, New York: Bantam, 1970

54 Goetzl, J. et al. "Enhancement of Random Migration and Chemotactic Response of Human Leukocytes by Ascorbic Acid," *J. Clin. Invest.*, 1974, 5:813-818

55 Blode, G. "Vitamin C and Cancer: Epidemiologic Evidence of Reduced Risk" *Ann. New York Acad Sci.*, 1992, 669:280-92

56 Howe, G.R. et al. "Dietary Factors and Risk of Breast Cancer: Combined Analysis of 12 Case Control Studies," *J. Nat'l. Cancer Inst.*, 1990, 82:561-9

57 Cameron, E. and Pauling, L. "Supplemental Ascorbate in the Supportive Treatment of Cancer: Prolongation of Survival Times in Terminal Human Cancer," *Proc. Nat. Acad. Sci.*, 1976, 73(10): 3685-3689

58 Spittle, C. "The Action of Vitamin C on Blood Vessels," *Amer. Heart J.*, 1974, 88(3):387-388

59 Thoa, N.B. et al. "A Deficient Binding Mechanism for Norepinephrine in Hearts of Scorbutic Guinea Pigs," *Proc. Soc. Exp. Biol. Med.*, 1966, 121: 267-270

60 Ginter, E. "Cholesterol: Vitamin C Controls Its Transformation to Bile Acids," *Science*, 1973, 179:702-704

61 Spittle, C. "Atherosclerosis and Vitamin C," *Lancet*, 1971, 2: 1280-1281

62 Sprince, H. et al. "L-ascorbic Acid in Alcoholism and Smoking: Protection against Acetaldehyde Toxicity as an Experimental Model," *Int. J. Vit. Nutr. Res.*, 1977, 47 (suppl. 1G):185-212

63 Harrison, H.E. "Phosphorus," *Present Knowledge in Nutrition*, Washington, D.C.: Nutrition Foundation, 1976, p. 244

64 Shute, W. op. cit.

65 Pearson, D. "Mechanism of Aging and Life Extension," an address to the 8th annual convention of the Northern California Food Association, September 1982, Reno,

Nevada. Recorded on tape by Audio Recording Services, Las Vegas, Nevada

66 Shute, W. op. cit.

67 Fredericks, C. op. cit.

68 Stampfer, M.J. et al. "Vitamin E Consumption and the Risk of Coronary Disease in Women," *New Engl. J. Med.*, 1993, 328:1444-9 Rimm, E.B. et al. "Vitamin E Consumption and the Risk of Coronary Heart Disease in Men," *New Engl. J. Med.*, 1993, 328:1450-56

69 Knekt, P. et al. "Serum Vitamin E and Risk of Cancer Among Finnish Men During a 20-year Follow-up"; *Amer. J. Epid.*, 1988, 127:28-41 Gridley, F. et al. "Vitamin Supplement Use and Reduced Risk of Oral and Pharyngeal Cancer", *Amer. J. Epid.*, 1992, 135:1083-92

70 Shute, W. op. cit.

71 Shamberger, R. et al. "Carcinogen-induced Chromosomal Breakage Decreased by Antioxidants," *Proc. Nat. Acad. Sci.*, 1973, 1:1461-1463

72 Pelletier and Keith. "Bioavailability of Synthetic and Natural Ascorbic Acid," *J. Amer. Diet. Assn.*, 1974, 64:271-275

73 Afanasev, I.G, Dorozhko, A.I. et al. "Chelating and Free Radical Scavenging Mechanisms of Inhibitory Action of Rurin and Quercetin in Lipid Peroxidation," *Biochemical Pharmacology*, 1989, vol. 38, no. 11 pp. 1763-1769

74 Della Loggia, R., et al. "Anti-inflammatory Activity of Benzopyrones that are Inhibitors of Cyclo-and Lipo-Oxygenase," *Pharmacol. Res. Commun.* 1988, 20:S91-S94

75 Timofeev, A.A. et al. "The Use of Quercetin Granules for Treating Suppurative Soft-Tissue Wounds of the maxillofacial Area and Neck," *Stomatologiia* (USSR), 1989, 68:11-13

76 Kaul, T.N. Middleton, E. Jr, and Ogra, P.L. "Antiviral Effect of Flavonoids on Human Viruses," *J. Med. Virology*, 1985, 15:71-79

77 Scambia, G. et al. "Quercetin Inhibits the Growth of a Multidrug-Resistant Estrogen-Receptor-Negative MCF-7 Human Breast-Cancer Cell Line Expressing Type II Estrogen-Binding Sites," *Cancer Chemother. Pharmacol.* (Germany), 1991, 28:255-258

78 Scambia, G. et al. "Synergistic Antiproliferative Activity of Quercetin and Cisplatin on Ovarian Cancer Cell Growth," *Anticancer Drugs* (England), 1990, 1:45-48

79 Larocca, L.M. et al. "Antiproliferative Activity of Quercetin on Normal Bone Marrow and Leukaemic Progenitors," *Brit. J. Haematol.*, 1991, 79:562-566

80 Middleton, E., et al. "Quercetin: An Inhibitor of Antigen-Induced Human Basophil Histamine Release," *J. Immunol.*, Aug. 1981, vol. 127, 2:546-560

81 Varma, S.D. et al. "Diabetic Cataracts and Flavonoids," *Science*, 1977, 195:87-89

82 Hill C.S.T. and Howell, S.L. "Effects of Flavonoids on Insulin Secretion and Calcium Handling in Rat Islets of Langerhans," *J. Endocrinol.*, 1985, 107:1-8

83 Williams, R. op. cit., p. 41

CHAPTER 4

1 Beattie, A.D. et al. "Role of Chronic Low-level Exposure in the Etiology of Mental Retardation," *Lancet*, 1975, 1:589

2 Schroeder, H.A. *The Trace Elements and Man*, Old Greenwich, Conn.: Devin-Adair, 1978, p. 116

3 Schroeder, H.A. *The Poisons Around Us*, New Canaan, Conn.: Keats, 1974, p. 130

4 Lal, S. et al. "Effect of Copper Loading on Various Tissue Enzymes and Brain Monoamines in the Rat," *Toxicol. Appl. Pharmacol.*, 1974, 28:394-405

5 Pfeiffer, C. and Iliev, V. "A Study of Zinc Deficiency and Copper Excess in the Schizophrenias," *Intern. Rev. Neurobiol. Supp.*, 1972, 1:141-165

6 Schroeder, H.A. *The Poisons Around Us*, op. cit., p. 96

7 Crapper, D.R. et al. "Brain Aluminum Distribution Alzheimer's Disease and Experimental Neurofibrillary Degeneration," *Science*, 1973, 180:511-513

8 Passwater, A.R. *Selenium as Food and Medicine*, New Canaan, Conn.: Keats, 1980, pp. 3-9

9 Mertz, W. "Chromium Occurrence and Function in Biological Systems," *Phys. Rev.*, 1969, 49:163

10 Raylor, R. *Hunza Health Secrets*, Englewood Cliffs, N.J.: Prentice-Hall, 1964. Also McCarrison, R. *Studies in Deficiency Diseases*, Milwaukee, Wis.: Lee Foundation for Nutritional Research, 1945

11 Tolmasoff, L. et al. "Superoxide Dismutase: Correlation with Life-Span and Specific Metabolic Rate in Primate Species," *Proc. Nat. Acad. Sci.*, 1980, 77(5):2777-2781

12 Ellis, W. "Protect your Family against Radiation," *Health Express*, April 1982, p. 12

13 Green, G.M. "Cigarette Smoke: Protection of Alveolar Macrophages by Glutathione and Cysteine," *Science*, 1968, 162:810-811

14 Griffin, A.C. "Role of Selenium in the Chemoprevention of Cancer," *Advan. Cancer Res.*, 1979, 29:424

15 Miller, P.D. and John J. "Chelation: A New Approach to the Practice of Medicine," *J. Appl. Nutr.*, 15(3&4):193

16 Koltz, C. "Calcium Deficiency," *Let's Live*, November 1982, p. 85

17 Flach, F.F. "Calcium Metabolism in States of Depression," *Brit. J. Psychiat.*, 1964, 110:588-593

18 Smith, L. *Feed Your Kids Right*, New York: Dell, 1980, p. 211

19 Rusoff, L.L. "The Role of Milk in Modern Nutrition," *Borden's Review of Nutrition Research*, 1964, 25(2-3):37

20 Kosman, M.E. "Management of Potassium Problems During Long-Term Diuretic Therapy," *J. Amer. Med. Assn.*, 1974, 230:5

21 Wade, C. *Magic Minerals*, New York: Arco, 1976, p. 22

22 Rodale, J.I. *Sex and a Healthy Prostate*, Herts, England: Rodale Press, 1968, pp. 53-66

23 Fredericks, C. *Nutrition Handbook*, Canoga Park, CA: Major Books, 1977, p. 102

24 Barbeau, A. and Donaldson, J. "Zinc, Taurine and Epilepsy," *Arch. Neurol.*, 1974, 30:52

25 Muirden, K.D. "The Anemia of Rheumatoid Arthritis: The Significance of Iron Deposits in the Synovial Membranes," *Aust. Ann. Med.*, 1970, 2:97-104

26 Prout, G.R. Sierp, M. and Whitmore, W.F. "Radioactive Zinc in the Prostate," *J. Amer. Med. Assn.*, 1959, 169(15):1703-1710

27 Hoare, R., Delory, G.E. and Penner, D.W. "Zinc and Acid Phosphatase in the Human Prostate," *Cancer*, 1956, 9:721-726

28 Statistical Bulletin of the Metropolitan Life Insurance Co., December 1964

29 Sullivan, J.F. and Lankford, H.G. "Urinary Excretion of Zinc in Alcoholism and Postalcoholic Cirrhosis," *Amer. J. Clin. Nutr.*, 10:153-157

30 Pfeiffer, C. and Iliev, V. op. cit.

31 Pories, W.J. et al. "Acceleration of Wound Healing with Zinc Sulfate," *Ann. Surg.*, 1967, 165:432

32 Kozloff, L.M. and Lute, M. "The Role of Zinc in Bacteriophage Invasion," *J. Biol. Chem.*, 1957, 228:529-535

33 Vorhees, J.G. et al. "Zinc Therapy and Distribution in Psoriasis," *Arch. Derm.*, 1969, 100:669-673

34 Caldwell, D.F. et al. "Behavioral Impairment in Adult Rats Following Acute Zinc Deficiency," *Proc. Soc. Exp. Biol. Med.*, 1970, 133:1417

35 Hussey, H.H. "Taste and Smell Deviations: Importance of Zinc," *J. Amer. Med. Assn.*, 1974, 228:1669-1670

36 Schroeder, H.A. *The Trace Elements and Man*, op. cit., p. 64

37 Pfeiffer, C. *Mental and Elemental Nutrients*, New Canaan, Conn.: Keats, 1976, pp. 326-336

38 Pfeiffer, C. and Iliev, V. op. cit.

39 Everson, G.J. and Shrader, R.E. "Abnormal Glucose Tolerance in Manganese-Deficient Guinea Pigs," *J.Nutr.*, 1968, 94:89

40 Hurley, L.S. "Disproportionate Growth in Offspring of Manganese-Deficient Rats," *J. Nutr.*, 1961, 74:274

41 Schroeder, H.A. *The Trace Elements and Man*, op. cit., p. 60

42 Ibid. p. 80

43 Ibid. p. 152

44 Evans, G.W. "The Picolinates," *Keats Publishing*, New Canaan, Conneticut, 1989, p. 1.

45 Evans, G. "The Effect of Chromium Picolinate on Insulin Controlled Parameters in Humans," *Int. J. Biosoc. Med. Res.*, 1989, 11:163-180

46 Kaats, G.R. et al. "The Effects of Chromium Picolinate Supplementation on Body Composition in Different Age Groups," *Amer. Aging Assoc.*, 21st Ann. Mtg. Denver, Oct 12, 1991. Page, T.C. et al. "Effects of Chromium Picolinate on Growth and Carcass Characteristics of Growing-Finishing Pigs," *Animal Sci.*, Suppl. 1, 1991, 69:356

47 Bogardus, C. et al. "Familial Dependence of the Resting Metabolic Rate," *New Engl. J. Med.*, 1986, 315:96-100

48 Blundell, J.E. "Serotonin and Appetite," *Neuropharmacology*, 1984, 23:1537-1551

49 Ibid. p. 77

50 Ibid. p. 64

51 Greer, M.A. and Astwood, E.B. "The Antithyroid Effect of Certain Foods in Man as Determined with Radioactive Iodine," *Endocrinology*, 1948, 43:105-119

52 Rotruck, J.T. et al. "Selenium: Biochemical Role as a Component of Glutathione Peroxidase," *Science*, 1973, 179:588-590

53 Levander, O.A. et al. "Comparative Effects of Selenium and Vitamin E in Lead-poisoned Rats," *J. Nutr.*, 1977, 107(3):378-382

54 Rastogi, S.C. et al. "Selenium and Lead: Mutual Detoxifying Effects," *Toxicology*, 1976, 6:377

55 Ganther, H.E. et al. "Selenium: Relation of Decreased Toxicity of Methylmercury Added to Diets

Containing Tuna," *Science*, 1972, 175:1122

56 Ibid.

57 Shamberger, R.J. "Relationship of Selenium to Cancer: Inhibitory Effect of Selenium on Carcinogenesis," *J. Nat. Cancer Inst.*, 1970, 44(4):931-936

58 Crary, E. 2nd International Symposium on Selenium in Biology and Medicine, Texas Tech University, Lubbock, Texas, May 1980

59 Wallach, J. and Garmaise, B. Proceedings of the 13th Annual Conference on trace Substances in Environmental Health, University of Missouri, June 1978, pp. 469-476

60 Shamberger, R.J. op. cit.

61 Passwater, A.R. op. cit., p. 9

62 Schroeder, H.A. *The Trace Elements and Man*, op. cit., p. 63

63 Ibid. p. 51

64 Guyton, A.C. *Textbook of Medical Physiology*, Philadelphia: W.B. Saunders, 1971, 4th ed., p. 935

65 Fredericks, C. op. cit., p. 229

66 Inkovaara, J. et al. "Prophylactic Fluoride Treatment and Aged Bones," *Brit. Med. J.*, 1975, 3: 73-74

67 Rodale, J.I. *Complete Book of Minerals for Health*, Herts, England: Rodale Press, 1965, pp. 367-370

68 Brody, J.E. "Dietary Factors Linked to Cancer of Digestive Tract," *New York Times*, September 29, 1972, p. 24

69 Levine, S.A. and Kidd, P.M. "Oxygen Nutrition for Super Health," *J. Orthomolecular Med.*, 1986, 1(3):145-148

70 Levine, S. and Huntington, K. "Organic Germanium: Restoring Health Through Increased Oxygenation," *Total Health*, 1986, 18

71 Ishida, N., et al. "Organo-Germanium Induction of Interferon

Production," United States Patent No. 4, 473, 581, 1984

72 Aso, H. et al. "Induction of Interferon and Activation of NK Cells and Macrophages in Mice by Oral Administration of Ge-132, an Organic Germanium Compound," *Microbiol. Immunol.*, 1985, 20: 65-74

73 Badger, A.M. et al. "Generation of Suppressor Cells in Normal Rats by Treatment with Spiro-Germanium, a Novel Heterocyclic Anticancer Drug." *Immunopharmacology*, 1985, 10:201-207

74 Mizushima, Y. et al. "Restoration of Impaired Immunoresponse by Germanium in Mice," *Int. Arch. Allergy Appl. Immunol.*, 1980, 63:338-339

75 Lekim, D/. Samochowiec, L. and Gieldanowski, J. "Results of Studies on Antineoplastic Activity of Sanumgerman Preparation," First International conference on Germanium, Hanover, October 1984, Lekim and Samochowiec (eds.), Semmelweis-Verlag, 1985

76 Kumano, N. et al. "Antitumour Effect of the Organogermanium Compound Ge-132 on the Lewis Lung Carcinoma (3LL) in C57BL/6 (B6) Mice," *Tohoku J. Exp. Med.*, 1985, 146:97-104

77 Samochowiec, L. "Experience with Sanumgerman in Poland and Germany," First International Conference on Germanium, Hanover, October 1984, Lekim and Samochowiec (eds.), Semmelweis-Verlag, 1985

78 Schein, P.S. "The Clinical Pharmacology of Spirogermanium, A Unique Anti Cancer Agent," First International Conference on Germanium, Hanover, October 1984, Lekim and Samochowiec (eds.) Semmelweis-Verlag, 1985

79 DiMartino, M.J. et al. "Antiarthritic and Immuno-regulatory Activity of Spirogermanium," *J. Pharmacol. Exp. Ther.*, 1986, 236:103

80 Badger, A.M. et al. op. cit.

81 Walker, C.M. et al. "CD8 Lymphocytes can Control HIV Infection in Vitro by Suppressing Virus Replication," *Science*, 1986, 234:1563-1566

82 Schroeder, H.A. and Balassa, J.J. "Abnormal Trace Metals in Man: Germanium," *J. Chron. Dis.*, 1967, 20:211-224

83 Asai, K. *Miracle Cure: Organic Germanium*, Tokyo, Japan: Japan Publications Inc., 1980

84 Hunt C.D. and Nielsen, F.H. "Interaction between Boron and Cholecalciferol in the Chick." In: McC Howell J. Gawthorne J.M. White C.L. editors. *Trace Element Metabolism in Man and Animals*, vol. 4, Canberra: Australian Academy of Science, 1981, 597-600

85 Nielsen, F.H. et al. "Effect of Dietary Boron on Mineral, Estrogen, and Testosterone Metabolism in Postmenopausal Women," *Fed. Amer. Soc. Exp. Biol. (FASEB)*, 1987, 1(5):394-397

86 Newnham, R.E. "Arthritis or Skeletal Fluorosis and Boron," Letter, *Int'l Clin. Nutr. Rev.*, 1991, 11(2):68-70

87 Newnham, R.E. "Boron Beats Arthritis," *Proc anzaas*, Australian Academy of Science, Canberra, Australia, 1979

88 Botsford, R.A. "Lead in Pet Food and Processed Organ Meats: A Human Problem," *J. Amer. Med. Assn.*, 1975, 231:484-485

89 Schroeder, H.A. *The Poisons Around Us*, op. cit., p. 38

90 Michaelson, A. and Sauerhoff, M. "Hyperactivity and Brain Catecholamines in Lead-Exposed Developing Rats," *Science*, 1973, 182:725-727

91 Beattie, A.D. et al. op. cit.

92 Davis, L.E. et al. "Central Nervous System Intoxication from Mercurous Chloride Laxatives," *Arch. Neurol.*, 1974, 30:428

93 Six, K.M. and Goyer, R.A. "Experimental Enhancement of Lead Toxicity by Low Dietary Calcium," *J. Lab. Clin. Med.*, 1970, 76:933-942

94 Airola, P. *How to Get Well*, Phoenix, AZ: Health Plus, 1979, p. 70

95 Schroeder, H.A. *The Poisons Around Us*, op. cit., p. 66

96 Ibid. p. 92

97 Ibid. p. 84

CHAPTER 5

1 Scott, C. *Crude Black Molasses*, Northamptonshire, England: Athene, 1974, p. 3

2 Schroeder, H. *The Poisons Around Us*, New Canaan, Conn.: Keats, 1974, p. 125

3 Scott, C. op. cit.

4 Krueger, H. "The Wulzen Calcium Dystrophy Syndrome in Guinea Pigs," *Amer. J. Phys. Med.*, 1955, 34:1. Also Clark, L. *Get Well Naturally*, New York: ARC Books, 1972, p. 175

5 Hauser, G. *New Treasury of Secrets*, Greenwich, Conn.: Fawcett, 1974, p. 183

6 Jarvis, D.C. *Folk Medicine*, Greenwich, Conn.: Fawcett, 1958, p. 67

7 Hanssen, M. *Cider Vinegar*, Northamptonshire, England: Thorsons, 1974, pp. 27-62

8 Scott, C. *Cider Vinegar*, Northamptonshire, England: Athene 1968

9 Jarvis, D.C. op. cit., pp. 47-52

10 Davis, A. *Let's Get well*, New York: Harcourt Brace Jovanovich, 1965, p. 315

11 Airola, P. "Controversial Yeast," *Let's Live*, September, 1976, p. 72

12 Rorty, J. and Phillip, N. *Tomorrow's Food*, New York: Devin-Adair, 1955, p. 162

13 Reinshagen, B. "Yeast is not the Least," *Let's Live*, August 1982, p. 92

14 Lazncka, M. "Beer Yeast in Treatment of Liver Cirrhosis," *Nutritional Abstracts and Reviews*, 1958, 29:281-282

15 Bagshaw, J.M. and Leslie, G.G. "The Effects of Three Food Supplements on Feeding and Growth Rate in the Rat," *Laboratory Animals*, 1974, 8: 189-197

16 Hauser, G. op. cit., p. 182

17 Johnson, R.E. et al. "The Effects of a Diet Deficient in Part of the Vitamin B complex Upon Men Doing Manual labor," *J. Nutr.*, 1942, 24(6):585-595

18 Davis, A. op. cit., p. 231

19 Passwater, R. *Selenium as Food and Medicine*, New Canaan, Conn.: Keats, 1980, p. 185

20 Rabinowitz, R. et al. "Neuromuscular Disorders Amenable to Wheat Germ Oil Therapy," *J. Neurol. Neurosurg, Psychiat.*, 1951, 14:95

21 Alfin-Slater, R.B. "Factors Affecting EFA Utilization," a paper presented at the Symposium on Drugs Affecting Lipid Metabolism, Amsterdam, Holland: Elsevier, 1960, p. 111

22 Cureton, T.K. *The Physiological Effects of Wheat Germ Oil on Humans in Exercise*, Springfield, Ill.: Charles C. Thomas, 1972

23 Bruno, B. "Wheat Germ Oil Boosts Performance," *Prevention*, July 1974, p. 33

24 Marion, G.B. *J. Dairy Sci.*, 1962, 45:904

25 *Proc. Soc. Exp. Biol. Med.*, 1963, 112:331

26 Silbernagel, W.M. "The Role of Wheat Germ Oil Concentrate in Postpartum Care," *J. Int'l College of Surgeons*, 1961, 35:335

27 Fredericks, C. *Nutrition Handbook*, Canoga Park, CA: Major Books, 1977, p. 117

28 Pearson, D. "Mechanisms of Aging and Life Extension," an address to the Northern California Foods Association, 8th annual convention, Reno, Nevada, Sept. 1982. Recorded on tape by Audio Recording Services, Las Vegas, Nevada

29 Pearson, D. and Shaw, S. *Life Extension*, New York: Warner, 1982, p. 54

30 *Magazine Digest*, September 1951, pp. 36-39

31 Hauser, G. op. cit., p. 40

32 Fredericks, C. op. cit., p. 99

33 Taub, J.T. "Kelp can Guard Against Radiation," *Prevention*, February 1973, p. 42

34 Fredericks, C. op. cit., p. 21

35 Siedler, A.J. "Nutritional Contributions of the Meat Group to an Adequate Diet," *Borden's Review of Nutrition Research*, 1963, 24(3):39

36 Stadel, B.V. "Dietary Iodine and Risk of Breast, Endometrial, and Ovarian Cancer," *Lancet*, 1976, 1:890

37 "Seaweed Yields Fallout Protection," *Medical World News*, 1964, 5(14):25

38 Wiltshire, H.W. "The Value of Germinated Beans in the Treatment of Scurvy," *Lancet*, 1918, 2:811-813

39 Oliver, M. *Add a Few Sprouts*, New Canaan, Conn.: Keats, 1975, p. 8

40 Burkholder, P.R. and McVeigh, I. "Vitamin Content of Some Mature

and Germinated Legume Seeds," *Plant Physiol.*, 1945, 20:301-306

41 Oliver, M. op. cit., pp. 47-49

42 Clark, L. *Stay Young Longer*, New York: Pyramid, 1976, p. 246

43 Sreenivasan, A. and Wandrekar, S.D. "Biosynthesis of Vitamin C During Germination: Effects of Various Environmental and Cultural Factors," *Proc. Ind. Acad. Sci.* Sect. B, 1950, 32: 143-163

44 Kuppuswamy, S. et al. "Ascorbic Acid in Germinating Seeds of Sesbania Grandiflora Pers," *Current Sci.*, 1958, 27:343-345

45 Adkins, D.M. "Digestility of Germinated Beans," *J. Biochem*, 1920, 14:637-641

46 Adams, R. *Miracle Medicine Foods*, New York: Parker, 1977, p. 18

47 *In touch*, University of Rhode Island Newsletter, September/October 1981

48 Varon, S. "Medical Student Discovers Curative Powers of Garlic," *Heritage*, 1987, p. 28

49 Block, E. et al. "Ajoene: a Potent Antithrombotic Agent from Garlic," *J. Amer. Chem. Soc.*, 1984, 106:8295. Also Yoshida, S. "Antifungal Activity of Ajoene Derived from Garlic," *Appl. Environ. Microbiol.*, 1987, 53:615

50 Hirao, Y. et al. "Activation of Immunoresponder Cells by the Protein Fraction from Aged Garlic Extract," *Phytotherapy Res.*, 1987, 1:161

51 Fujiwara, M. and Nakata, T. "Induction of Tumor Immunity with Tumor Cells Treated with Extract of Garlic (Allium Sativum)," *Nature*, 1967, 216:83

52 Adetumbi, M.A. et al. "Allium Sativum (garlic) Inhibits Lipid Synthesis by Candida Albicans," *Antimicrob. Agents Chemother*, 1986, 30:499

53 Takasugi, N. et al. "Effect of Garlic on Mice Exposed to Various Stresses," *Oyo Yakuri Pharmacometrics*, 1984, 28:991

54 Lau, B. *Garlic for Health*, Wilmot, Wisconsin: Lotus Light Publications, 1988, p. 29

55 Bordia, A. "Effect of Garlic on Blood Lipids in Patients with Coronary Heart Disease," *Amer. J. Clin. Nutr.*, 1981, 34:2100-2103

56 Bordia, A. et al. "Effects of Essential Oil of Onion and Garlic on Experimental Atherosclerosis in Rabbits," *Atherosclerosis*, 1977, 26(3):379-386

57 Loeper, M. and Debray, M. "Antihypertensive Action of Garlic Extract," *Bull. Soc. Med.*, 1921, 37:1032

58 Zheziang Institute of Traditional Chinese Medicine. "The Effect of Essential Oil of Garlic on Hyperlipidemia and Platelet Aggregation," *J. Trad. Chinese Med.*, 1986, 6:117

59 Bordia, A. and Bansal, H.C. "Essential Oil of Garlic in Prevention of Atherosclerosis," *Lancet*, 1973, 2:1491

60 "Garlic: Powerful Medicine," an interview with Dr. Julius Fakunle on his garlic studies, *Prevention*, November 1982, p. 46

61 Jain, R.C. et al. "Hypoglycaemic Action of Onion and Garlic," *Lancet*, 1973, 2:1491

62 Walker, M. "Taking Garlic to the Heart," *Health Express*, October 1982, p. 84

63 Airola, P. *How to Get Well*, Phoenix, AZ: Health Plus, 1974, p. 160

64 O'Rourke, J. "Update on Garlic," *Let's Live*, May 1980, p. 119

65 Davis, A. op. cit., p. 50

66 Morrison, L.M. "Serum Cholesterol Reduction with Lecithin," *Geriatrics*, 1958, 13:12

67 Ibid.

68 Cheraskin, E. and Ringsdorf, W.M. *Psychodietetic Foods as the Key to Emotional Health*, New York: Stein & Day, 1974, p. 164

69 Martin, D.W., Mayes, P.A. and Rodwell, V.W. *Harper's Review of Biochemistry*, Los Altos, CA: Lange, 1981, p. 532

70 Mann, G.V. and Andrus, S.B. "Xanthomatosis and Atherosclerosis Produced by Diet in an Adult Rhesus Monkey," *J. Lab. Clin. Med.*, 1956, 48:533

71 Simons, L.A. et al. "Treatment of Hypercholesterolemia with oral Lecithin," *Australian & New Zealand J. Med.*, 1977, 7:262

72 Carew, T.E. et al. "A Mechanism by which High-Density Lipoproteins May Slow the Atherosenic Process," *Lancet*, 1976, 1:1315-1317

73 Martin, D.W. Mayes, P.A. and Rodwell, V.W. op cit.

74 Toouly, J. et al. "Gallstone Dissolution in Men Using Cholic Acid and Lecithin," *Lancet*, 1975, 2:1124

75 Gross, P. and Kesten, B.M. "The Treatment of Psoriasis as a Disturbance of Lipid Metabolism," *New York State J. Med.*, 1950, 50(2):2686

76 Sitaram, N. et al. "Human Serial Learning: Enhancement with Arecholine and Choline and Impairment with Scopolamine," *Science*, 1978, 201-274

77 Brunette, M. Gaiti, A. and Porcellati, G. "Synthesis of Phosphatidylcholine Phosphatidylethanolamine at Different Ages in the Rat Brain in Vitro," *Lipids*, 1979, 14:925

78 Cohen, B.M. et al. "Lecithin in Mania: A Preliminary Report," *Amer. J. Psychiat.*, 1980, 137-242.

Also Carrol, A.J. et al. "Cholinergic Reversal of Manic Symptoms," *Lancet*, 1973, 1:424. *Also Growdon, J.H. et al. "Lecithin can Suppress Tardive Dyskinesia," New Engl. J. Med.*, 1978, 298:1029. Also Barbeau, A. "Lecithin in Movement Disorders," *Choline and Lecithin in Brain Disorders*, Barbeau, A. Growdon, J.H. Wurtman, R.J. (eds), New York: Raven Press, 1979

79 Hill, R. *Bran*, Northamptonshire, England: Thorsons, 1976, p. 22

80 Walker, A.R.P. "The Effect of Recent Changes of Food Habits on Bowel Motility," *South African Med. J.*, 1947, 21: 590-596

81 Walker, A.R.P. et al. "Appendicitis, Fibre Intake and Bowel Behaviour in Ethnic Groups in South Africa," *Postgraduate Med. J.*, 1973, 49: 243-249

82 Burkitt, D.P. "Diverticular Disease of the Colon: A Deficiency of Western Civilization," *Brit. Med. J.*, 1971, 2:450-454

83 Burkitt, D.P. "Varicose Veins, Deep Vein Thrombosis and Haemorrhoids: Epidemiology and Suggested Aetiology," *Brit. Med. J.*, 1972, 2:556-561

84 Walker, A.R.P. "Overweight and Hypertension in emerging Populations," *Amer. Heart J.*, 1964, 68:581-585

85 Doll, R. "The Geographical Incidence of Cancer," *Brit. J. Cancer*, 1960, 23:1-8

86 Schire, V. "Heart Disease in Southern Africa with Special Reference to Ischaemic Heart Disease," *South African Med. J.*, 1971, 45:634-644

87 Hill, M.J. "Bacteria and Aetiology of Cancer of the Large Bowel," *Lancet*, 1971, 1:95-100

436 COMPLETE NUTRITION

88 Heinerman, J. *Science of Herbal Medicine*, Orem, Utah: Bi-World, 1980, p. 262

89 Ibid. p. 262

90 Koester, S. Wm. "It's All in the Pollen," *Let's Live*, June 1979, p. 59

91 Hanssen, M. *The Healing Power of Pollen*, Northamptonshire, England: Thorsons, 1979, p. 24

92 Ibid. pp. 39–41

93 Ibid. p. 36

94 Ibid. pp. 33–34

95 Taub, H. "How Pollen Helps in Prostatitis," *Prevention*, 1974, 16(7):75–80

96 Binding, G.J. *About Pollen*, Northamptonshire, England: Thorsons, 1976, p. 51

97 Franklin, B. "Pollen - The Bees," *Let's Live*, July 1982, p. 28

98 Hanssen, M. op. cit., p. 20

99 Clement, G. et al. "Amino Acid Composition and Nutrition Value of the Alga Spirulina Maxima," *J. Sci., Food and Agriculture*, 18:497–501

100 Laquerbe, B. et al. "Mineral Composition of Two Cyanophcea, Spirulina Platensis and Spirulina Geitleri," *Comptes Rendues Acad. Sci. ser. D.*, 270(17):2130–2132

101 Hanssen, M. *Spirulina*, Northamptonshire, England: Thorsons, 1982, p. 30

102 Challem, J.J. *Spirulina*, New Canaan, Conn.: Keats, 1981, p. 16

103 Ibid.

104 Ibid. p. 19

105 Passwater, R. *Evening Primrose Oil*, New Canaan, Conn.: Keats, 1981, p. 3

106 Ibid. p. 7

107 Ibid. p. 5

108 Kamen, B. "An Interview with Dr. David Horrobin on Prostaglandins and Essential Fatty Acids," *Let's Live*, October 1981, pp. 66–74

109 Vaddadi, K.S. and Horrobin, D.F. "Weight Loss Produced by Evening Primrose Oil. Administration in Normal and Schizophrenic Individuals," *J. Med. Sci.*, 1979, 7:52

110 Pearson, D. and Shaw, S. *Life Extension*, op. cit., p. 108

111 McCormick, J.N. et al. "Immunosuppressive Effect of Linoleic Acid," *Lancet*, 1977, 2:508

112 Horrobin, D.F. et al. *Medical Hypotheses*, 1980, 6:469–486

113 Ibid.

114 Horrobin, D.F. "Schizophrenia: Reconciliation of the Dopamine, Prostaglandin, and Opioid Concepts and the Role of the Pineal," *Lancet*, 1979, 1:529–531

115 Swank, R.L. "Multiple Sclerosis: Twenty Years on a Low Fat Diet," *Arch. Neurol.*, 1970, 23:460

116 Colquhoun, V. and Bunday S. "A Lack of Essential Fatty Acids as a Possible Cause of Hyperactivity in Children," *Medical Hypotheses*, 1980, 7:681–686

117 Horrobin, D.F. and Manku, M.S. "Possible Role of Prostaglandin E1 in the Affective Disorders and in Alcoholism," *Brit. Med. J.*, 1980, 280:1363–1366

118 Horrobin, D.F. and Cunnane, S.C. *Medical Hypotheses*, 1980, 6:277–296

119 Shreeve, C. *The Premenstrual Syndrome*, Northamptonshire, England: Thorsons, 1983, pp. 109–132

120 Carpenter, M. *Curing PMT*, Century Publishing, London, 1985, p. 6

121 Schopf, J. William. "Precambrian Micro-organisms and Evolutionary Events Prior to the Origin of Vascular Plants," *Biol. Rev.*, 1970, 45:319–352

122 Bewicke, D. and Potter, B. *Chlorella, The Emerald Food,*

Berkeley, California: Ronin Publishing, 1984

123 Hughes, J.H. and Latner, A.L. "Chlorophyll and Haemoglobin Regeneration after Haemorrhage." *J. Physiol.*, 1936, 86:388-395

124 Burgi, E. "Das Chlorophyll als Wachstumsstoff," *Klinische Wochenzeitschrift*, 1930, 9:789

125 Burgi, E. "Ueber die Wirkung von Chlorophyll auf die Wundheilung," *Schweizer Medical Wochenzeitschrift*, 1938, 68:483-485

126 Gahan, E. et al. "Chlorophyll in the Treatment of Ulcers," *Arch. Dermatol. Physiol.*, 1943, 49:849-851

127 Yoshida, A. et al. "Therapeutic Effect of Chlorophyll-A in the Treatment of Patients with Chronic Pancreatitis," *Gastroenterologia Japonica*, 1980,15(1):49-61

128 Kojima, M. et al. "A New Chlorella Polysaccharide and Its Accelerating Effects on the Phagocytic Activity of the Reticuloendothelial System," *Recent Adv. R.E.S., Res.*, 1973, 13:11

129 Matsueda, S. "Studies on Antitumor Active Glycoprotein from Chlorella Vulgaris," *Yajugaku-Zasshi*, 1982, 102:447-451

130 Tanaka, K.F. et al. "Augmentation of Antitumor Resistance by a Strain of Unicellular Green Algae, Chlorella Vulgaris," *Cancer Immunol. Immunother.*, 1984, 17:90-94

131 Yamaguchi, N.S. et al. "Immunomodulation by Single Cellular Algae (Chlorella Pyrenoidosa) and Antitumor Activities for Tumor-Bearing Mice," a paper presented at the Third International Congress of Developmental and Comparative Immunology, Reims, France, July 7-13, 1985

132 Sassen, A. et al. *Cytobiologie*, 1970, 1:273-382

133 Yoshiro, T. *Chlorella - Its Basis and Application*, Tokyo, Japan: Gakushu Kenku-Sha, 1971

134 Okamoto, K. et al. "Effects of Chlorella Alkali Extract on Blood Pressure in SHR, "*Japan Heart J.*, 1978, 19(4):622-623

135 Young, R.W. and Beregi, J.S. "Use of Chlorophyllin in the Care of Geriatric Patients," *J. Amer. Geriat. Soc.*, 1980 XXVIII(1):46-47

136 Hunter, B. and Batham, P. Huntington Research Centre, Toxicology Report, November 1972. Paper submitted to the FDA for approval of chlorella as a food substance

137 *N.Y. Acad. Sci. Ann.*, 719:146-158, 1994

138 *J. Pineal Res.*, 18:28-31, 1995

139 *Life Sci.*, 23:2257-2274, 1978

140 *Biol. Psychiatry*, 23:405-425, 1988

141 Reiter, R.J. et al. "A Review of the Evidence Supporting Melatonin's Role as an Antioxidant," *J. Pineal Res.*, 1995, 18:11
Tan, D. et al., "Melatonin: A Potent, Endogenous Hydroxyl Radical Scavenger." *Endocrine Journal*, 1993, 1:57-60.

142 Tan, D. et al. "The Pineal Hormone Melatonin Inhibits DNA-Adduct Cancer Letters, 1993, 70:65-71.

143 Vijayalaxmi, B.Z. et al. "Melatonin Protects Human blood Lymphocytes from Radiation Induced Chromosome Damage," *Mutation Research*, 1995, 346(1):23-31.

144 Abe, M., Reiter, R.J., and Poeggeler, B., "Inhibitory Effect of Melatonin on Cataract Formation in Newborn Rats: Evidence for an Antioxidative Role for Melatonin," *J. Pineal Res.*, 1994, 17(2):94-100

145 Reiter, R.J., "Oxidative Processes and Antioxidative Defense

Mechanisms in the Aging Brain," *Amer. Soc. Exp. Biol.* (FASEB), 1995, 9(7):526-533.

146 Pieri, C. et al. "Melatonin: A Peroxyl Radical Scavenger More Effective than Vitamin E," *Pergamon*, 1994, 55(15):271-276

147 Reiter, R.J. et al. "The Role of Melatonin in the Pathophysiology of Oxygen Radical Damage," *Advances in Pineal Research*, vol. 8, ed. M. Moller and P. Pévet (London: John Libbey & Co., 1994), p. 278

148 Caroleo, M.C. Frasca, D. and Doria, G., "Melatonin as Immunomodulator in Immunodeficient Mice," *Immunopharmacology*, 1992, 23:81-89

149 Ben Nathan, D. Maestroni, G.J. and Conti, A. "Protective Effects of Melatonin in Mice Infected with Encephalitis Viruses," *Archives of Virology*, 1995, 140:223-230

150 Wilson, S.T. Blask, D.E. and Lemus-Wilson, A.M. "Melatonin Augments the Sensitivity of MCF-7 Human Breast Cancer Cells to Tamoxifen in Vitro" *J. Clin. Endo. Metab.*, 1992, 75(2):669-670

151 Brugger, P. Marktl, W. and Herold, M. "Impaired Nocturnal Secretion of Melatonin in Coronary Heart Disease," *Lancet*, 1995, June 3, 345:1408

152 Kawashima, K. Nagakura, A. and Spector, S., "Melatonin in Serum and the Pineal of Spontaneously Hypertensive Rats," *Clinical and Experimental Hypertension-Theory and Practice*, 1984, A6(8):1517-1528

153 Vacas, M. Del Zar, M. and Cardinali, D. "Inhibition of Human Platelet Aggregation and Thromboxane B2 Production by Melatonin. Correlation with Plasma Melatonin Levels," *Munksgaard*, 1991, 135-139. (B-small 2)

154 Cavallo, A. Holt, K.G. and Meyer, W.J. "Melatonin Circadian Rhythm in Childhood Depression," *Journal of the American Academy of Child and Adolescent Psychiatry*, 1987, 26(3):395-399

155 Parry, B.L. Berga, S.L. and Gillin, J.C. *Chronobiology: Its Role in Clinical Medicine, General Biology and Agriculture. Melatonin and Phototherapy in Premenstrual Depression* (Wiley-Liss, 1990), pp. 35-43

156 Hajak, G. et al. "The Influence of Intravenous L-Tryptophan on Plasma Melatonin and Sleep in Men," *Pharmacopysychiatry*, 1991, 24:17-20

157 Maestroni, G.J. Conti, A. and Pierpaoli, W. "Pineal Melatonin, Its Fundamental Immunoregulatory Role in Aging and Cancer," *Annals of the N.Y. Academy of Sciences*, 1988, 521:140-148

158 Touitou, Y. Fevre-Montagne, M. and Nakache, J.P. "Age and Sex-Associated Modification of Plasma Melatonin concentration in Man. Relationship to Pathology, Malignant or Not, and Autopsy Findings," *Acta Endocrinologica*, 1985, 108:135-144

159 Espiritu, R.C. Kripke, D.F. and Kaplan, O.J. "Low Illumination Experienced by San Diego Adults: Association with Atypical Depressive Symptoms," *Biological Psychiatry*, 1994, 35:403-407

160 Danziger, L. "Read It and Sleep," *Allure*, Oct. 1994, pp. 110-112

161 Drovanti, A. et al. "Therapeutic Activity of Oral Glucosamine Sulfate in Osteoarthritis: A Placebo-Controlled Double-Blind Investigation," *Clin. Ther.*, 1980, 3:260-272

162 Feature Article, "Glucosamine Sulfate: Effective Osteoarthritis

Treatment," *Amer. J. Natur. Med.*, 1994, 1(1):10

163 Ibid.

164 Crolle, G. and D'este, E. "Glucosamine Sulfate for the Management of Arthrosis: A Controlled Clinical Examination," 1980, *Curr. Med. Res. Opin.*, 7:104-109

165 Vaz, A.L. "Double-Blind Clinical Evaluation of the Relative Efficacy of Ibuprofen and Glucosamine Sulfate in the Management of Osteoarthritis of the Knee in out-patients," 1982, *Curr. Med. Res. Opin.*, 8:145-149

166 Shield, M.J. "Anti-Inflammatory Drugs and their Effect on Cartilage Synthesis and Renal Function," *Eur. J. Rheumatol. Inflam.*, 1993, 13:7-16

167 Setnikar, I. et al. "Pharmacokinetics of Glucosamine in the Dog and Man," Arzneim Forsch, 1986, 36(4):729-735

168 Tapadinhas, M.J. et al. "Oral Glucosamine-Sulfate in the Management of Arthrosis: Report on a Multi-Centre Open Investigation in Portugal," *Pharmatherapeutica*, 1982, 3:157-168

169 Feature Article, op. cit.

170 Oski, F.A. "Don't Drink Your Milk!", TEACH Services, Inc, New York, p. 3

171 Epstein, S. et al. *International Journal of Health Services*, January 1996, 26(1):173-185

172 Committee on Nutrition, American Academy of Pediatrics: "Should Milk Drinking by Children be Discouraged?", *Pediatrics*, 1974, 53:576

173 Bayles, T.M. and Huang, S. "Recurrent Abdominal Pain due to Milk and Lactose Intolerance in School Aged Children," *Pediatrics*, 1971, 47:1029

Bart, R.G. et al. "Recurrent Abdominal Pain of Childhood due to Lactose Intolerance," *N. Engl. J. Med.*, 1979, 300:1449

174 Oski, F.A. op. cit., p. 10

175 Steinmetz K.A. Potter, J.D. "Vegetables, Fruit, and Cancer," II. Mechanisms., Cancer Causes and Control, 1991, 2:427-442

176 Troll, W. et al. "Soybean Diet Lowers Breast Tumor Incidence in Irradiated Rats," *Carcinogenesis*, 1980, 1:469-472
Troll, W. et al., "Inhibition of Carcinogenesis by Feeding Diets Containing Soybeans," *Proc. Amer. Assoc. Cancer Res.*, 1979, 20:265 (abstract 1075)

177 Weed, H.G. et al. "Protection against Dimethylhydrazine-Induced Adenomatous Tumors of the Mouse Colon by the Dietary Addition of an Extract of Soybeans Containing the Bowman-Birk Protease Inhibitor," *Carcinogenesis*, 1985, 6:1239-1241

178 Witschi, H., Kennedy, A.R. "Modulation of Lung Tumor Development in Mice with the Soybean-derived Bowman-Birk Protease Inhibitor," *Carcinogenesis*, 1989, 10:2275-2277

179 Shamsuddin, A.M. "Phytate and Colon-Cancer Risk," *Amer. J. Clin. Nutr.* 1992, 55:478-485

180 Raicht, R.F. et al. "Protective Effect of Plant Sterols against Chemically Induced Colon Tumors in Rats," *Cancer Res.* 1980, 40:403-405

181 Nakashima, H. et al. "Inhibitory Effect of Glycosides like Saponin from Soybean on the Ineffectivity of HIV in vitro," *AIDS* 1989, 3:655-658

182 Tang, B.Y. Adams, N.R. "Effect of Equol on Oestrogen Receptors and on Synthesis of DNA and Protein in

the Immature Rat Uterous," *J. Endocrinol*. 1980, 85:291-297

183 Akiyama, T. Ogawara, H. "Use and Specifity of Genistein as Inhibitor of Protein-Tyrosine Kinases," *Meth Enzymol*, 1991, 201:362-370

184 Kritchevsky, D. "Dietary Protein, Cholesterol and Atherosclerosis: a Review of the Early History," *J. Nutr*. 1995, 125:suppl:589S-593S

185 Anderson, J.W. et al. "Meta-Analysis of the Effects of Soy Protein Intake on Serum Lipids," *N. Engl. J. Med*. 1995, 333:276-282

186 Kito, M. et al. "Changes in Plasma Lipids in Young Healthy Volunteers by Adding an Extruder Cooked Soy Protein to Conventional Meals," *Biosci. Biotech. Biochem*. 1993, 57:354-355

187 Tranter, H.S. et al. "The Effect of the Olive Phenolic Compound, Oleuropein, on Growth and Enterotoxin B Production by Staphylococcus Aureus," *J. Appl. Bacteriol*., 1993, 74:253-259

188 Pasquale, A.D. et al. "HPLC Analysis of Oleuropein and Some Flavonoids in the Leaf and Bud of Olea Europaea L.," *Farmaco*, 1991, 46:803-815

189 Renis, H.E. "In Vitro Antiviral Activity of Calcium Elenolate," *Antimicrobial Agents and Chemotherapy*, 1970, pp. 167-168

190 Tassou, C.C. et al. "Effect of Phenolic Compounds and Oleuropein on the Germination of Bacillus Cereus T Spores," *Biotechnol. Appl. Biochem*., 1992, 13:231-237

191 Fleming, H.P. et al. *Applied Microbiology*, 1969, 18:859-860 Rutz-Barba, J.L. et al. *Syst. Appl. Microbiol*., 1990, 13:199-205

192 Vaughn, R.H., in *Industrial Fermentations* (Underkotler, L.A. and Hickery, R.J. Eds.) 1954, vol. 2, New York Chemical Publishing

193 Visioli, F., and Galli, C., "Oleuropein Protects Low Density Lipoprotein from Oxidation," *Life Sciences*, 1994, 55(24):1965-1971

194 Hertog, M.G.L. et al. *Lancet*, 1993, 342:1007-1011

195 Gao, Y.T. McLaughlin J.K., et al.: "Reduced Risk of Esophageal Cancer Associated with Green Tea Consumption," *J. Nat. Cancer Inst*. 1994, 86:11, June 1

196 Muramatsu K. et al. "Effect of Green tea Catechins on Plasma Cholesterol Level in Cholesterol-Fed Rats," *J. Nutr. Sci. Vitaminol*., 1986, 32:623-622

197 Sano, M. et al. "Effect of Tea on Lipid Peroxidation in Rat Liver and Kidney: a Comparison of Green and Black Tea Feeding," *Biol. Pharm. Bull*. 1995, 18(7):1006-1008

198 Kanaya, S. et al. "The Physiological Effect of Tea Catechins on Human Volunteers," Seirei Mikatabara General Hospital, 3453 Mikatabara, Hamamatsu, Japan

199 Steinman, D. "Why You Should Drink Green Tea," -Natural Pharmacy. Natural Health magazine, 1994, March/April

200 Nestler, J.N. et al. "DHEA the "Missing Link" Between Hyperinsulinemia and Atherosclerosis?" FASEB J., 6(12):3073-3075

201 Shafagoj, J. et al. "Dehydroepiandrosterone Prevents Dexamethasone-Induced Hypertension in Rats," 1992, *Amer. J. Physiol*., 263(2 pt 1):210-213

202 Gordon, G.B. et al. "Reduction of Atherosclerosis by Administration of Dehydroepiandrosterone (DHEA). A Study in the Hypercholesterolemic New Zealand White Rabbit with Aortic Intimal

Injury," *J. Clin. Invest.*, 82(2):712-720

203 Giona, F. et al. "Gonadal, Adrenal, Androgen and Thyroid Functions in Adults Treated for Acute Lymphoblastic Leukemia," 1994, *Haematologica*, 79(2):141-147. Also: Bhatavdekar, D.D. et al. "Levels of Circulating Peptide and Steroid Hormones in Men with Lung Cancer," *Neoplasma*, 1994, 41(2):101-103

204 Williams, D.P. et al. "Relationship of Body Fat Percentage and Fat Distribution with Dehydroepiandrosterone Sulfate in Premenopausal Females," 1993, *J. Clin. Endocrinol. Metab.*, 77(1):80-85

205 Singh, V.B. et al. "Intracranial Dehydro-Epiandrosterone Blocks the Activation of Tryptophan Hydroxylase in Response to Acute Sound Stress," 1994, *Mol. Cell. Neurosci.*, 5(2):176-181

206 Melchior, C.L. and Ritzman, R.F. "Dehydroepiandrosterone is an Anxiolytic in Mice on the Plus Maze," *Pharmacol. Biochem. Behav.*, 1994, 47(3):437-441

207 Wolkowitz, O.M. et al. "Antidepressant and Cognition-Enhancing Effects of DHEA in Major Depression," Dehydroepiandrosterone (DHEA) and Aging, New York Academy of Sciences Meeting, 1995, June 17-19

208 Buffington, C.K. et al. "Case Report: Amelioration of Insulin-Resistance in Diabetes with Dehydroepiandrosterone," *Amer. J. Med. Sci.*, 1993, 306(5):320-324. Also: Coleman, D.L. et al. "Therapeutic Effects of Dehydroepiandrosterone Metabolites in Diabetic Mice," 1984, *Endocrinology*, 115:239-243

209 Barrett-Connor, E. et al. "A Prospective Study of Dehydroepiandrosterone Sulfate, Mortality and Cardiovascular Disease," *New Engl. J. Med.*, 1986, 315(24):1519-1524

210 Bulbrook, R.D. et al. "Relation Between Urinary Androgen and Corticoid Excretion and Subsequent Breast Cancer," *Lancet*, 1971, II:395-398

211 Cacciari, E. et al. "Effects of Sport (Football) on Growth: Auxological, Anthropometric and Hormonal Aspects," *Eur. J. Appl. Physiol.*, 1990, 61:149-158

212 Turturro, A. and Hart, R.W. "Longevity-Assurance Mechanisms and Caloric Restriction," *Annals New York Acad. Sci.*, 1991, 621:363-372

213 Glaser, J.L. et al. "Elevated Serum Dehydroepiandrosterone Sulfate levels in Practitioners of Transcendental Meditation (TM)and TM-Siddhi Program," *J. Behav. Med.*, 1992, 15(4):327-341

214 Seminars in Arthritis and Rheumatism, 1987, 17:2 (Suppl.)

215 Whitaker, J. *Health and Healing*, 1992, 2:6

216 D'Amore, P. "Antiangiogenesis as a strategy for Antimetastasis," Seminars in Thrombosis and Homeostasis, 1988, 14:113-177. Also: Blumberg, N. "Tumor Angiogenesis Factor: Speculations on an Approach to Cancer Chemotherapy," *Yale J. Biol. Med.*, 1974, 47:71-84

217 Prudden, J.F. et al. "Acceleration of Wound Healing with Cartilage-1," *Surgery, Gynecology & Obstetrics*, 1957, 105:283

218 Kirchhof, D. and Kirchhof, E. "The Successful Use of Bovine Tracheal Cartilage in the Treatment of Cancer," 1995, Kriegel & Associates Publishers, Belgrade, Montana 59714, p. 6

219 Prudden, J.F. "The Treatment of Human Cancer with Agents Prepared from Bovine Cartilage," 1985, *Journal of Biological Responses Modifiers*, 4:583

220 Prudden, J.F. Summary of Bovine Tracheal Cartilage Research Programs, 1993, 5

221 Durie, Brian G.M. et al. "An Assessment of the Anti-Mitotic Activity of Catrix-S in the Human Stem Cell Assay," *Journal of Biological Response Modifiers*, 1985, 4:590-595

222 Lane, I.W. "Sharks Don't Get Cancer," 1993, A very Publishing Company, Garden City park, New York, p. 102

223 Morrison, M.L. "Reduction of Ischemic Coronary heart Disease by Chondroitin Sulfate A," *Angiology*, 1971, 22:165

CHAPTER 6

1 Schroeder, H. *The Poisons Around Us*, New Canaan, Conn.: Keats, 1978, p. 112

2 Fredericks, C. *Nutrition Handbook*, Canoga Park, CA: Major Books, 1977, p. 209

3 Vanderkamp, H.A. "A Biochemical Abnormality in Schizophrenia Involving Ascorbic Acid," *Inter. J. Neuropsychiat.*, 1966, 2:204

4 Albrecht, W.A. "Physical, Chemical and Biologic Changes in the Soil Community," *Man's Role in Changing the Face of the Earth*, Thomas, W.L. (ed.), University of Chicago Press, 1956, p. 671

5 Rodale, R. *Prevention*, April 1978

6 Raymond, B. *The Organic Revolution in Nutrition*, The Lee Foundation for Nutritional Research, Milwaukee, Wis.

7 Chesley, F.F. et al. "The Vitamin B Complex and Its Constituents in Functional Digestive Disturbances," *Amer. J. Digest. Dis.*, 1940, 7:25

8 Ludwig, H. et al. "Report on Distillation Product Industry," Eastman Kodak Affiliate Publication, September 1962

9 Karie, E. *Vitamins: A Shelter against Disease*, Tel-Aviv, Israel: Reshafim, 1975, p. 62

10 Shute, W. "An Update on Vitamin E," an address to the 42nd annual convention of National Nutritional Foods Association (NNFA), 1979. Recorded on tape by Audio Recording Services, Las Vegas, Nevada

11 Pauling, L. "Nutrition Research for Optimum Health," an address to the 42nd annual convention of the National Nutritional Foods Association, 1979. Recorded on tape by Audio Recording Services, Las Vegas, Nevada

12 Pfeiffer, C. *Mental and Elemental Nutrients*, New Canaan, Conn.: Keats, 1976, pp. 118-120

13 Schroeder, H. op. cit., p. 130

14 Airola, P. *How to Get Well*, Phoenix, AZ: Health Plus, 1979, p. 172

15 Schroeder, H. *Trace Elements and Man*, Old Greenwich, Conn.: Devin-Adair, 1973, p. 89

16 Passwater, R. *Selenium as Food and Medicine*, New Canaan, Conn.: Keats, 1980, p. 13

17 Rusoff, L.L. "The Role of Milk in Modern Nutrition," *Borden's Review of Nutrition Research*, 1964, 25(2-3):37

18 Airola, P. op. cit., p. 170

CHAPTER 7

1 Orton, J.H. and Neuhaus, O.W. *Biochemistry*, St. Louis, Mo.: C.V. Mosby, 1970, pp. 182-184

2 Steen, E. and Montagu, A. *Anatomy and Physiology*, New York: Barnes and Noble, 1959, vol. 1, p. 177

3 Ibid. p. 192

4 Ingelfinger, F.J. et al. "Diet as Related to Gastrointestinal Function," *J. Amer. Diet. Assn.*, 1961, 38:425

5 Steen and Montagu. op. cit., p. 186

6 Ibid. p. 155

7 Ibid. p. 162

8 Ibid.

9 Vannini, V. and Pogliani, G. *The New Atlas of the Human Body*, London, U.K.: Transworld Publishers, 1980, p. 86

10 Taber, C.W. & Assoc. *Cyclopedic Medical Dictionary*, Philadelphia: Davis Co., 4th ed., pp. B23-B24

11 Steen and Montagu. op. cit., p. 163

12 Ibid.

13 Ibid. p. 182

CHAPTER 8

1 Steen, E. and Montagu, A. *Anatomy and Physiology*, New York: Barnes and Noble, 1959, vol. 1, p. 193

2 Mindell, E. *Vitamin Bible*, New York: Rawson Wade, 1980, p. 146

3 Ibid. p. 220

4 Colimore, B. and Colimore, S.S. *Nutrition and Your Body*, Los Angeles, CA: Light Wave Interprises, 1978, p. 215

5 Ibid.

6 Brolus, T. "Nutrition for Adults," *Let's Live*, February 1980, 48(2):112

7 Dale, A. "Why the Balanced Diet Doesn't Work for Everyone," an address to the 45th annual convention of the national Nutritional Foods Association (NNFA), 1983, Denver, Co. 1983. Recorded on tape by Audio Recording Services, Las Vegas, Nevada

8 Donsbach, K. "Basic Nutrition Facts," *Nutrition in Action*, Huntington Beach, CA: Int'l Ins. Nat. Health Sci., 1977, p. 26

9 Yano, S. et al. "The Etiology of Caffeine-Induced Aggravation of Gastric Lesions in Rats Exposed to Restraint," *J. Pharmacobiodyn.*, 1982, 5(7):485-494

10 Veleber, D.M. et al. "Effects of caffeine on Anxiety and Depression," *J. Abnorm. Psychol.*, 1984, 93(1):120-122

11 Whitsett, T.L. et al. "Cardiovascular Effects of Coffee and Caffeine," *Amer. J. Cardiol.*, 1984, 53(7):918-922

12 Kurppa, K. et al. "Coffee Consumption During Pregnancy and Selected Congenital Malformations: A Nationwide Case-Control Study," *Amer. J. Public Health*, 1983, 73(12):1397-1399

13 Wilcox, A. et al. "Caffeinated Beverages and Decreased Fertility," *Lancet*, 1988, 2:1453-6

14 Minton, J.P. et al. "Caffeine and Unsaturated Fat Diet Significantly Promotes DMBA-Induced Breast Cancer in Rats," *Cancer*, 1983, 51(7):1249

15 Marrett, L.D. et al. "Coffee Drinking and Bladder Cancer in Connecticut," *Amer. J. Epidemiol.*, 1983, 117(2):113

16 Aitken, R.J. et al. "Influence of Caffeine on Movement Characteristics, Fertilizing Capacity and Ability to Penetrate Cervical Mucus of Human Spermatozoa," *J. Reprod. Fertil.*, 1983, 67(1):19-27

17 Schauss, G.A. An address to the South West Health Organization

(SWHO), Fort Worth, Texas, February 1983. Recorded on tape by Audio Recording Services, Las Vegas, Nevada

18 Olsson, A.G. and Eklund, B. "Studies in Asymptomatic Primary Hyperlipidemia. Vascular Peripheral Circulation," *Acta Med. Scand.*, 1975, 198(3): 197-206

19 Barakat, M.H. et al. "Cigarette Smoking and Duodenal Ulcer Healing," *Digestion*, 1984, 29(2):85-89

CHAPTER 9

1 Thurston, E. *The Parents' Guide to Better Nutrition for Tots to Teens*, New Canaan, Conn.: Keats, 1979, p. 139

2 Kaplan, R. "Cytotoxic Testing," *Let's Live*, January 1982, p. 64

3 Coca, A. *The Pulse Test*, New York: Lyle Stuart, 195, p. 17

4 Fredericks, C. *Nutrition Handbook*, Huntington Beach, CA: Int'l Ins. Nat. Health Sci., 1977, p. 80

5 Randolph, T.G. "The Descriptive Features of Food Addiction," *Quarterly J. of Studies on Alcohol*, June 1956, 17:2. Also Kittler, F.J. and Baldwin, D.G. "The Role of Allergic Factors in the Child with Minimal Brain Dysfunction," *Ann. Allergy*, May 1970, vol 28. Also Speer, F. *Allergy of the Nervous System*, Springfield, Ill.: Charles C. Thomas, 1970

6 Frazier, C.A. "What is new and Important in Food Allergy?" *Medical Tribune and Medical News*, 1975, 16(16):5

7 Thurston, E. op. cit., p. 142

8 Mindell, E. *Vitamin Bible*, New York: Rawson Wade,1980, p. 146

9 Clark, L. *Get Well Naturally*, New York: ARC Books, 1972, p. 158

10 Fredericks, C. op. cit., p. 81

11 Hemmings, W.A. and Williams, E.W. "Transport of Large Breakdown Products of Dietary Protein Through the Gut Wall; *Gut*, 1974, 19:715

12 Walleer, W.A. "Uptake and Transport of Macromolecules by the Intestine - Possible Role in Clinical Disorders," *Gastroenterology*, 1974, 67:531

13 Grusley, F.L. "Gastrointestinal Absorption of Unaltered Protein in Normal Infants," *Pediatrics*, 1955, 16:763

14 Ibid. p. 79

15 Thurston, E. op. cit., p. 142

16 Ibid. p. 10

17 Smith, L. *Feeds Your Kids Right*, New York: Delta, 1979, pp. 96-97

18 Fredericks, C. op. cit., p. 80

19 Pfeiffer, C. *Mental and Elemental Nutrients*, New Canaan, Conn.: Keats, 1976, p. 417

20 Ibid., p. 416. Also Egger, J. et al. "Is Migraine Food Allergy?" *Lancet*, 1983, 2:865-869

21 Egger, J. et al. op. cit.

22 Kaplan, R. op. cit., p. 60

23 Pfeiffer, C. op. cit., p. 418

24 Coca, A. op. cit.

25 Frazier, C.A. op. cit.

26 Kaplan, R. op. cit., p. 60

27 Fredericks, C. op. cit., p. 81

28 Irvine, W.T. "The Liver's Role in Histamine Absorption from the Alimentary Tract," *Lancet*, 1959, 1:1064

29 Clark, L. op. cit., p.157

30 Mindell, E. op. cit., p. 192

31 Airola, P. *How to Get Well*, Phoenix, AZ: Health Plus, 1979, p. 34

32 Mindell, E. op. cit., p. 146

33 Airola, P. op. cit., p. 34

34 Fredericks, C. op. cit., p. 83

CHAPTER 10

1 Airola, P. *Hypoglycemia - A Better Approach*, Phoenix, AZ: Health Plus, 1977, p. 27

2 Fredericks, C. *Low Blood Sugar and You*, New York: Grosset and Dunlap, 1969, p. 2

3 Ibid. p. 1

4 Egeli, E.S. and Berkmen, R.B. "Action of Hypoglycemia on Coronary Insufficiency and Metabolism of ECG Alterations," *Amer. Heart J.*, 1960, 59:527

5 Fredericks, C. *Nutrition Handbook*, Canoga Park, CA: Major Books, 1977, p. 60

6 Ibid. p. 61

7 Colimore, B. and Colimore, S.S. *Nutrition and Your Body*, Los Angeles, CA: Light Wave Enterprises, 1978, p. 53

8 Fredericks, C. *Nutrition Handbook*, op. cit., p. 81

9 Ibid. p. 58

10 Airola, P. op. cit., p. 29

11 Pearson, D. and Shaw, S. *Life Extension*, New York: Warner, 1982, p. 372

12 Airola, P. op. cit., p. 22

13 *Psychopharmacological Bulletin*, 1989, 20(1):45-59

14 Ibid. p. 60

15 Abrahamson, E.M. *Body, Mind and Sugar*, New York: Avon Books, 1951, p. 118

16 Ibid. p. 136

17 Airola, P. op. cit., p. 66

18 Ibid. pp. 67-69

19 Davis, A. *Let's Get Well*, New York: Harcourt Brace Jovanovich, 1972, p. 311

20 Siperstein, M.D. "Inter-Relationship of Glucose and Lipid Metabolism," *Amer. J. Med.*, 1959, 26(5):685-702

21 "Nutrient Intake and Its Association with HDL and LDL Cholesterol in Selected US and USSR Subpopulations. The US-USSR Steering Committee for Problem Area I: The Pathogenesis of Atherosclerosis," *Amer. J. Clin. Nutr.*, 1984, 39(6):942-952

22 Antar, M.A. et al. "Changes in Retail Market Food Supplies in the U.S. in the Last Seventy years in Relation to the Incidence of Coronary Heart Disease, with Special Reference to Dietary Carbohydrates and Essential Fatty Acids," *Amer. J. Clin. Nutr.*, 1964, 14:169-177

23 Atkins, R. *Super Energy Diet*, New York: Crown, 1977, p. 55

24 Ibid. p. 69

25 Airola, P. op. cit., p. 76

26 "Vascular Research Laboratory," report in *Amer. Med. Assn News Release*, June 21, 1965

27 Visek, W. "Report on Cornell University Research," *Los Angeles Times*, March 29, 1973

28 Airola, P. op. cit., p. 72

29 Ibid.

CHAPTER 11

1 Leevy, C.M. et al. "Protein Tolerance in Liver Disease," *Amer. J. Clin. Nutr.*, 1962, 10:46

2 McKibbin, F. and J. *Cookbook of Foods from Bible Days*, Pennsylvania: 1972, p. 101

3 Davis, J.G. and Latto, D. "Yogurt in Gastro-Enteritis of Infancy," *Lancet*, 1957, 1:274

4 Ibid.

5 Reddy, G.V. et al. "Inhibitory Effect of Yogurt on Ehrlich Ascites Tumor-Cell Proliferation," *J. Nat. Cancer Inst.*, 1973, 50(3):815-817

6 *Medical World News*, September 28, 1962

7 Mann, G.V. "A Factor in Yogurt Which Lowers Cholesteremia in Man," *Atherosclerosis*, 1977, 26:335-336

8 Hepner, G. et al. "Hypocholesterolemia Effect of Yogurt and Milk," *Amer. J. Clin. Nutr.*, 1979, 32:19-24

9 Davis, A. *Let's Get Well*, New York: Harcourt Brace Jovanovich, 1972, p. 144

10 Clark, L. *Get Well Naturally*, New York: ARC Books, 1972, p. 250

11 Mitsuoka, T. et al. "Effect of Fructo-digosaccharides on Intestinal Microflora", *Die Nahrung*, 31 (1987) 5-6,427-36

12 Ibid.

13 Yamashita, K. et al. "Effects of fructo-oligosaccorides on Blood Glucose and Serum Lipids Diabetic subjects," *Nutrition Research*, 1984, vol. 4, pp 961-66

14 Thurston, E. *The Parents' Guide to Better Nutrition for Tots to Teens*, New Canaan, Conn.: Keats, 1979, p. 86

15 Mendeloff, A.I. "Dietary Fiber," *Present Knowledge in Nutrition*, New York: The Nutrition Foundation, 1976, pp. 396-397

16 Wells, A.F. and Ershoff, B.H. "Beneficial Effects of Pectin in Prevention of Hypercholesterolemia and Increase in Liver Cholesterol in Cholesterol-Fed Rats," *J. Nutr.*, 1961, 74:87-92

17 Orton, J.H. and Neuhaus, O.W. *Biochemistry*, St. Louis, Mo: C.V. Mosby, 1970, p. 17

CHAPTER 12

1 Lundberg, (ed.) *Autoxidation and Antioxidants*, New York: Wiley Interscience, vols. 1 and 2

2 Sherwin, E. "Antioxidants for Food Fats and Oils," *J. Amer. Oil Chem. Soc, (JAOCS)*, 1972, 49(8):468-472. Also Braco, J. et al. "Production and Use of Natural Antioxidants," 1981, *JAOCS*, 58(6):686-690

3 Lewis, W.H. and Elvin-Lewis, M.P.F. *Medical Botany*, New York: Wiley Interscience, 1977, p. 292

4 Weil, A.T. "Nutmeg and Other Psychoactive Groceries," in Gunckel, J.E. (ed.), *Current Topics in Plant Science*, New York: Academic Press, 1969, pp. 356-366

5 Der Marderodian, A. "Current Status of Hallucinogens in the Cactaceae," *Amer. J. Pharm.*, 1966, 138:204-212. Also Bergman, R.L. "Navajo Peyote Use: Its Apparent Safety," *Amer. J. Psychiatr.*, 128: 695-699

6 Hocking, G.M. "Plant Flavor and Aromatic Values in Medicine and Pharmacy," in Gunckel, J.E. (ed.), *Current Topics in Plant Science*, New York: Academic Press, 1969, pp. 273-288

7 Lewis, W.H. and Elvin-Lewis, M.P.F. op. cit., p. 318

8 Withering, W. "An Account of the Foxglove, and Some of Its Medical Uses," with Swinney, M. "Practical Remarks on Dropsy, and Other Diseases," reprinted in *Med. Classics*, 1937, 5(4):303-443

9 Chung, E.K. "The Current Status of Digitalis Therapy," *Mod. Treat.*, 1971 8(3):641-714. Also Fisch, C. and Surawicz, B. (eds), *Digitalis*, New York and London: Grune & Straton, 1969, p. 230

10 Huebner, C.F. and Link, K.P. "Studies on the Hemorrhagic Sweet Clover Disease," VI, *J. Biol. Chem.*, 1941, 138:529-534

11 Bordia, A. et al. "Effects of Essential Oil of Onion and Garlic on Experimental Atherosclerosis in Rabbits," *Atherosclerosis*, 1977, 26(3):379-386

12 Reis, E.D. "The Treatment of Primary Hypertension," *Mod. Med.*, 1968, 36(6):86-91

13 Yamaguchi, K. et al. "The Mechanism of Purgative Action of Geniposide, an Iridoid Glucoside of the Fruit of Gardenia, in Mice," *Planta Medica*, 1976, 30:39-47

14 Govindachari, T.R. "Chemical and Biological Investigations on Indian Medicinal Plants," *New Natural Products and Plant Drugs with Pharmacological, Biological or Therapeutical Activity*, New York: Wagner and Wolff, 1977, p. 222

15 Sircus, W. "Progress Report: Carbenoxolone Sodium," *Gut*, 1972, 13:816-824

16 Cheney, G. et al. "Vitamin U Therapy of Peptic Ulcer: Experience at San Quentin Prison," *Calif. Med.*, 1956, 84:39-42

17 Ahronson, Z. et al. "Hypoglycemic Effect of the Salt Bush (Artiplex Halimus) - A Feeding Source of the Sand Rat," *Diabetologia*, 1969, 5:379-383

18 Veleber, D.M. et al. "Effects of Caffeine on Anxiety and Depression," *J. Abnorm. Psychol.*, 1984, 93(1):120-122

19 Yano, S. et al. "The Etiology of Caffeine-Induced Aggravation of Gastric Lesions in Rats Exposed to Restraint," *J. Pharmacobiodyn.*, 1982, 5(7):485-494

20 Scully, V. *A Treasury of American Indian Herbs*, New York: Crown, 1970, p. 306

21 Steinberg, N.P. "Cat's Claw (*Unadegato*) a Wondrous Herb from the Amazon Rain Forest," *The Herb Quarterly*, Winter 1994, p. 20

22 Ibid.

23 Heinerman, J. *Science of Herbal Medicine*, Orem, Utah: Bi-World, 1983, p. 111

24 Hills, L.D. *Comfrey-Fodder, Food and Remedy*, New York: University Books, 1976, pp. 200-203

25 Luettig, B. et al. "Macrophage Activation by the Polysaccharide Arabinogalactan Isolated from Plant Cell Cultures of Echinacea Purpurea," *J. Nat'l. Cancer Inst.*, 1989, 81(9):669-675

26 Lersch, C. et al. "Stimulation of Immunocompetent Cells in Patients with Gastrointestinal Tumors During an Experimental Therapy with Low Dose Cyclophosphamide, Thymostimulin, and Echinacea Purpurea Extract (Echinacin), 1992, *Mordiagen Ther*, 13:115-120 (In German)

27 Blumenthal, M. "The History and Modern Day Uses of Echinacea," *Whole Foods*, March 1992, p. 24

28 Foster, S. "*Echinacea*: The Cold and Flu Remedy," *Alternative and Complementary Therapies*, June/July 1995, pp. 254-257

29 Coeugniet, E.G. and Kuhnast, R. "Recurrent Candidiasis: Adjuvant Immunotherapy with Different Formulations of Echinacin," *Therapiewoche*, 1986, 36:3352-3358

30 Foster, S. op. cit.

31 Johnson, E.S. et al. "Efficacy of Feverfew as Prophylactic Treatment of Migraine," *Brit. Med. J.*, 1985, 6495(291):569-573

32 Heinerman, J. *Science of Herbal Medicine*, Bi-World Publishers, Orem, Utah, 1983, pp. 129-130

33 *Indian J. Psychiat.*, 1973, 19(4):54-59

34 Mowrey, D.B. "The Effects of Capsicum, Gotu Kola and Ginseng on Activity: Further Evidence," *The Herbalist*, 1976, 1(1):51-54

35 Presse Medicale, 1933; 1958, 66. Also: *Minerva Med.*, 1960, 15:1235

36 *Gazet. Med. France*, 1975, 82:4579

37 Wilmshurst, P. and Crawley, J.C.W. "The measurement of Gastric Transit Time in Obese Subjects Using 24-Na and the Effects of Energy Content and Guar Gum on Gastric Emptying Time and Satiety," *Brit. J. Nutr.*, 1980, 44:1-6

38 Blackburn, N.A. and Johnson, I.T. "The Influence of Guar Gum on the Movements of Insulin, Glucose and Fluid in Rat Intenstine during Perfusion in Vivo," *Pflugers, Arch.*, 1983, 397:144-148

39 Tuomilehto, J.E. et al. "Effect of Guar Gum on Body Weight and Serum Lipids in Hypercholesterolemic Females," *Acta Med. Scand.*, 1980, 209:45-48

40 Keung, W.M. and Vallee, B.H. "Daidzin and Daidzein Suppress Free-choice Alcohol Intake by Syrian Golden Hamsters," *Proc. Nat'l. Acad. Sci.*, U.S.A., 1993, 90:10008-12

41 Heinerman, J. op. cit., p. 107

42 Koster, M. and David, G.K. "Reversible Severe Hypertension due to Licorice Ingestion," *New Engl. J. Med.*, 1968, 278:1381-1383. Also Robinson, H.J. et al. "Cardiac Abnormalities Due to Licorice Intoxication," *Penn. Med.*, 1971, 74:51-54

43 Copeman, W.S. "Historic Aspects of Gout," *Clin. Orthop.*, 1970, 71:14-22

44 Vogel, G. "Natural Substances with Effects on the Liver," *New Natural Products and Plant Drugs with Pharmacological, Biological or Therapeutical Activity*, New York: Wagner and Wolff, 1977, pp. 249-262

45 Herrman, E.C. and Kucera, L.S. "Antiviral Substances in Plants of the Mint Family (Labiatae), Peppermint (Mentha Piperita) and other Mint Plants," *Proc. Soc. Exp. Biol. Med.*, 1967, 124:874

46 Anand, C.L. "Effect of Avena Sativa on Cigarette Smoking," *Nature*, 1971, 233:496

47 Bordia, A. et al. "The Protective Action of Essential Oils of Onion and Garlic in Cholesterol-fed Rabbits," *Atherosclerosis*, 1975, 22(1):103-109

48 "New Help for Slipped Discs," *TIME* magazine, December 6, 1982

49 Hazum, J. et al. "Morphine in Cow and Human Milk: Could Dietary Morphine Constitute a Ligand for Specific Morphine Receptors?" *Science* 1981, 213:1010-1012

50 Ahronson, Z. et al. op. cit.

51 Grieve, M. *A Modern Herbal*, New York: Dover Publications, 1971, 2:712-714

52 Champault, G. et al. "A Double-Blind Trial of an Extract of the Plant Serenoa Repens in Benign Prostatic Hyperplasia," *Brit. J. Clin. Pharm.*, 1984, 18:461-462

53 Tripodi, V. et al. "Treatment of Prostatic Hypertrophy with Serenoa Repens Extract," *Med. Praxis*, 1983, 4:41-46

54 Emili, E. et al. "Clinical Trial of a New Drug for Treating Hypertrophy of the Prostate (Permixon)," *Urologia*, 1983, 50:1042-1048

55 Tyler, V.E. "Herbs of Choice: The Therapeutic Use of Phytomedicinals," Pharmaceutical Products Press, 1994

56 Moore, M. "Medicinal Plants of the Mountain West," Museum of New Mexico Press, 1979

57 Heinerman, J. *Science of Herbal Medicine*, 1983, Bi-World Publishers, Orem, Utah, p. 220

58 Lewis, W.H. and Elvin-Lewis, M.P.F. op. cit., p. 318

59 Shaffer, W. *Wild Yam - Birth Control Without Fear*, Provo, Utah: Woodlands Books, 1986, pp. 2–4

CHAPTER 13

1 Cheraskin, E. *Diet and Disease*, New Canaan, Conn.: Keats, 1968, p. 11

2 Atkins, R. *Super Energy Diet*, New York: Crown, 1977, p. 101

3 Mayer, J. "Obesity," *Post Graduate Medicine*, 1972, 51(6):65-75

4 Bruch, H. "Psychiatric Aspects of Obesity," *Metabolism*, 1957, 6:461

5 Taitz, L.S. "Infantile Overnutrition Among Artificially Fed Infants in the Sheffield Region," *Brit. Med. J.*, 1971, 1:315-316

6 Atkins, R. op. cit., p. 100

7 Ibid. p. 67

8 Airola, P. *How to Get Well*, Phoenix, AZ: Health Plus, 1979, p. 136

9 Atkins, R. op. cit., p. 115

10 Pearson, D. and Shaw, S. *Life Extension*, New York: Warner, 1982, p. 288

11 Merimee, J. et al. "Arginine-initiated Release of Human Growth Hormone," *New Engl. J. Med.*, 1969, 280(26):1434-1438

12 Katz, L.N. Stamler, J. and Pick, R. *Nutrition and Atherosclerosis*, Philadelphia: Lea and Febiger, 1958, pp. 16-20

13 Cheraskin, E. op. cit., p. 308

14 Pfeiffer, C. *Mental and Elemental Nutrients*, New Canaan, Conn.: Keats, 1976, p. 52

15 Airola, P. op. cit., p. 138

16 Williams, R. *Nutrition Against Disease*, Huntington Beach, CA: Int'l. Ins. Nat. Health Sci., p. 93

17 Meyer, J. "Genetic, Traumatic and Environmental Factor in the Etiology of Obesity," *Physiol. Rev.*, 1953, 33:472

18 Pfeiffer, C. op. cit., p. 382

19 Williams, R. op. cit., p. 102

20 Yudkin, J. "The Practical Treatment of Obesity," *Proc. Royal Soc. Med.*, 1965, 58:200

21 Williams, R. op. cit., p. 102

22 Cohn, C. and Joseph, C. "Changes in Body Composition Attendant on Force Feeding," *Amer. J. Physiol.*, 1959, 196:965

23 Gwinup, G. et al. "Effect of Nibbling Versus Gorging on Serum Lipids in Man," *Amer. J. Clin. Nutr.*, 1963, 13:209

24 Stunkard, A.J. et al. "The Night Eating Syndrome: Patterns of Food Intake Among Certain Obese Patients," *Amer. J. Med.*, 1955, 19:78

25 Smith, E., Gibbs, J.G. and Young, L. "Cholecystokinin and Intestinal Satiety in the Rat," *Fed. Proc.*, 1974, 33(5):1146-1149

26 Nelson, G. "Appecurb Clinical Weight Loss Study," Kal Memo, August 30, 1984, issued by makers of Kal Inc., P.O. Box 4023, Woodland Hills, CA 91365-4023

27 Williams, R.H. "Relation of Obesity to the Function of Thyroid Gland," *J. Clin. Endocrinol.*, 1948, 8:257. Also Cleghorn, R.A. "The Interplay Between Endocrine and Psychological Dysfunction," in Wittkower, E. and Cleghorn, R. (eds.), *Recent Development in Psychosomatic Medicine*, Philadelphia: Lippincott, 1954. Also Robinson, A.M. and Norton, J.M. "Estimation of Corticosteroid-Like Substances in Human Urine," *Endocrinology*, 1950, 7:321

28 Atkins, R. op. cit., p. 62
29 Freyburgh, R.H. "A Study of the Value of Insulin in Undernutrition," *Amer. J. Med. Sci.*, 1955, 190:28
30 Stunkard, A.J. et al. "The Mechanism of Satiety: Effect of Glucagon on Gastric Hunger Contractions in Man," *Proc. Soc. Exp. Biol. Med.*, 1955, 89:258
31 Pfeiffer, C. op. cit., p. 474
32 Ballin, J.C. and White, P.L. "Fallacy and Hazard," *J. Amer. med Assn.*, 1974, 230:5
33 Mowrey, D. *Fat Management: The Thermogenic Factor*, Victory Publications, Utah, 1994
34 *The Journal of Biological Chemistry*, 1971, 246(3):629-632
35 *Phytochemistry*, 1965, 4:619-625
36 The Useful Plants of India, 1873, p. 220
37 *The Journal of Biological Chemistry*, 1977, 252(21):7583-7590
38 *Lipids*, 1974, 9(2):121-128
39 "The Diet and Health Benefits of HCA," Keats Publishing, Inc. New Canaan, Conneticut, 1994
40 *Lipids*, 1974, 9(2):129-134
41 *The American Journal of Clinical Nutrition*, 1977, 30(5):767-776
42 Federation Proceedings, 1985, 44(1):139-144
43 Williams, R. *Biochemical Individuality*, New York: Wiley Interscience, 1956, pp. 48-49
44 Passwater, R. *The Easy No-Flab Diet*, New York: Richard Marek, 1979, pp. 20-22
45 Yudkin, J. *Sweet and Danterous*, New York: Bantam, 1979, p. 125
46 Passwater, R. op. cit., p. 202

CHAPTER 14

1   Fredericks, C. *Nutrition Handbook*, Canoga Park, CA: Major Books, 1977, p. 39
2   Ibid.
3   Ibid. p. 40
4   Burke, R.S. et al. "Nutrition Studies During Pregnancy (4)," in "Relation of Protein Content of Mother's Diet during Pregnancy to Birth Defects, Birth Weight and Condition of Infant at Birth," *J. Pediat*, 1943, 23:506
5   Williams, R. *Nutrition Against Disease*, Huntington Beach, CA: Int'l. Ins. Nat. Health Sci., p. 51
6   LeFevres-Boisselot, J. "The Influence of a Slight Pantothenic Acid Deficiency on the Results of Gestation in the Rat," *Comptes Rendues*, 1954, 238:2123
7   Hale, F. "Pigs Born Without Eyeballs," *J. Heredity*, 1933, 24:105
8   Williams, R. op. cit., p. 58
9   Caldwell, D.F. et al. "Behavioral Impairment in Adult Rats Following Acute Zinc Deficiency," *Proc. Soc. Exp. Biol. Med.*, 1970, 133:1417
10 Prasad, A.S. *Zinc Metabolism*, Springfield, Ill: Charles, C. Thomas, 1966
11 Stone, M.L. "Folic Acid Metabolism in Pregnancy," *Amer. J. Obstet. Gynecol.*, 1967, 99:638
12 Williams, R. op. cit., p. 60
13 Challem, J.J. and Lewin, R. "Folic Acid: The Little B Vitamin with a Big Job to do," *Let's Live*, July 1985, pp. 26-28
14 Thurston, E. *The Parents Guide to Better Nutrition from Tots to Teens*, New Canaan, Conn.: Keats, 1979, pp. 15-24
15 Reiser, R. and Sidelman, Z. "Control of Serum Cholesterol

Homeostasis by Cholesterol in the Milk of the Suckling Rat," *J. Nutr.*, 1972, 102(8): 1009-1016

16 Smith, L. *Feed Your Kids Right*, New York: Dell, 1979

17 Ibid. p. 117

18 Thurston, E. op. cit., p. 36

19 Ibid. p. 38

20 Ibid. p. 36

21 Wade, N. "Bottle-Feeding: Adverse Effects of a Western Technology," *Science*, 1974, 184:45-48

22 Smith, L. op. cit., p. 91

23 Ibid. p. 92

24 Ibid. p. 10

25 Schauss, G.A. An address to the South West Health Organization, Fort Worth, Texas, February 1983. Recorded on tape by Audio Recording Services, Las Vegas, Nevada

26 Benton, D. and Roberts, G. "Effect of Vitamin and Mineral Supplementation on Intelligence of a Sample of Schoolchildren," *Lancet*, 1988, 8578(1):140-143

CHAPTER 15

1 Stoneycypher, D. "Old Age need Not Be Old," *New York Times*, August 18, 1957

2 Kugler, H. *Dr. Kugler's Seven Keys to a Longer Life*, New York: Stein & Day, 1978, p. 21

3 Ibid.

4 McCann, A. *The Science of Keeping Young*, New York: Doubleday, 1926

5 Williams, R. *Nutrition Against Disease*, Huntington Beach, CA: Int'l. Ins. Nat. Health Sci., 1977, p. 138

6 Kugler, H. op. cit. p. 24

7 Hauser, G. *New Treasury of Secrets*, Greenwich, Conn.: Fawcett, p. 24

8 McCarrison, R. *Studies in Deficiency Diseases*, Milwaukee, Wis.: Lee Foundation for Nutritional Research, 1945

9 Abrams, L. "The Healthy Maya," *Family News*, March 1960, 7:3

10 De Vries, A. *Primitive Man and His Food*, Chicago, Ill.: Chandler Books, 1952

11 Tobe, J. *Junza*, Emmaus, Pa.: Rodale Press, 1960

12 Clark, L. *Stay Young Longer*, New York: Pyramid Books, 1976, p. 37

13 Tappel, A.L. "Will Antioxidant Nutrients Slow Aging Processes?" *Geriatrics*, 1968, 23:97-104. Also Curtis, H.J. "Radiation and Aging," *Soc. Exp. Biol. Symposia*, 1967, 21:51

14 Mann, D.M.A. and Yates, P.O. "Lipoprotein Pigments -Their Relationship to Aging in the Human Nervous System: The Lipofuscin Content of Nerve Cells," *Brain*, 1974, 97:481-488

15 Rodale, J.I. *Sex and the Healthy Prostate*, Herts., England: The Rodale Press, 1968

16 Merimee, J. et al. "Arginine-initiated Release of Human Growth Hormone," *New Engl. J. Med.*, 1969, 280(26): 1434-1438

17 Barbul et al. "Arginine: A Thymotropic and Wound-Healing Promoting Agent," *Surgical Forum*, 1977, 28:101-103

18 Hansen, M. "Serum Growth Hormone Response to Exercise in Non-Obese and Obese Normal Subjects," *Scand. J. Clin. Lab. Invest.*, 1973, 31(2):175-178

19 Prinz, A. et al. "Growth Hormone Levels During Sleep in Elderly Males," a paper presented at the 29th Annual Gerontological Society Conference, October 13, 1976

20 Hansen, M. op. cit.

21 Harman, D. "Role of Free Radicals in Mutation, Cancer, Aging, and the maintenance of Life," *Rad. Res.*, 1962, 16:753-764

22 Demopoulos, H. et al. "The Possible Role of Free Radical Reactions in Carcinogenesis," *J. Environ. Pathol. Toxicol.*, 1980, 3(4):273-303

23 Sokoloff, B. et al. "Aging, Atherosclerosis and Ascorbic Acid Metabolism," *J. Amer. Geriat. Soc.*, 1966, 14(12):1239-1260. Also Ross and Glomset. "Atherosclerosis and the Arterial Smooth Muscle Cell," *Science*, 1973, 180:1332-1339

24 Demopoulos, H. et al. "The Free Radical Pathology and the Microcirculation in the Major Central Nervous System Disorders," *Acta Physiol. Scand. Suppl., 1980, 492:91-119*

25 Mann, D.M.A. and Yates, P.O. op. cit.

26 Walford, E. "Immunologic Theory of Aging: Current Status," *Fed. Proc.*, 1974, 33(9:2020-2027

27 Bjorksten, J. "The Crosslinkage Theory of Aging," *J. Amer. Geriatr. Soc.*, 1968, 16:408-427

28 Kirk and Chieffic. "Variation with Age in Elasticity of Skin and Subcutaneous Tissue in Human Individuals," *J. Derm., 1962, 17:373-380*

29 Bellows and Bellows, "Crosslinkage Theory of Senile Cataracts," *Ann. Ophthal.*, February 1976, pp. 129-135

30 Pearson, D. and Shaw, S. *Life Extension*, New York: Warner, 1982, p. 100

31 Schuckit, E. and Rayses, A. "Ethanol Ingestion: Differences in Blood Acetaldehyde Concentrations in Relatives of Alcoholics and Controls," *Science* 1979, 203(5): 54-55

32 Sprince, H. et al. "Protectants Against Acetaldehyde Toxicity: Sulfhydryl Compounds and Ascorbic Acid," *Fed. Proc.*, March 1974, 33(3), pt. 1

33 Tomalsoff, E. et al. "Superoxide Dismutase: Correlation with Life-span and Specific Metabolic Rate in Primate Species," *Proc. Nat. Acad Sci.*, 1980, 77(5):2777-2781 (USA)

34 McCord, J.M. "Superoxide Radical May Play a Role in Arthritis," paper presented at the Third Biennial Conference on Chemical Education, Pennsylvania State University, August 1, 1974

35 Sunde and Hoekstra. "Structure, Synthesis, and Function of Glutathione Peroxidase," *Nutr. Rev.*, 1980, 38(8):265-273

36 Pearson, D. and Shaw, S. op. cit., p. 280

37 *Prev. Med.* 1992, 21:329,*Cancer Res.* 1992, 52: 1162,*Cell Biophys.* 1989, 14:175

38 *Arch. Biochem. Biophys.* 1989, 274:532

39 Shaw, S. An address to the 8th Annual Convention of the national Nutritional Foods Association (NNFA), September 1982, Reno, Nevada. Recorded on tape by Audio Recording Services, Las Vegas, Nevada

40 Spector, H. "Vitamin Homeostasis in the Central Nervous System," *New Engl. J. Med.*, 1977, 296:1393

41 Fridovich, M. "Oxygen:Boon and Bane," *Amer. Scientist*, 1975, 63: 54-59

42 Beutler, E. "Glutathione Reductase: Stimulation in Normal Subjects by Riboflavin Supplementation," *Science*, 1969, 165:613-615

43 Coker, J. et al. "Thromboxane and Prostacyclin Release from Ischaemic Myocardium in Relation to

Arrhythmias," *Nature*, 1981, 291:323-324

44 Pearson, D. "Mechanisms of Aging and Life Extension," an address to the 8th annual convention of the Northern California Foods Association, September 1982, Reno, Nevada. Recorded on tape by Audio Recording Service, Las Vegas, Nevada

45 Vorberg, G. "Ginkgo Biloba Extract (GBE): A Long Term Study of Chronic Cerebral Insufficiency in Geriatric patients," *Clin. Trials J.*, 1985, 22(2):149

46 Anonymous. "Extrait supplémentaire consacré à l'Extrait de Ginkgo Biloba," *La Presse Médicale*, 1986, 31:25-29

47 Taillandier J. et al. "Traitement des Troubles du Vieillissement cérébral par l'Extrait de Ginkgo Biloba. Etude longitudinale multicentrique à double insu face au placébo," *La Presse Médicale*, 1986, 31: 1583

48 Pincemail, J. and Deby, C. "Propriétés antiradicalaires de l'Extrait de Ginkgo Biloba," *La Presse Médicale*, 1986, 31:1475

49 Doly, M. et al. "Effet de l'Extrait de Ginkgo Biloba sur l'Électrophysiologie de la Rétine isolée de Rat diabétique," *La Presse Médicale*, 1986, 31: 1480

50 Folkers, K. et al. "New Progress on the Biomedical and Clinical Research on Coenzyme Q," *Biomedical and Clinical Aspects of Coenzyme Q, Elsevier/North Holland Biomedical Press, 1981, 3:399-412*

51 Ernster, L. et al. "Functions of Coenzyme Q," ibid. pp. 159-167

52 Mortensen, M. et al. "Long Term Coenzyme Q10 Therapy: A Major Advance in the Management of Resistant Myocardial Failure," *Drugs Under Experimental and Clinical Research*, 1985, 11(8):581

53 Folkers, K. et al. "Observations of Significant Reductions of Arrhythmias in Treatment with Coenzyme Q10 of Patients having Cardiovascular Disease," *IRCS Medical Science*, 1982, 10:348-349

54 Yamagami, T. et al. "Bioenergetics in Clinical Medicine. Studies on Coenzyme Q10 and Essential Hypertension," *Research Communications in Chemical Pathology and Pharmacology*, 1975, 11(2):273-288

55 Kamikawa, T. et al. "Effects of Coenzyme Q10 on Exercise Tolerance in Chronic Stable Angina Pectoris," *Amer. J. Cardiol.*, 1985, 56:247-251

56 Tsuyasaki, T. et al. "Mechanocardiography of Ischemic or Hypertensive Heart Failure," *Biomedical and Clinical Aspects of Coenzyme Q*, Elsevier/North Holland Biomedical Press, 1980, 2:273-288

57 Iwamoto, Y. et al. "Clinical Effects of Coenzyme Q10 on Periodontal Disease," *Biomedical and Clinical Aspects of Coenzyme Q*, op. cit., 1981, 3:109-119. Also Wilkinson, E.G. et al. "Bioenergetics in Clinical Medicine. II. Adjunctive Treatment with Coenzyme Q in Periodontal Therapy," *Res. Comm. Chem. Clin. Pharm.*, 1975, 12(1)

58 Wilkinson, E.G. and Folkers, K. "Measuring Changes in the Health of the Human Periodontum and Other Oral Tissues," *Biomedical and Clinical Aspects of Coenzyme Q*, op. cit., 1981, 3:93-102

59 Van Gaal, L. et al. "Exploratory Study of Coenzyme Q10 in Obesity," *Biomedical and Clinical Aspects of Coenzyme Q*, op. cit., 1984, 4:369-373

60 Folkers, K. et al. "Increase in Levels of IgG in Serum of Patients Treated

with Coenzyme Q10," *Res. Comm Chem. Pathol. Pharm.*, 1982, 38(2)

61 Gregory, M. "Life Extension Benefits of Coenzyme Q10, 1981, 3

62 Lenaz, G. et al. "Multiple roles of Ubiquinone in Mammalian Cells," *Drugs, Exp. Res.*, 1984, X(7):481-490

63 Hutschenecker, A.A. *The Will to Live*, New Jersey: Prentice-Hall, 1958

64 Roberts, E.E. Indian *Handark Medical Digest*, January 1958

65 Sweetland, B. *Grow Rich While You Sleep*, Hollywood, CA: Wilshire Books, 1977, p. 189

66 Clark, L. op. cit., p. 332

67 Meares, A. "Stress, meditation and the Regression of Cancer," *Practitioner*, 1982, 226:1607-1609

68 Stein, M. Miller, A.H. and Trestman, R.L. "Depression, the Immune System, and Health and Illness," Archives of General Psychiatry, 1991, 48:171-177

69 Rogers, M.P. Dubey, D. and Reich, P. "The Influence of the Psyche and the Brain on Immunity and Disease Susceptibility: A Critical Review," *Psychosomatic medicine*, 1979, 41:147-165

70 Bennett, H.T. and Cohen, S. "Stress and Immunity in Humans: A Meta-Analytic Review," *Psychosomatic Medicine*, 1993, 55:364-379

71 Stokkan, K.A. Reiter, R.J. and Vaughan, M.K. "Food Restriction Retards Aging of the Pineal Gland," *Brain Research*, 1991, 545:66-72

72 McMillen, S.I. *None of These Diseases*, Old Tappan, NJ: Fleming H. Revell, 1973

73 Ralli, E.P. and Dumm, M.E. "Relation of Pantothenic Acid to Adrenal Cortical Function," *Vitamins & Hormones*, 1953, 11:135

74 Pfeiffer, C. *Mental and Elemental Nutrients*, New Canaan, Conn: Keats, 1976, p. 138

75 Ibid. p. 125

76 Flach, F.F. "Calcium Metabolism in States of Depression," *Brit. J. Psychiat.*, 1964, 110:588-593

77 *Prevention*, November 1980, 23(11):35

78 Ibid.

CHAPTER 16

1 Peale, N.V. *The Power of Positive Thinking*, New York: Fawcett, 1956, p. 159

2 Davis, A. *Let's Get Well*, New York: The New American Library, 1972, p. 19

3 Peale, N.V. op. cit., p. 160

4 Ibid.

5 Meyerowitz, S. "The Continuing Investigation of Psychosocial Variables in Rheumatoid Arthritis," *Modern Trends in Rheumatology*, Hill, A.G. (ed.), 2nd ed., New York: Appleton-Century-Crofts, 1966, pp. 92-105

6 Davis, A. op. cit., p. 111

7 LeShan, L. "Psychological States as Factors in the Development of Malignant Disease: A Critical Review," *Nat. Cancer Inst. J.*, 1959, 22:1-18

8 McMillen, S.I. *None of These Diseases*, New York: Fleming H. Revel, 1973

9 Benson, H. *The Relaxation Response*, New York: William Morrow, 1975

10 Ibid.

11 Klerman, G.L. "Psychotropic Drugs as Therapeutic Agents," *Hastings Center Studies 2*, 1974, 1:8

12 Peale, N.V. op. cit., p. 144

13 Ibid. p. 147

14 Peale, N.V. op. cit., p. 149

15 Frank, J. "The Faith that Heals," *Johns Hopkins University Med. J.*, 1975, 137:127-131

16 Beecher, H.K. "The Powerful Placebo," *J. Amer. Med. Assn.*, 1955, 159(17):1602-1606

17 Klopfer, B. "Psychological Variables in Human Cancer," *J. of Projective Techniques*, 1957, 21:337-339

18 Peale, N.V. op. cit., p. 149

CHAPTER 17

1 Null, G. *The New Vegetarian*, New York: William Morrow, 1978, p. 42

2 Fisher, I. *Advanced Nutrition Reader*, N.I.A. Special Research Project on Protein, 1975, p. 8

3 National Livestock and Meat Board, *Meat Board Reports*, January 1977, 10(1):9

4 Hardinge, M.G. and Crooks, H. "Nonflesh Dietaries," *J. Amer. Diet. Assn.*, 1964, 45:541

5 Pfeiffer, C. *Mental and Elemental Nutrients*, New Canaan, Conn.: Keats, 1976, p. 102

6 Ibid. p. 110

7 Marshall, J. "A Dietary Breakthrough," *The American Chiropractor*, October-November, 1981

8 Greer, M.A. and Astwood, E.B. "The Antithyroid Effect of Certain Foods in Man as Determined with Radioactive Iodine," *Endocrinology*, 1948, 43:105-119

9 Clark, L. *Stay Young Longer*, New York: Pyramid Books, 1976, p. 205

10 McClure, J.A. *The Meateaters are Threatened: An Insider's Exposé of Conditions in America's Meat Markets*, New York: Pyramid Books, 1973

11 Pfeiffer, C. op. cit., p. 35

12 Ibid. p. 36

13 Hardinge, M.G. and Stare, F.J. *Modern Medicine*, April 15, 1965, p. 99

14 Pfeiffer, C. op. cit., p. 111

15 Hardinge, M.G. et al. "Nutritional Studies of Vegetarians," *Amer. J. Clin. Nutr.*, 1958, 6(5):523-525

16 Clark, L. op. cit., p. 57

17 Fisher, I. op. cit.

18 Rodale, J.L. *The Healthy Hunzas*, Emmaus, Pa: Rodale Press, 1949

19 Wokes, F. "Proteins," *Plant Foods for Human Nutrition*, 1968, 1(1):32

20 Lappe, F.M. *Diet for a Small Planet*, New York: Ballantine, 1975, p. 78

21 Ibid. p. 79

22 Ibid. p. 363

23 Ibid.

24 Altschul, A.M. *Proteins, Their Chemistry and Politics*, New York: Basic Books, 1965, p. 115

25 Lappe, F.M. op. cit., p. 101

CHAPTER 18

1 Airola, P. *How to Get Well*, Phoenix, AZ: Health Plus, 1979, p. 284

2 Martin, D.W., Mayes, P.A. and Rodwell, V.W. *Harper's Review of Biochemistry*, Los Altos, CA: Lange, 1981, pp. 524-526

3 Steen, E. and Montagu, A. *Anatomy and Physiology*, New York: Barnes and Noble, 1959, 1:223

4 Airola, P. op. cit., p. 284

5 Ibid.

6 Ibid.

7 Ibid.

8 Ross, S. *Fasting: The Super Diet*, New York: Ballantine, 1976, p. 38

9 Cott, A. *Fasting as a Way of Life*, New York: Bantam, 1977, p. 7

10 Catt, W. "Growth Hormone," *Lancet*, 1:933-939

11 Cott, A. op. cit., p. 3

12 Ross, S. op. cit., p. 40

13 Cott, A. op. cit., p. 104

14 Airola, P. op. cit., p. 215

15 Ross, S. op. cit., p. 31

16 Clark, L. *Get Well Naturally*, New York: ARC Books, 1972, p. 366

17 Ross, S. op. cit., p. 40
18 Lust, J.B. *Raw Juice Therapy*, Northamptonshire, England: Thorsons, 1974, p. 16
19 Airola, P. op. cit., p. 219
20 Hauser, G. *New Treasury of Secrets*, Greenwich, Conn.: Fawcett, 1976, p.386

CHAPTER 19

1 Fredericks, C. *Nutrition Handbook*, Canoga park, CA: Major Books, 1977, p. 36
2 Ibid.
3 Pfeiffer, C. *Mental and Elemental Nutrients*, New Canaan, Conn.: Keats, 1976, pp. 469-472
4 Airola, P. *Sex and Nutrition*. Information Inc., New York, 1970
5 Greer, M.A. and Astwood, E.B. "The Antithyroid Effect of Certain Foods in Man as Determined with Radioactive Iodine," *Endocrinology*, 1948, 43:105-119
6 Tui, C.J. "Review: The Fundamentals of Clinical Proteinology," *Amer. J. Clin. Nutr.*, 1953, 1:232
7 Forbes, J.C. "Effect of Thyroxine on the Neutral Fat and Cholesterol Content of the Body and Liver of Rats," *Endocrinology*, 1944, 35:126
8 Gosmani, M.N.D. and Knox W.E. "An Evaluation of the Role of Ascorbic Acid in the Regulation of Tyrosine Metabolism," *J. Chron. Dis.*, 1963, 16:363-370
9 Fredericks, C. op. cit., p. 21
10 Davis, A. *Let's Eat Right to Keep Fit*, New York: Harcourt Brace Jovanovich, 1970, pp. 159-160
11 Steen, E. and Montagu, A. *Anatomy and Physiology*, New York: Barnes and Noble, 1959, 2:187
12 Rosenkrantz, H.J. "Studies in Vitamin E Deficiency -The Estimation of Tissue Tocopherol with Phosphomolybdic Acid," *J. Biol. Chem.*, 1957, 224:165-174
13 Hurley, L.S. and Morgan, F.A. "Carbohydrate Metabolism and Adrenal Cortical Function in the Pantothenic-Acid Deficient Rat," *J. Biol. Chem.*, 1952, 195(2):583-589 Also Cole, D.R. et al. "Studies on Pituitary Lactogenic Hormone," *J. Biol. Chem.*, 1957, 224:399-404
14 Guggenheim, K. and Olson, R.E. "Studies of Lipogenesis in Certain B Vitamin Deficiencies," *J. Nutr.*, 1952, 8:345
15 Williams, R. *Nutrition Against Disease*. Huntington Beach, CA: Int'l. Ins. Nat. Health Sci., 1976, p. 56
16 Gelenberg, A. et al. "Tyrosine for the Treatment of Depression," *Amer. J. Psychiat.*, 1980, 137(5):622-623
17 Prout, G.R. Sierp, M. and Whitmore, W.F. "Radioactive Zinc in Prostate," *J. Amer. Med. Assn.*, 1959, 169(15):1703-1710
18 Ronaghy, H.A. and Halsted, J.A. "Zinc Deficiency Occurring in Females," *Amer. J. Clin. Nutr.*, 1975, 28:831-836
19 Yates, J. "Is Sex in Your Diet?" an interview with Dr Ali Abbasi, *Prevention*, March 1980, p. 33
20 Ibid.
21 Ibid.
22 Lucas, L. "Zinc and Your Love Life," an interview with Dr. Parviz Rabbani, *Prevention*, February 1981, p. 58
23 McLardy, T. "Hippocampal Zinc and Structural Deficit in Brain from Schizophrenics and Chronic Alcoholics," presented at the Trace Elements and Brain Function Symposium, Princeton, New Jersey, 1973
24 Rodale, J.I. *Sex and a Healthy Prostate*, Berkhamsted, England: Rodale Press, 1968, p. 123

25 "Diet can Improve Sexual Health," *Prevention*, October 1974, p. 62

26 Van Thiel, D.H. et al. "Ethanol Inhibition of Vitamin A Metabolism in the Testes: Possible Mechanism for Sterility in alcoholics," *Science*, 1974, 186:941

27 Ibid.

28 Rodale, J.I. op. cit., p. 68

29 Masters, W.H. and Johnson, V.E. *Human Sexual Inadequacy*, Boston, MA: Little, Brown, and Co., 1970. Also Masters, W.H. and Johnson, V.E. *Human Sexual Response*, Boston, MA: Little, Brown, and Co., 1966

30 *Insider's Newsletter for Women*, May 30, 196

CHAPTER 20

1 Pfeiffer, C. *Mental and Elemental Nutrients*, New Canaan, Conn.: Keats, 1976, p. 57

2 Kavanash, T. et al. "Influence of Exercise and Life-Style Variables Upon High Density Lipoprotein Cholesterol after Myocardial Infarction," *Arteriosclerosis*, 1983, 3(3):249-259

3 Morris, J. et al. "Vigorous Exercise in Leisure Time and the Incidence of Coronary Heart Disease," *Lancet*, 1973, 1:333-338

4 Wood, P.D. and Haskell, W.L. "The Effect of Exercise on Plasma High Density Lipoprotein," *Lipids*, 1979, 14:417

5 Wyndham, C.H. "The Role of Physical Activity in the prevention of Ischaemic Heart Disease," *South African Med. J.*, 1979, 56:7

6 Greenberg, M.A. et al. "The Role of Physical Training in Patients with Coronary Heart Disease," *Amer. Heart J.*, 1979, 97:527

7 Redwood, D.R. et al. "Circulatory and Symptomatic Effects of Physical Training in Patients with Coronary Artery Disease and Angina Pectoris," *N. Engl. J. Med.*, 1972, 286:959

8 Black, H.R. "Nonpharmacologic Therapy for Hypertension," *Amer. J. Med.*, 1979, 66:837

9 Engerbreston, D.L. "The Effects of Exercise Upon Diabetic Control," *J. Assos. Phys. Ment. Rehab.*, 1965, 19:74

10 "What's a Joint Like That Doing in a Nice Person Like You?" *Prevention*, May, 1974

11 De Vries, H. "Exercise Intensity Threshold for Improvement of Cardiovascular/Respiratory Function in Older Men," *Geriatrics*, 1971, 26:94-101

12 Kugler, H. *Dr. Kugler's Seven Keys to a Longer Life*, New York: Steen and Day, 1978, p. 52

13 Ibid. p. 54

14 Pfeiffer, C. op. cit., p. 271

15 Ratcliff, J.D. "The Miracle of Muscle," *Today's Health*, January 1956

16 Pfeifer, C. op. cit., p. 76

17 Yudkin, J. *Sweet and Dangerous*, New York: Bantam, 1972, p. 95

18 Ibid.

19 Copper, K.H. *The New Aerobics*, New York: Bantam, 1981, p. 150

20 Morehouse, L.E. and Gross, L. *Total Fitness in 30 Minutes a Week*, New York: Granada, 1976, p. 148

CHAPTER 21

1 Hundley, J.M. *Statistics of Health, USDA Yearbook on Food, 1959, pp. 175-180*

2 Davis, A. *Let's Get Well*, New York: Harcourt Brace Jovanovich, 1972, p. 335

3 Antar, M.A. et al. "Changes in Retail Market Food Supplies in the U.S. in the Last Seventy Years in Relation to the Incidence of

Coronary Heart Disease, with Special Reference to Dietary Carbohydrates and Essential Fatty Acids," *Amer. J. Clin. Nutr.*, 1964, 14:169-177. Also Dilling, K. *Nat. Health Fed. Bull.*, 1964, 10:23

4 Hundley, J.M. op. cit.

5 Fredericks, C. *Nutrition Handbook*, Canoga Park, CA: Major Books, 1977, p. 12

6 Scrimshaw, N.S. "Synergistic and Antagonistic Interaction of Nutrition and Infections," *Fed. Proc.*, 1966, 25:1679-1681

7 Holvey, N.D. (ed.) *The Merck Manual of Diagnosis and Therapy*, 12th edition. Rahway, N.J. Merck, Sharp and Dohme Laboratories, 1972

8 Gordon, J.E. "Synergism of Malnutrition and Infectious Diseases," *Nutrition in Preventive Medicine*, Geneva, WHO, 1976

9 Ibid.

INDEX

brewer's yeast 101, 149–52, 212
   complete protein 28
   sexual hormones 396
   supplements 224
   vegetarians 374
   zinc 397
bronchitis 128
brown rice 35
   thyroid function 395
bruising 90
BSE *see* Mad Cow Disease
buchu (*Borosma betulina*), uses 285
bulk minerals 97–140
burns
   pollen 176
   vitamin E 86, 217
bursitis, PABA 72
buttermilk 88, 218

cabbage
   iodine content 394
   uses 274
cadmium (Cd) 27, 139–40
   calcium 104
   dangers of 98
caffeine
   actions 270, 275, 277
   dangers of 234
   diuretic qualities 235
   hypoglycaemia 249, 251
   maté 299
   weight loss 321
calcium (Ca) 38, 97, 102–5
   absorption 23, 103
   allergy alleviation 243
   best natural sources 105
   bones 22, 83, 102–4, 126–7, 342, 403
   brewer's yeast intake 152
   choline 76
   deficiency symptoms 104, 106, 342
   individual requirements 8
   lead neutralizing properties 137
   mercury protection 139
   non-aerobic exercise 403
   self-check kits 53

   supplements 214–15, 219
   teeth 22, 82, 102–4, 125–6
   yogurt 258
calcium pangamate 71
calcium-phosphorus balance 76, 105–6
calorie counting, weight loss 323
calorie intake
   exercise 408–11
   fats 38
   obesity 313, 324–5
   restriction 358–9
camomile tea 235
cancer 12, 20
   alcohol 37
   bladder 234
   breast 14, 76–7, 91, 160, 191, 196, 204,
      234, 332
   chlorella 187–8
   colon 253, 261, 375
   DHEA 201
   emotionally induced 364
   evening primrose oil 180–1, 183
   free radicals 42, 344, 350
   germanium treatment 132
   high protein diets 315
   inhibition of 196–7, 203–4
   laboratory animals 3
   melatonin 190–1
   methionine 185
   mortality 414–15
   obesity 311
   oesophageal 129, 200
   ovarian 160
   overheated fats 41
   prevention 26, 55–6, 71, 125, 132
   prostate 16
   quercetin 91
   risk reduction 124, 199–200
   terminal patients, vitamin C 217
   trace elements 101
   tumour inhibition 166–7
   vitamin A 56
   vitamin C 80, 217
   vitamin E 86, 217
   yogurt 258